Bone Response to Dental Implant Materials

Related titles

Materials Science for Dentistry (text book)
(ISBN 978-1-84569-529-3)

Pre-prosthetic and Maxillofacial Surgery
(ISBN 978-1-84569-589-7)

Bioactive Glasses
(ISBN 978-1-84569-768-6)

Woodhead Publishing Series in Biomaterials

Bone Response to Dental Implant Materials

Edited by

Adriano Piattelli

ELSEVIER

AMSTERDAM • BOSTON • CAMBRIDGE • HEIDELBERG
LONDON • NEW YORK • OXFORD • PARIS • SAN DIEGO
SAN FRANCISCO • SINGAPORE • SYDNEY • TOKYO
Woodhead Publishing is an imprint of Elsevier

WP
WOODHEAD
PUBLISHING

Woodhead Publishing is an imprint of Elsevier
The Officers' Mess Business Centre, Royston Road, Duxford, CB22 4QH, United Kingdom
50 Hampshire Street, 5th Floor, Cambridge, MA 02139, United States
The Boulevard, Langford Lane, Kidlington, OX5 1GB, United Kingdom

ISBN: 978-0-08-100287-2 (print)
ISBN: 978-0-08-100288-9 (online)

Library of Congress Cataloging-in-Publication Data
A catalog record for this book is available from the Library of Congress

British Library Cataloguing-in-Publication Data
A catalogue record for this book is available from the British Library

For information on all Woodhead Publishing publications
visit our website at https://www.elsevier.com/

Publisher: Matthew Deans
Acquisition Editor: Laura Overend
Editorial Project Manager: Lucy Beg
Production Project Manager: Poulouse Joseph
Designer: Mark Rogers

Contents

List of contributors

H. Alexander Orthogen LLC, Springfield, NJ, United States

S. Anil Prince Sattam Bin Abdulaziz University, AlKharj, Saudi Arabia

L. Bagán-Debon University of Valencia, Valencia, Spain

J.V. Bagán-Sebastián University of Valencia, Valencia, Spain

J.L. Calvo-Guirado Universidad Católica San Antonio (UCAM), Murcia, Spain

E.P. Chalisserry Pukyong National University, Busan, Korea

A. De Sanctis University "G. d'Annunzio" of Chieti-Pescara, Pescara, Italy

J. Diaz-Marcos Scientific and Technological Centers of the University of Barcelona, Barcelona, Spain

J. Duyck KU Leuven, Leuven, Belgium; U.Z. St. Raphaël, Leuven, Belgium

A. Fontana University "G. d'Annunzio", Chieti, Italy

G. Frisardi Epochè – Orofacial Pain Centre, Rome, Italy; University of Sassari, Sassari, Italy

F. Frisardi Epochè – Orofacial Pain Centre, Rome, Italy

S.A. Gattone University "G. d'Annunzio" of Chieti-Pescara, Pescara, Italy

S. Gehrke Universidad Católica San Antonio (UCAM), Murcia, Spain

A. Giuliani Università Politecnica delle Marche, Ancona, Italy

F. Iaculli University "G. d'Annunzio", Chieti, Italy

G. Iezzi University "G. d'Annunzio", Chieti, Italy

O.T. Jensen University of Utah School of Dentistry, Salt Lake City, UT, United States

S.-K. Kim Pukyong National University, Busan, Korea

J.E. Maté Sánchez de Val Universidad Católica San Antonio (UCAM), Murcia, Spain

C. Murray European University College, Dubai, UAE

M. Peñarrocha-Diago University of Valencia, Valencia, Spain

V. Perrotti University "G. d'Annunzio", Chieti, Italy

A. Piattelli University "G. d'Annunzio", Chieti, Italy

R.L. Reuben Heriot-Watt University, Edinburgh, United Kingdom

J. Ricci New York University College of Dentistry, New York, NY, United States

M.S. Shim Incheon National University, Incheon, Republic of Korea

D. Soto-Peñazola University of Valencia, Valencia, Spain

E.M. Staderini Western Switzerland Universities of Applied Sciences, Geneva, Switzerland

P.P. Valentini University Tor Vergata, Rome, Italy

K. Vandamme KU Leuven, Leuven, Belgium; U.Z. St. Raphaël, Leuven, Belgium

J. Venkatesan Incheon National University, Incheon, Republic of Korea

I.-S. Yeo Seoul National University, Seoul, Korea

B. Zavan University of Padova, Padova, Italy

Introduction to bone response to dental implant materials

1

V. Perrotti, F. Iaculli, A. Fontana, A. Piattelli, G. Iezzi
University "G. d'Annunzio", Chieti, Italy

1.1 Introduction

1.1.1 Bone structure in the aspect of functionality

Bone tissue, originating from mesenchymal tissue, is a type of specialized connective tissue that functions as a support. It is involved in many processes, which are essential for the human body. Bone is uniquely designed for its role of providing mechanical stability to the skeleton, which is needed for load bearing, locomotion, and protection of internal organs; it presents characteristics such as strength, hardness, and resistance to pressure, traction, and torsion. Furthermore, the homeostasis of calcium level in blood is maintained because the mineral calcium, which is stored in the bone, is mobilized from the storage reserve to enter the blood. The diversity of the bone functionality can be attributed to its complex structure. Indeed, most of the unique properties of the bone are related to its specific constitution.

Bone is composed of cells and an intercellular matrix rich in organic compounds, mainly type I collagen fibers embedded in a ground substance consisting of proteoglycans, glycoproteins, as well as inorganic minerals. The collagen fibers form bundles or fibrils, which resist the pulling forces, whereas the minerals provide stiffness, which resists bending and compression. Bone minerals are mainly in the form of crystals of calcium phosphate—calcium hydroxyapatite (HA) and when associated with collagen fibers give the specific hardness to the bone.

Although the bone is populated by a variety of different cells, its functional integrity is guaranteed by four principal cell types: the osteoclasts (OCLs), bone-destroying cells; the osteoblasts (OBLs), bone-forming cells; the osteocytes (OCTs), bone-maintaining cells; and the endothelial cells (ECs), bone-related angiogenic cells. All of them have defined tasks and are thus essential for the maintenance of a healthy bone tissue.

OCLs are large, multinucleated cells formed by the self-fusion of macrophages (Fig. 1.1). They are located on the bone surface in shallow pits called resorption pits or Howship's lacunae. The main function of OCLs is resorption of the bone tissue. The OCLs are able to resorb the strong matrix by secreting acid and collagenase. Resorption plays a crucial role in the maintenance, repair, and remodeling of bones. OCLs are formed by the fusion of mononuclear precursors derived from the pluripotential hematopoietic stem cells and share more committed hematopoietic progenitors with cells of the mononuclear phagocyte system [1].

Bone Response to Dental Implant Materials. http://dx.doi.org/10.1016/B978-0-08-100287-2.00001-X

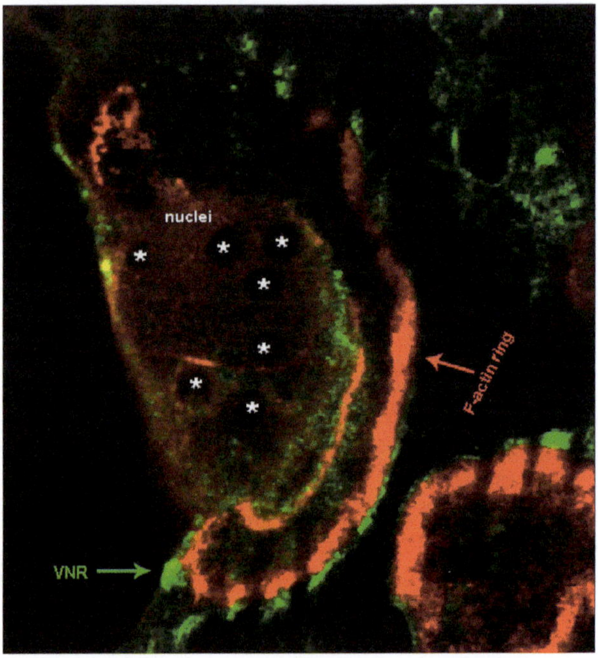

Figure 1.1 High-power *XY* view of a multinucleated OCL (asterisks) in peripheral blood mononuclear cell cultures of the bovine bone. Red indicates positive staining for F-actin—enriched patches and rings with phalloidin—tetramethylrhodamine B isothiocyanate (TRITC) indicating activated OCLs (*red arrows*). Green indicates positive staining for the monoclonal antibody 23C6 to detect human integrin alpha V beta 3 complex of the vitronectin receptor, scale bar ¼ 10 mm.

OBLs are mononucleate cells of mesenchymal origin that are responsible for the bone formation; they are located mostly on the surface of the bone, as a single layer of mononuclear cells (Fig. 1.2). Their function is to produce the organic components of the bone matrix. When active, they show high alkaline phosphatase activity. OBLs eventually become trapped in the matrix they produce and become OCTs.

OCTs are star-shaped cells that occupy the lacunae in the bone matrix and are the most common cell types in the bone (Figs. 1.3 and 1.4). They show thin cytoplasmic processes called filopodia that form a network of small canals called canaliculi. This network is essential for the exchange of nutrients and waste. OCTs are very long-living cells, with a half-life of 25 years, and are not capable of division. These cells have a mechanosensory activity, they have reduced synthetic activity, but are also able to break down the bone matrix through a mechanism called osteocytic osteolysis that releases calcium ions for calcium homeostasis and has an important role in phosphate metabolism. Besides these functions in molecular synthesis and modification, OCTs are able to transmit signal over long distances through canaliculi. There is growing evidence that OCTs are regulatory cells that control the function of OBLs and OCLs.

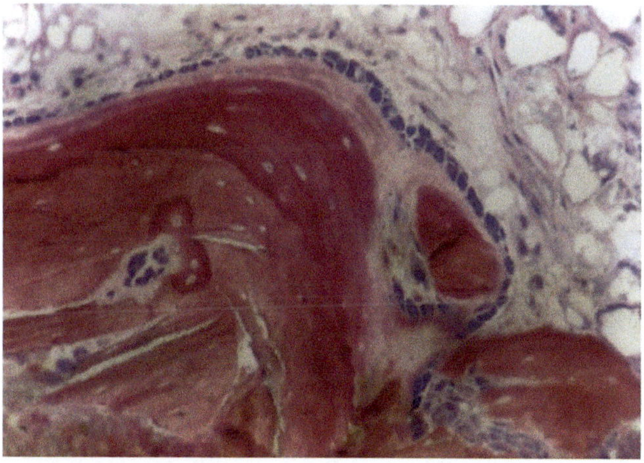

Figure 1.2 A rim of OBLs producing osteoid matrix. Toluidine blue and acid fuchsin staining; original magnification 200×.

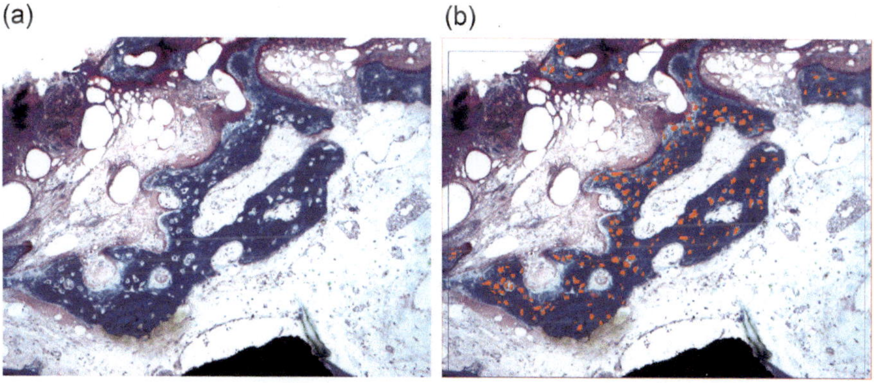

Figure 1.3 (a) Histological image showing OCTs in the peri-implant bone tissue of samples retrieved from humans after a loading period of 4 weeks−7 months. (b) Images showing how the count of the number of OCTs was undertaken. OCTs lacunae were highlighted in red. Toluidine blue and acid fuchsin staining; original magnification 100×.

ECs are very flat, they form pavement-like patterns on the inside of the vessels and are known to function in a variety of important physiological processes. Essentially, ECs secrete a number of mediators (factors), which may elicit biological responses by various signal-transduction mechanisms. Such mediators are implicated in regulating the permeability of the endothelium and can promote chemotactic responses, such as inflammation and blood clotting.

It is well established that bone formation is an angiogenesis-dependent process [2], and ECs have long been known for their role in the formation of blood vessels that supply oxygen and nutrients to the developing bone tissue. However, it has been

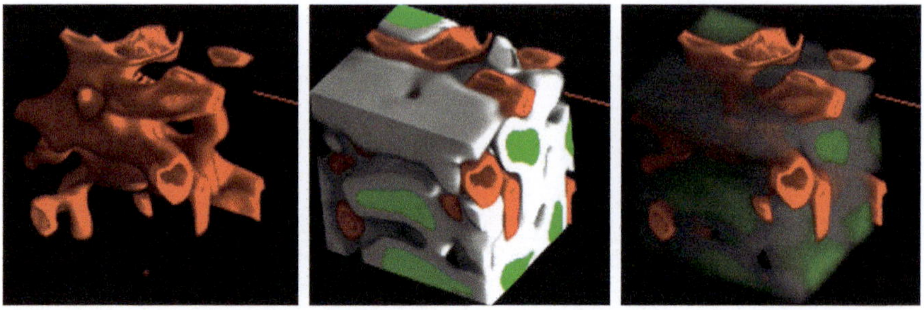

Figure 1.4 Regenerative potential of collagenated biomaterial grafts. Representative subvolume of a collagenated biomaterial as retrieved from in vivo test after 12 months and studied by synchrotron radiation–based, phase-contrast microtomography. Legend: *red phase*, regenerated vessels; *white phase*, newly formed bone and bone under remodeling; *green phase*, fully mineralized bone and residual scaffold.
Courtesy Dr. Alessandra Giuliani, Università Politecnica delle Marche, Ancona, Italy.

suggested, more recently, that ECs may play a more direct role in bone development and formation through their interactions with osteoprogenitor cells [3] and, under certain conditions, their production of specific bone-inductive factors [4].

At the macroscopic level, the bone is arranged in two architectural forms: dense compact bone (cortical, around 80% of the total skeleton) and cancellous (trabecular, around 20% of the total skeleton) bone (Fig. 1.5). Cortical bone is dense and made of multiple stacked layers with less than 10% porosity.

It is organized in cylindrical shaped elements called osteons, composed of concentric lamellae (Fig. 1.6).

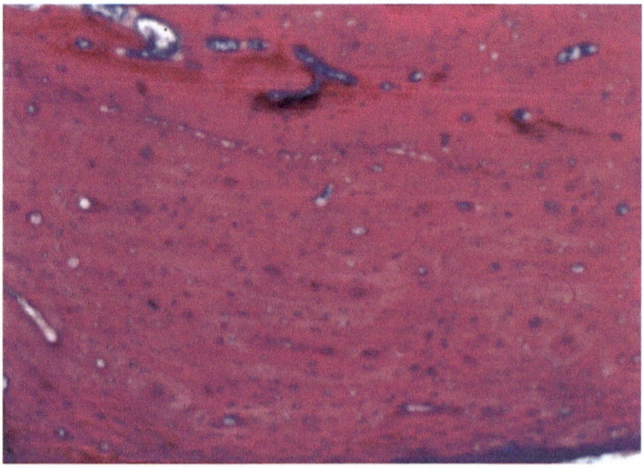

Figure 1.5 Histological image of the dense cortical bone tissue. Toluidine blue and acid fuchsin staining; original magnification 200×.

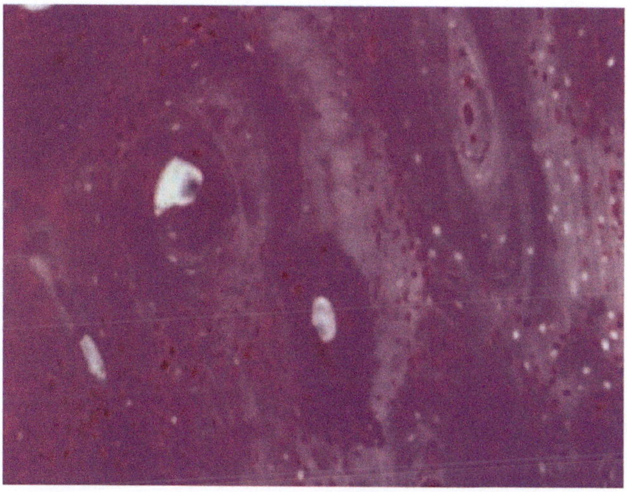

Figure 1.6 Histological image of osteons consisting of concentric layers, or lamellae, of compact bone tissue that surround a central canal, the Haversian canal. Toluidine blue and acid fuchsin staining; original magnification 100×.

The space between osteons is occupied by interstitial lamellae, which are remnants of osteons partially resorbed during bone remodeling. Osteons are cylindrical structures that are usually several millimeters long and around 0.2 mm in diameter.

The center of an osteon is made of a central canal, called the Haversian canal, that contains the bone's nerve and blood supply. On the surface of the osteon, the boundary is formed by the cement line (Fig. 1.7).

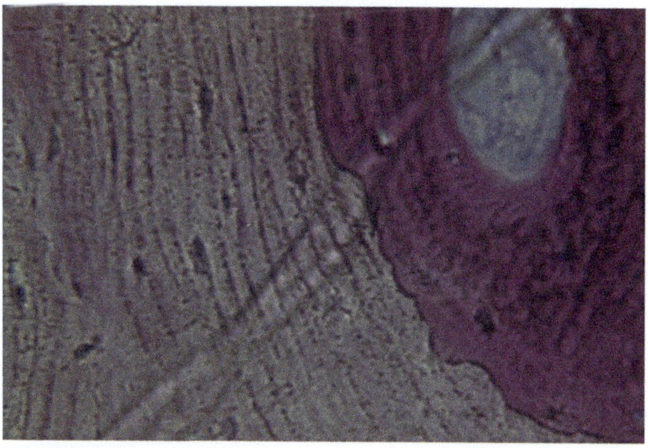

Figure 1.7 Histological image of a secondary osteon, showing the cement line formed as a result of bone remodeling process. Toluidine blue and acid fuchsin staining; original magnification 200×.

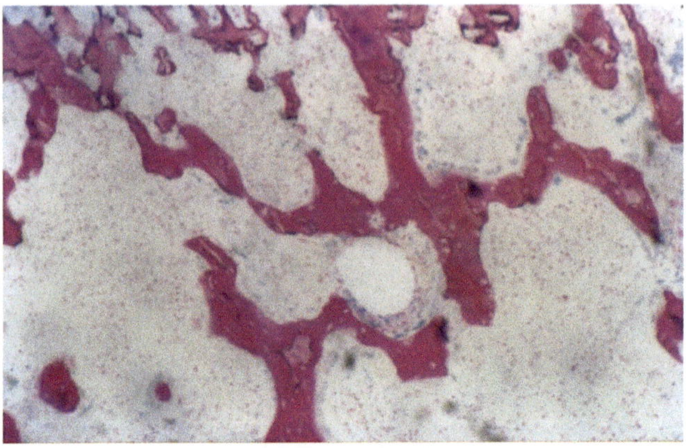

Figure 1.8 Histological image of the trabecular bone with wide marrow spaces. Toluidine blue and acid fuchsin staining; original magnification 100×.

Cortical bone is usually found on the surface of bones. In contrast, cancellous bone is organized in a porous sponge-like pattern (50–90% porosity) and it consists of a honeycomb of branching bars, plates, and rods of various sizes called trabeculae and oriented according to the direction of the physiological load (Fig. 1.8).

It is much softer, weaker, and more flexible than the cortical bone and therefore has a higher surface area to mass ratio, which makes it suitable for metabolic activity such as the exchange of calcium ions. It is found in most areas of the bone that is not under high mechanical stress. Cancellous bone makes up the bulk of the interior of most bones. The difference in tissue arrangement between the two types of bone provides increased resistance to torsion and bending; the resistance to torsion and bending by cortical bone is around 20 times superior compared to that by cancellous bone.

At the microscopic level, cortical and cancellous bone may consist of woven or lamellar bone. Woven bone is organized in a small number of randomly oriented collagen fibers and contains a high proportion of OCTs (four times the number of OCTs per unit of volume compared to lamellar bone; Fig. 1.9).

Lamellar bone is highly organized in concentric sheets filled with many collagen fibers parallel to other fibers in the same layer and contains a low proportion of OCTs. After a fracture, woven bone quickly forms and is gradually replaced by slow-growing lamellar bone through a process known as "bony substitution."

Bone is a dynamic, highly vascularized tissue with the unique capacity to heal and remodel without leaving a scar. The dynamics of bone formation involves three different processes:

- Growth
- Modeling
- Remodeling

During childhood and the early years of adulthood, while the epiphyses are still open, the skeleton grows in length (growth), the bones expand in diameter and achieve their external shape (modeling). During bone modeling, OBLs and OCLs work

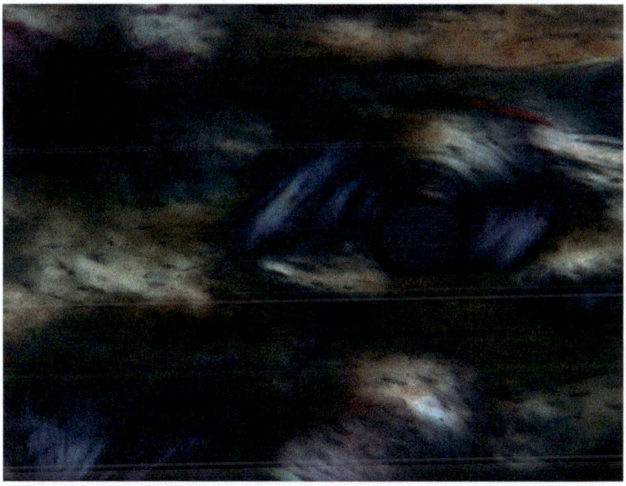

Figure 1.9 A light micrograph under the polarized light of human bone, where an osteon, typical of lamellar bone, is evident. Toluidine blue and acid fuchsin staining; original magnification 100×.

independently of each other and on different bone surfaces. The net balance is positive and it results in bone expansion, with the bone formation exceeding bone resorption. Bones reach their final external form and high bone density during this period. Both the growth and the modeling processes are controlled by hormones and mechanical forces. Following growth, bone volume remains static, with resorption and formation being in balance. Around the age 20–25 years, peak bone mass is achieved as a result of these processes. However, in later life resorption exceeds formation, leading to a slow decline in the bone mass. There is thus an unavoidable loss of the bone mass with age and a disruption of the trabecular network, which makes fortuitous osteoclastic perforations possible. Loss of the bone mass with age is unavoidable and is caused by the third process—bone remodeling. The latter process occurs once growth and modeling of the skeleton have been completed. It is likely that the major reason for remodeling is to enable the bones to respond and adapt to mechanical stresses, for example, as a result of physical exercise and during mechanical loading (e.g. orthodontic tooth movement or implant loading). Moreover, bone remodeling is designed to maintain a physiologically and mechanically competent skeleton and to repair areas of microdamage. Wolff's law states that bones develop a structure most suited to resist the forces acting upon them, adapting both the internal architecture and the external conformation to the change in external loading conditions. This change follows precise mathematical laws. When a change in loading pattern occurs, stress and strain fields in the bone are modified accordingly. Bone tissue detects the local change in strain and then adapts accordingly. The internal architecture is adapted in terms of change in density and disposition of trabeculae and osteons, the external conformation in terms of shape and dimensions. When strain is intensified, the new bone is formed. The process is complex and requires interaction between different cell phenotypes that are regulated by a variety of biochemical and mechanical factors.

Many oral conditions could lead to bone loss, such as infection, trauma, resorption after tooth extraction or surgical bone resection, and aging. It is imperative to restore the bone loss, which is the first step in any further prosthetic restoration. Various surgical solutions have been developed that allow the recovery of the lost bone. These techniques are combined with the use of biocompatible materials acting as scaffolds in supporting the bone regeneration.

1.1.2 Bone remodeling

The current concept of bone remodeling is based on the hypothesis that OCL precursors become activated and differentiate into OCLs and this begins the process of bone resorption. This step is followed by a bone formation phase. The number of sites entering the bone formation phase, called the activation frequency, together with the individual rates of the two processes, determines the rate of tissue turnover [5]. The signal that initiates bone remodeling has not been identified yet. Recently, it has been shown that mechanical stress can be sensed by OCTs and that these cells secrete paracrine factors such as insulin-like growth factor I (IGF-I) in response to mechanical forces [6]. Although IGF may act as a coupling factor in the bone remodeling cycle, the signal that initiates the cycle remains elusive. The sequence of events in the normal remodeling cycle is always the same, osteoclastic bone resorption, a reversal phase, followed by osteoblastic bone formation to repair the defect.

The termination of bone resorption and the initiation of bone formation in the resorption lacunae occur through a coupling mechanism [7]. The coupling process ensures that an equivalent amount of bone is laid down following the previous resorption phase. The detailed nature of the activation and coupling mechanism is still unknown, although the roles of some growth factors and proteinases such as transforming growth factor-β1 (TGF-β), IGF-I, IGF-II, and plasminogen activators have been indicated [8]. Whether the activation of OBLs begins simultaneously with OCLs' recruitment or at some later stage during the lacunar development is still not clear. Bone remodeling is regulated by systemic hormones and by local factors, which affect cells of both the OCL and OBL lineage and exert their effects on the replication of undifferentiated cells, the recruitment of cells, and the differentiated function of cells [9]. The end product of remodeling is the maintenance of a mineralized bone matrix and the major organic component of this matrix is collagen I (COL-1). The local factors are synthesized by skeletal cells and include growth factors, cytokines, and prostaglandins. Growth factors have effects on cells of the same class (autocrine factors) or on cells of another class within the tissue (paracrine factors).

Growth factors are also present in the circulation and may act as systemic regulators of skeletal metabolism, but the locally produced factors have more direct and important functions in cell growth. Growth factors may play a critical role in the coupling of bone formation to bone resorption and possibly in the pathophysiology of bone disorders.

Bone resorption is stimulated or inhibited by signals from other parts of the body, depending on the demand for calcium. Calcium-sensing membrane receptors in the parathyroid gland monitor calcium levels in the extracellular fluid. Low levels of calcium stimulate the release of parathyroid hormone (PTH) from chief cells of the parathyroid gland. In addition to its effects on the kidney and intestine, PTH also - increases the number and activity of OCLs to release calcium from the bone and thus stimulates bone resorption. High levels of calcium in the blood, on the other hand, leads to decreased PTH release from the parathyroid gland, decreasing the number and activity of OCLs, resulting in less bone resorption.

OBLs stimulate osteoclastic differentiation of OCL precursors through Wingless-related integration site 5a (Wnt5a) signaling. The matricellular signaling effected by TGF-β1 and IGF-1 is integrated with the Sema4D-Plexin B1-mediated OCL–OBL interaction. Sema4D, whose secretion by OCLs is stimulated by increased OCL differentiation factor receptor activator of nuclear factor kappa-B ligand (RANKL), inhibits OBLs' differentiation. OBLs are induced to migrate to the resorption sites and differentiate through the secretion of Wnt10b by OCLs at the end of the resorption phase. OBLs, in turn, inhibit osteoclastogenesis (and therefore bone resorption) via osteoprotegerin (OPG) and RANKL secretion.

OCTs regulate bone formation through the release of Wnt antagonists, Sclerostin and Dickkopf-related protein 1, which in turn are inhibited by mechanosignals and PTH. Wnt signaling in OCTs controls the production of OPG, a decoy receptor for the key RANKL. In the bone resorption cavity, calcium, TGF-β1, and IGF-1 are released in response to osteoclastic activity. A number of paracrine signals are stimulated in OCTs following changes in skeletal loading, including prostaglandin I2 and prostaglandin E2, nitric oxide, and IGF. Recent studies have raised the intriguing possibility that the OCT apoptosis may be part of the mechanism whereby OCLs are targeted to sites of bone resorption as it is elevated in the bone that is being remodeled. Estrogen suppression, a known stimulant of bone resorption, increases OCT apoptosis, and changes in bone loading are also associated with OCT apoptosis. The phenotype of the OCTs appears deficient in some receptors found on the OBL. However, the OCT is well adapted for its role in bone homeostasis and maintains intracellular signaling to respond to the unique demands of its location.

It is well established that the bone formation is an angiogenesis-dependent process [2], and ECs have long been known for their role in the formation of blood vessels that supply oxygen and nutrients to the developing bone tissue. However, it has been suggested, more recently, that ECs may play a more direct role in the bone development and formation, through their interactions with osteoprogenitor cells [3] and, under certain conditions, their production of specific bone-inductive factors [4]. ECs secrete a number of mediators (factors), which may elicit biological responses by various signal-transduction mechanisms. Such mediators are implicated in regulating the permeability of the endothelium and can promote chemotactic responses in a variety of important physiological processes, such as bone formation, remodeling, and healing. Indeed, it is the capillary that supplies oxygen and nutrients and removes calcium and waste products of resorption. One of the most important nutrients transported via the vasculature to the basic multicellular unit is oxygen. In the absence of oxygen, OBLs cannot produce collagen effectively and their proliferation is reduced. Cellular responses to changes in oxygen tension are directed through the activity of the hypoxia-inducible factor (HIF), which is capable of activating the gene transcription in response to low oxygen levels. OBL-specific knockdown of HIF1α or HIF2α has demonstrated important roles for HIF in controlling bone formation and vascularity. Furthermore, low oxygen environments encourage OCL HIF1α stabilization leading to increased OCL number.

1.1.3 The modern concept of biocompatibility

For over 50 years, biocompatibility consisted of implantable medical devices that should remain in contact with the tissues of the human body for a long time, without showing any adverse effect on those tissues from a chemical and biological point of view.

The first generation of implantable devices was designed and developed during the 1940s, and over the next few decades it became obvious that the best biological performance would be achieved with materials that showed the least chemical reactivity.

The selection criteria for implantable biomaterials included a list of events that had to be avoided, such as the local or systemic release of some products of corrosion or degradation, additives or contaminants of the main biomaterial, and their subsequent biological reaction. So, materials were selected if they were nontoxic, nonimmunogenic, nonthrombogenic, noncarcinogenic, and nonirritant.

Three important factors initiated a reevaluation of the biocompatibility concept:

1. The response to specific materials could vary from one application site to another, showing that the biocompatibility was dependent both on the material characteristics and on its application;
2. The material should specifically react with the surrounding tissues in a positive way, avoiding any adverse effect;
3. The material should degrade over time in the body rather than remain indefinitely.

Accordingly, biocompatibility was redefined in 1987 as follows: "Biocompatibility refers to the ability of a material to perform with an appropriate best response in a specific situation" [10]. Because this definition appeared to be too general, because specific mechanisms, such as individual involved processes or innovation of new biomaterials, were not provided, a modern approach defined biocompatibility as "a complex that depends on the characteristics of a material and on the biological host system."

Once grafted, the biomaterial should interact with cells of the host tissue, producing an appropriate response, which would lead to the desired clinical outcome through a combination of positive effects on critical cells and the avoidance of negative impact on others. The critical cells could be embryonic stem cells, ECs, or OBLs. The time scale may be minutes, hours, days, or years and the clinical outcome could be tissue replacement, functional support, tissue regeneration, etc. The biomaterial influences the events within the biological environment by either mechanical or molecular signaling processes, or more commonly by both. The biomaterial encounters macromolecules in the environment and becomes coated by an adsorbed layer typically composed of proteins, which may be coupled with biomaterial-derived ions or molecules. All subsequent interactions will take place between macromolecule-coated biomaterial and surrounding tissues. Although because a material may affect different biological systems in different ways, there is not a material with unique biocompatibility characteristics.

Bone substitute materials should have osteoconductive properties, become integrated in bone and replace it, allow ingrowth of blood vessels, and be easy to use as well as cost-effective. However, the modern concept of biocompatibility implicates that biomaterials, besides osteoconductivity, should also show osteoinductive and even osteogenic properties. Osteoconductive materials are composed of a matrix that acts as a scaffold for the bone deposition. Osteoinductive materials contain molecules that stimulate differentiation of progenitor cells into OBLs. Some biomaterials even contain osteogenic cells, OBLs, or OBL precursors, which are capable of forming bone if placed in the proper environment.

Autologous bone (AB) is the only material characterized by osteogenic properties with the best results in bone regeneration, although its limited availability and the need for an additional surgical procedure to harvest the bone are nowadays considered disadvantages in its use.

It is extremely important to evaluate the interaction of a biomaterial with the host in the attempt to establish its biocompatibility and investigate their interactions. A good biomaterial should stimulate some cells of the receiving site, such as OBLs, OCLs, cells of innate, and adaptive immunity and platelets. Therefore, the host cells can be divided into three groups [11]:

1. Target cells
2. Defensive cells
3. Interfering cells

The target cells are the cells at which the therapy is aimed. They could be OBLs in bone contacting device, stems cells in a tissue engineering bioreactor, or cancer cells in a polymer-chemotherapeutic agent [12,13]. The defensive cells are cells of innate and adaptive immunity and platelets. Their existence is based on the need to repel and remove adverse external agents. The interfering cells are those that are in their natural habitat and essentially get in the way and interfere with the response, for example, fibroblasts in the soft connective tissue [14] or OCLs in the bone [15]. The activity of these cells can lead to hyperplasia or tissue resorption, or other undesirable events.

The involvement of defensive cells in the entire process is inevitable and the critical question is whether their responses are controlled or uncontrolled. In the latter case, the cells of the immune system react to the presence of the biomaterial, resulting in the release of a variety of proinflammatory mediators. The combined cellular and humoral answer during the inflammatory process can lead to an accelerating and aggressive reaction that destructs both biomaterial and host tissue [16]. In other cases, the presence of the irritant biomaterial may lead to giant cell formation and granulation tissue generation [17]. Interfering cells form part of the normal anatomical structure into which the biomaterial may be grafted and their influence can have an important effect on the clinical outcomes. The biomaterial components are usually nonspecific and may induce uncontrolled response of both defensive and interfering cells, which may lead to excessive tissue growth, tissue loss, and the loss of function because of the perturbation of normal homeostasis [18].

Moreover, the biomaterial components can be uptaken by the surrounding cells through a variety of mechanisms such as phagocytosis, pinocytosis, endocytosis, or the direct transit through the plasma membrane. Once inside the cell, the component can directly affect some cellular metabolic pathways or it can be degraded in endosomes and lysosomes or be altered by the cell enzymes. The products of these processes also influence the cell metabolism. The generation of reactive oxygen species could be induced and, together with alterations in organelle function, can result in cell damage or interfere with apoptotic and necrotic pathways [19].

1.2 Biomaterials

Several different biomaterials have been used in bone regeneration procedures and all of them seem to be able to favor the formation of a significant amount of vital bone.

A biomaterial should act as a scaffold for the formation of bone, possesses pore volume, pore interconnectivity, and pores size adequate to allow the invasion of osteogenic cells and blood vessels, and have mechanical features similar to the tissues to be regenerated. Biomaterials should, moreover, present a biologic stability, help in the volume maintenance, and allow for bone remodeling. Macro- and microporosity and the interconnecting porous structure of the grafted biomaterial play a relevant role in supporting the penetration, proliferation, and differentiation of OBLs and the ingrowth of newly formed blood vessels into the biomaterial particles.

Some researchers believe that a biomaterial should be completely resorbed and replaced by newly formed bone.

1.2.1 Autologous bone

AB is the golden standard of the grafting material due to the presence of vital OBL and growth factors. It has osteogenic, osteoinductive, and osteoconductive capabilities. Histology shows that it is a highly osteoconductive material, and most of the particles are partially and/or completely surrounded by newly formed bone, in tight contact with the particles. A complete absence of inflammatory cells, multinucleated giant cells, or foreign body reaction cells should be noted. However, its main disadvantage is related to its quantity obtained from intraoral sources, and often an additional surgical procedure is required, with a higher morbidity. Furthermore, AB can present a rapid and unpredictable resorption [20].

1.2.2 Porous phycogenic hydroxyapatite

Porous phycogenic hydroxyapatite (PHA) derived from calcifying maritime algae (*Coralline officialis*) is a biologic HA, prepared by the hydrothermal conversion of the calcium carbonate in the presence of ammonium phosphate at about 700°C. This process helps in preserving the porous structure of the biomaterial. Its composition is pure inorganic calcium phosphate. The pores have a mean diameter of 5–10 μm with a periodical septation with a mean length of 50–100 μm and interconnected by means of small perforations with a mean diameter of 1–3 μm. Every pore is lined by fluorhydroxyapatite crystallites, with a size of 25–35 nm [11]. The particles are interconnected by microperforations, having a mean diameter of 1 μm. Its elevated microporosity should be helpful in the ingrowth of osteogenic cells and blood vessels.

PHA is a biocompatible, osteoconductive, and resorbable biomaterial. Most of the biomaterial particles appeared to be surrounded by newly formed bone, and in a few fields some particles seemed to be partially resorbed and substituted by newly formed bone. No inflammatory cell infiltrate or foreign body reaction cells were present; the bone was always in tight contact with the biomaterial particles with no intervening gaps (Figs. 1.10 and 1.11). Bone was present inside many biomaterial particles [21,22].

1.2.3 Collagenized porcine biomaterial

Collagenized porcine biomaterial is composed of carbonated nanocrystalline HA, containing organic material.

Most of the grafted biomaterial particles were surrounded by the newly formed bone with large OCT lacunae, always in tight contact with the particles, and no gaps were observed at the bone–biomaterial interface. No inflammatory cells and multinucleated giant cells were present. Some of the grafted particles were bridged and cemented by the newly formed bone. Many bone trabeculae were undergoing remodeling. Porcine bone is a highly osteoconductive biomaterial. It undergoes resorption, with the presence of active resorption signs (Fig. 1.12). OBLs and newly formed bone were commonly found on the surface of the biomaterial particles [23–25].

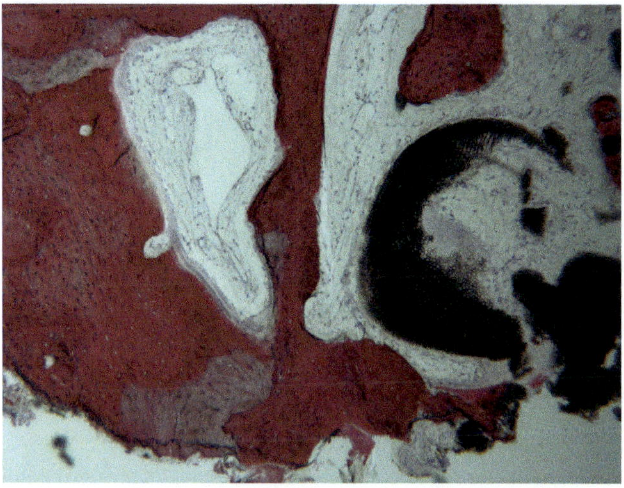

Figure 1.10 Histological image of a sample retrieved 6 months after a sinus lift in a human subject. Newly formed bone with remodeling areas and residual porous PHA material can be observed. Toluidine blue and acid fuchsin staining; original magnification 40×.

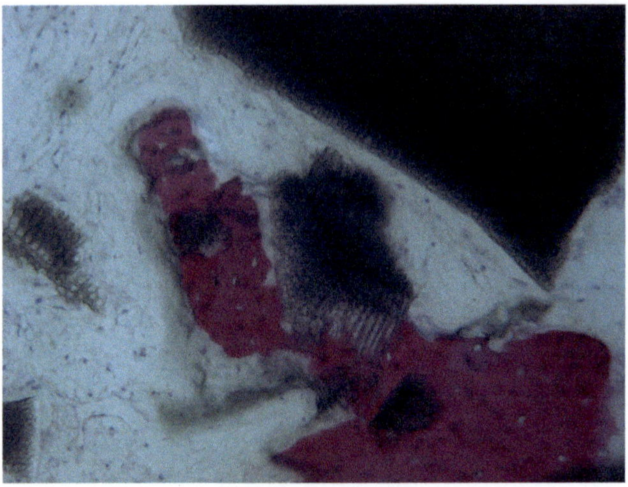

Figure 1.11 High-power histological image of porous PHA particles partially surrounded by the newly formed bone. Toluidine blue and acid fuchsin staining; original magnification 100×.

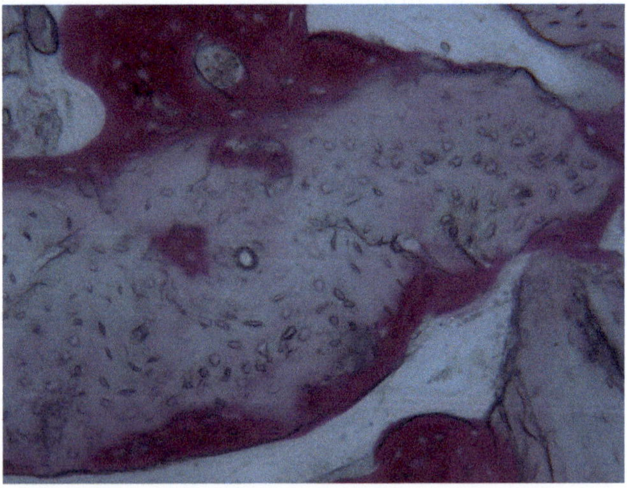

Figure 1.12 Histological image of a collagenized porcine material used to regenerate a postextraction socket in humans. The sample was retrieved after a 3-month healing time. The biomaterial particle is surrounded by the newly formed bone, which can be seen also in the inner part of the granule. The material's margin appears indented. Toluidine blue and acid fuchsin staining; original magnification 100×.

1.2.4 Anorganic bovine bone

Anorganic bovine bone (ABB) is a deproteinized bovine bone with a 75–80% degree of porosity and a size of the crystals of about 10 nm. It presents large pores and a high connectivity. ABB is one of the most used biomaterials and it has shown good osteoconductive properties. No inflammatory cell infiltrate, foreign body response, and other adverse effects are present. A high quantity of new bone formation has been reported with the use of ABB. Usually, ABB particles seem to be almost completely surrounded by the newly formed bone. No gaps or connective, fibrous tissue were observed at the bone–biomaterial interface. Some particles seemed to be bridged by the newly formed bone. Due to its low resorption rate, ABB may significantly contribute in the prevention of volume tissue loss in grafted sites opposing, for example, the sinus pressure due to repneumatization. The ABB particles and the newly formed bone produce a dense hard tissue supportive, also over the long term, of loaded implants (Fig. 1.13). This biomaterial has, thus, a long-term, three-dimensional stability [26,27].

1.2.5 Biphasic calcium phosphate

Biphasic calcium phosphate (BCP) is composed of a combination of HA and tricalcium phosphate (TCP) and used in bone regeneration procedures. It has different ratios of HA/TCP, giving rise to balanced phases of activity, a more stable phase of HA, and a more soluble phase of TCP. The resorption rate of the material is dependent on the HA/TCP ratio (a higher TCP means a higher solubility); this material gradually dissolves in the body, determining the new bone formation by the release of calcium and phosphate ions. BCPs are highly biocompatible, and they do not provoke a foreign body or a toxic response. Most of the grafted BCP particles were partially surrounded by the newly formed bone with no gaps (Fig. 1.14). Some particles were bridged by the newly formed bone. Resorption was observed at the surface of some particles [28,29,30].

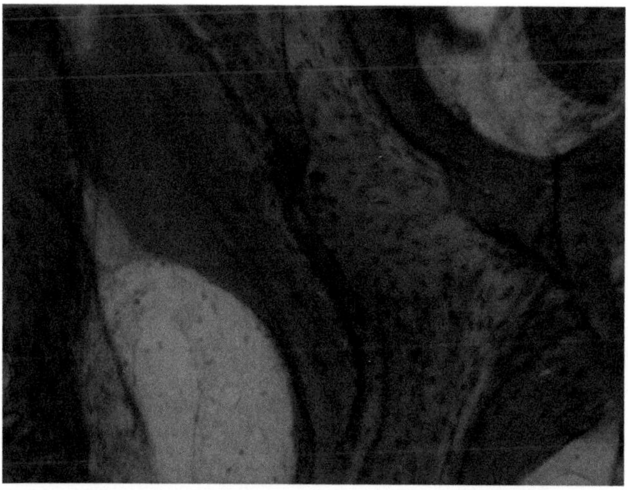

Figure 1.13 Histological image of an ABB particle integrated into the bone tissue and bridging the newly formed bone trabeculae. Toluidine blue and acid fuchsin staining; original magnification 100×.

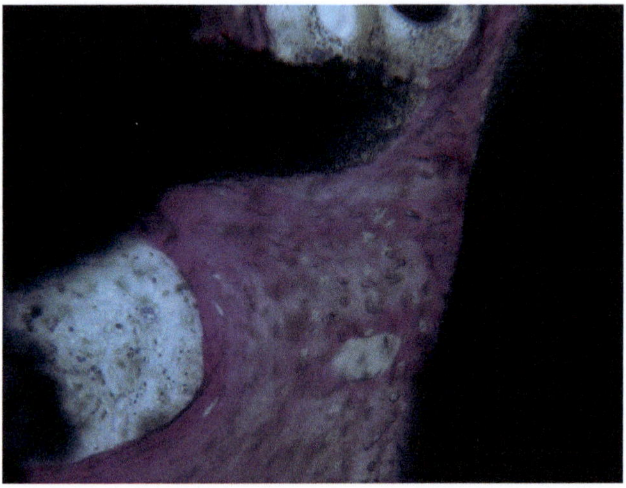

Figure 1.14 Histological image of BCP material retrieved 6 months after a sinus augmentation procedure in humans. In some portions, both next to newly formed bone and to a marrow space, signs of dissolution of the biomaterial particles can be observed. Toluidine blue and acid fuchsin staining; original magnification 100×.

1.2.6 Calcium carbonate

Different types of corals (aragonite or calcite forms of calcium carbonate) have been successfully used as a bone grafting biomaterial. They have a porous structure (150–500 μm), similar to the cancellous bone. These biomaterials can combine good mechanical properties with an open porosity. Their interconnected porous architecture, high compressive breaking stress, good biocompatibility, and resorbability, suggest their use as scaffolds for bone tissue engineering. Newly formed bone, with wide marrow spaces and wide OCT lacunae, was usually found around many biomaterial particles and some were bridged by the newly formed bone (Fig. 1.15). No inflammatory cell infiltrate, foreign body reaction, and fibrous connective tissue at the interface were observed [31,32].

1.3 Challenges and further trends

1.3.1 Graphene

Graphene is a flat monolayer of carbon atoms in a two-dimensional (2D) honeycomb lattice with high aspect ratio layer geometry and a very high specific surface area. It has attracted attention in recent years due to its exceptional thermal, mechanical, and electrical properties. Indeed, although graphene was originally developed for nanoelectronics applications, research interests in this material are continuously expanding to other fields, such as biomedicine and regenerative engineering.

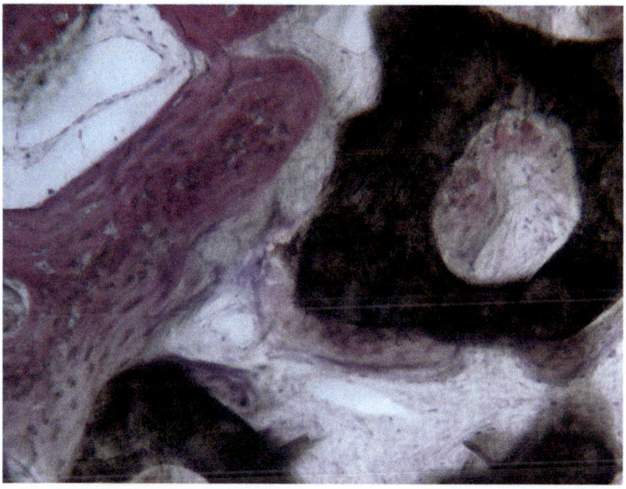

Figure 1.15 Histological image of calcium carbonate, where newly formed bone and osteoid matrix next to the particle can be observed. Toluidine blue and acid fuchsin staining; original magnification 100×.

Chemical bonding and structure were described during the 1930s. Philip Russell Wallace was the first who calculated in 1949 the electronic band structure, although the scientists did not pay special attention to this material until 2004. Andre Geim and Konstantin Novoselov, professor and doctoral student at the University of Manchester, respectively, isolated the first samples of graphene from graphite by mechanical exfoliation process [33]. Graphene can be obtained following both the bottom-up and the top-down approaches. Examples of the synthesis from simpler molecular entities (i.e. bottom-up) are chemical vapor deposition [34], anodic bonding [35], growth on silicon carbide [36], molecular beam epitaxy [37], unzipping of carbon nanotubes [38], self-assembly and polymerization of elected surfactants [39], and chemical syntesis [40]. Liquid-phase exfoliation [41] and mechanical exfoliation [33] of graphite are examples of cost-effective top-down strategies for the preparation of graphene.

Graphene, due to its 2D nature, owns unique electronic properties and is the thinnest ever tested material with an extremely high effective surface area ($\sim$2600 m^2/g). Graphene is a carbon allotrope in which each atom is connected with the neighboring carbon through a strong C–C covalent bond and shares with one of the two neighboring carbons one electron to form a π bond. Defect-free samples of graphene have a Young's modulus of 1.0 TPa and a superior intrinsic strength of $\sim$130 GPa. Graphene is one of the strongest materials known with a breaking strength over 100 times greater than a hypothetical steel film of the same thickness. With the functionalization of graphene, there is a reduction of mechanical robustness due to the introduction of defects. Thus, the mechanical properties of functionalized graphene are still much better than those of various traditional materials. Due to the out-of-plane quadratic dispersion of phonon, graphene possesses superior thermal transport properties and the intrinsic thermal conductivity (K) of this material is found to be as high as 5000 W m/K; thus, the graphene is a heat conductor one order better than copper.

Thanks to its 2D structure, each carbon atom can undergo chemical attack from both sides with respect to its plane resulting in the most reactive and lightest among all carbon allotropes and allowing to tune graphene properties at will. The possibility to favor its hydrophilicity (i.e. graphene oxide, GO) or tune its affinity to different materials via functionalization of the high exposed surface is responsible for the potential use of graphene in biological and medical applications. Particularly attractive appears to be the adaptability of graphene to flat or irregular surfaces due to its capacity to bend and its elasticity, and, therefore, its ability to be incorporated into any tissue or on any surface and scaffold (such as chitosan or HA), whether it is solid, in the form of hydrogels, or three dimensional. Moreover, worth noting is its transparency that differentiates graphene from black carbon analogs such as graphite, carbon nanotubes, and amorphous carbon. All these properties as well as the low cost of production process, playback on a large scale, and the availability of graphene makes it a really valuable and an exceptional additive for biomaterials.

1.3.2 Biomedical applications

Several studies have been conducted to study possible applications of graphene in the field of biomedicine. Studies clearly indicate that graphene and its related substrates are excellent nanoplatforms for promoting the adhesion, proliferation, and differentiation of various cells, such as human mesenchymal stem cells [42] and demonstrated that graphene synthesized by chemical vapor deposition was biocompatible with human OBL as well as mesenchymal stem cells, stimulating cell differentiation and growth [43]. Other interesting studies in the same line have been performed by other researchers [44–46], who demonstrated that graphene-based sheets were not harmful for human mesenchymal stem cells and concluded that those sheets accelerated their specific differentiation to bone cells (OBL) hypothesizing a great potential for this material in the field of bone regeneration. Also [47,48], in their studies in mice defects in which four types of scaffolds were used (titanium, titanium with bone morphogenetic protein 2 (BMP-2), titanium with GO, and titanium with BMP-2 and GO), the researchers concluded that Ti covered with GO allows a major amount of BMP-2 dose adhesion and its major liberation without modifying its structure and bioactivity. This enables a better human mesenchymal stem cell differentiation into OBLs and, therefore, a better bone neoformation in comparison with the other three scaffolds (Ti, Ti and GO, and Ti and BMP-2).

The exceptional physical properties of graphene certainly have a huge potential when combined with sophisticated derivatives and composites to provide functional, biologically active surfaces. The capability of biofunctionalization of graphene and its derivative, GO, has brought these nanomaterials under the spotlight and has drawn intense attention for a plethora of applications in biotechnology including bioassays, drug delivery, biosensors, photothermal anticancer therapy, and electrical stimulation of cells [49]. Several researchers have also evaluated the potential of graphene in neural and bone regeneration; however, few studies evaluated the ability of graphene to be biocompatible, osteoinductive, and osteoconductive when added to biomaterials.

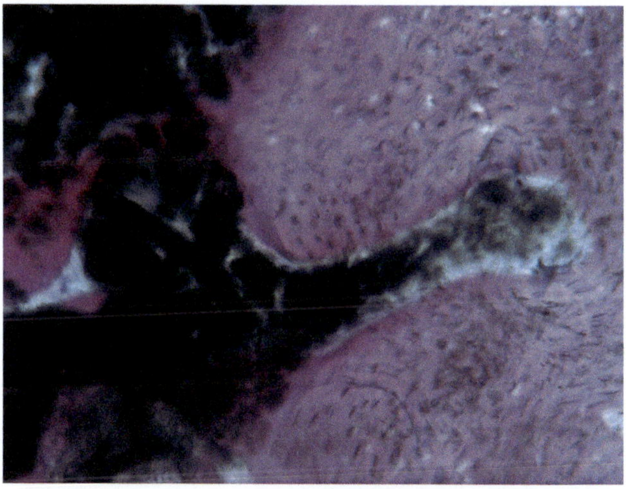

Figure 1.16 Histological image of a sample of PB coated with 50 μg/mL graphene oxide retrieved from sheep. Newly formed bone in contact with remnants of the graphene oxide coating can be observed. Toluidine blue and acid fuchsin staining; original magnification 100×.

Nowadays, the majority of biomaterials able to act as bone substitutes are limited to be osteoconductive and then only in part failed from the point of view of the processes of bone regeneration [50]. Studies report that graphene-HA are promising composites for scaffolds' fabrication in bone tissue engineering due to their ability to support proliferation and differentiation of human fetal osteoblastic (hFOB) cells [51]. Scientists developed a new effective procedure for the production of GO-coated porcine bone (PB) granules and analyzed their in vitro and in vivo potential. The results showed no toxic effects of GO-coated PB samples on primary human gingival fibroblasts and no inflammatory response around the grafted particles when implanted in vivo. Newly formed bone was detected around GO-coated PB particles (Fig. 1.16), although a small loss of GO was observed (Fig. 1.17), suggesting to use less GO concentrated samples.

In order for graphene to be used in biological and medical fields, biocompatibility as well as toxicological and ecological tests has been performed. It has been demonstrated that the in vivo effect of graphene-based materials (GBM) depends on their physical–chemical properties, concentration, time of exposure, and administration route, and also on the characteristics of the animals used. Most studies report no occurrence of adult animal death; however, there are some reports of GBM accumulation and histological findings associated with inflammation, and, more rarely, fibrosis.

In conclusion, before clinical applications, a systematic comparative study, for example, a deep meta-analysis, is highly desired to address the relative safety concerns (subtracting false-negative and false-positive effects) of graphene and derivatives. Although cell viability in vitro is not affected, graphene nanocytoxicity in a clinical setting using humans remains unknown, and further studies are needed to better evaluate the potential applications of this wonderful material.

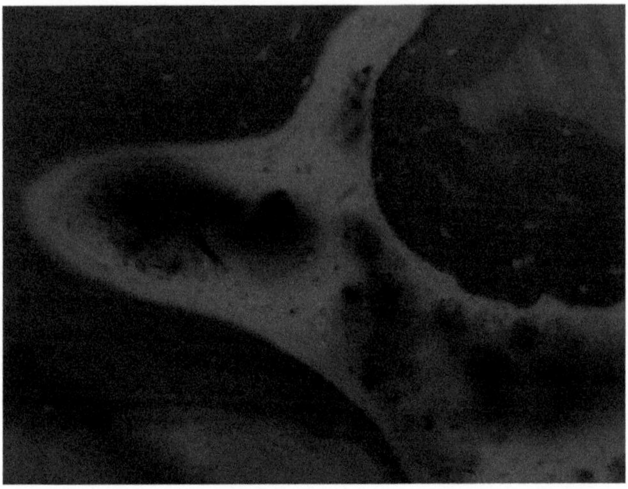

Figure 1.17 Histological image of a sample retrieved from sheep where PB particles coated with 50 μg/mL graphene oxide were used to fill bone defects. It is evident how the coating, although detached from the particles, is biocompatible as osteoblasts are depositing osteoid matrix next to the remnants of the coating. Toluidine blue and acid fuchsin staining; original magnification 200×.

Acknowledgment

This work has been supported by PRIN20102ZLNJ5 financed by Ministry of Education, University and Research (MIUR) Italy.

References

[1] Fujikawa Y, Quinn JM, Sabokbar A, McGee JO, Athanasou NA. The human osteoclast precursor circulates in the monocyte fraction. Endocrinology 1996;137(9):4058–60.

[2] Gerber HP, Vu TH, Ryan AM, Kowalski J, Werb Z, Ferrara N. VEGF couples hypertrophic cartilage remodeling, ossification and angiogenesis during endochondral bone formation. Nat Med 1999;5:623–8.

[3] Villars F, Guillotin B, Amedee T, Dutoya S, Bordenave L, Bareille R, et al. Effect of HUVEC on human osteoprogenitor cell differentiation needs heterotypic gap junction communication. Am J Physiol Cell Physiol 2002;282:775–85.

[4] Bouletreau PJ, Warren SM, Spector JA, Peled ZM, Gerrets RP, Greenwald JA, et al. Hypoxia and VEGF up-regulate BMP-2 mRNA and protein expression in microvascular endothelial cells: implications for fracture healing. Plast Reconstr Surg 2002;109: 2384–97.

[5] Siddiqui JA, Partridge NC. Physiological bone remodeling: systemic regulation and growth factor involvement. Physiology (Bethesda) 2016;31(3):233–45.

[6] Mikuni-Takagaki Y. Mechanical responses and signal transduction pathways in stretched osteocytes. J Bone Min Metab 1999;17(1):57–60 (review).

[7] Florencio-Silva R, Sasso GR, Sasso-Cerri E, Simões MJ, Cerri PS. Biology of bone tissue: structure, function, and factors that influence bone cells. Biomed Res Int 2015;2015:421746.
[8] Sims NA, Martin TJ. Coupling the activities of bone formation and resorption: a multitude of signals within the basic multicellular unit. Bonekey Rep 2014;3:481.
[9] Capulli M, Paone R, Rucci N. Osteoblast and osteocyte: games without frontiers. Arch Biochem Biophys 2014;561:3–12.
[10] Williams DF. Consensus and definitions in biomaterials. Adv Biomaterials 1988;8:11–6.
[11] Williams DF. There is no such thing as a biocompatible material. Biomaterials 2014; 35(38):10009–14.
[12] Park JH, Olivares-Navarrete R, Wasilewski CE, Boyan BD, Tannenbaum R, Schwartz Z. Use of polyelectrolyte thin films to modulate osteoblast response to microstructured titanium surfaces. Biomaterials 2012;33(21):5267–77.
[13] Ghaedi M, Mendez JJ, Bove PF, Sivarapatna A, Raredon MS, Niklason LE. Alveolar epithelial differentiation of human induced pluripotent stem cells in a rotating bioreactor. Biomaterials 2014;35(2):699–710.
[14] Eckes B, Zigrino P, Kessler D, Holtkötter O, Shephard P, Mauch C, et al. Fibroblast-matrix interactions in wound healing and fibrosis. Matrix Biol 2000;19(4):325–32 (review).
[15] Costa DO, Prowse PD, Chrones T, Sims SM, Hamilton DW, Rizkalla AS, et al. The differential regulation of osteoblast and osteoclast activity by surface topography of hydroxyapatite coatings. Biomaterials 2013;34(30):7215–26.
[16] Franz S, Rammelt S, Scharnweber D, Simon JC. Immune responses to implants—a review of the implications for the design of immunomodulatory biomaterials. Biomaterials 2011; 32(28):6692–709.
[17] Anderson JM, Rodriguez A, Chang DT. Foreign body reaction to biomaterials. Semin Immunol 2008;20(2):86–100.
[18] Schoen FJ. Mechanisms of function and disease of natural and replacement heart valves. Annu Rev Pathol 2012;7:161–83.
[19] Singh N, Manshian B, Jenkins GJ, Griffiths SM, Williams PM, Maffeis TG, et al. NanoGenotoxicology: the DNA damaging potential of engineered nanomaterials. Biomaterials 2009;30(23–24):3891–914.
[20] Soardi CM, Spinato S, Zaffe D, Wang HL. Atrophic maxillary floor augmentation by mineralized human bone allografts in sinuses of different size: an histologic and histomorphometric analysis. Clin Oral Implants Res 2011;22:560–6.
[21] Ewers R. Maxilla sinus grafting with marine algae derived bone forming material: a clinical report of long-term results. Oral Maxillofac Surg 2005;63:1712–23.
[22] Thorwarth M, Wehrhan F, Srour S, Schultze-Mosgau S, Felszeghy E, Bader RD, et al. Evaluation of substitutes for bone: comparison of microradiographic and histological assessments. Br J Oral Maxillofac Surg 2007;45:41–7.
[23] Barone A, Ricci M, Covani U, Nannmark U, Azarmehr I, Calvo-Guirado JL. Maxillary sinus augmentation using prehydrated corticocancellous porcine bone: hystomorphometric evaluation after 6 months. Clin Implant Dent Relat Res 2012;14:373–9.
[24] Calvo-Guirado JL, Ramirez Fernandez MP, Negri B, Delgado Riuz RA, Sanchez De-Val JEM, Gomez-Moreno G. Experimental model of bone response to collagenized xenografts of porcine origin (Osteobiol® MP3): a radiological and histomorphometric study. Clin Implant Dent Relat Res 2013;15:143–51.
[25] Ramirez Fernandez MP, Calvo-Guirado JL, Arcesio-Delgado Ruiz R, Maté Sanchez De-Val JE, Ortega VV, Olmes LM. Bone response to hydroxyapatites with open porosity of animal origin (porcine [OsteoBiol mp3] and bovine [Endobon]): a radiological and histomorphometric study. Clin Oral Implants Res 2011;22:767–73.

[26] Sartori S, Silvestri M, Forni F, Icaro Cornaglia A, Tepei P, Cattaneo V. Ten-year follow-up in a maxillary sinus augmentation using anorganic bovine bone (Bio-Oss). A case report with histomorphometric evaluation. Clin Oral Implants Res 2003;14:369–72.
[27] Polyzois I, Renvert S, Bosshardt DD, Lang NP, Claffey N. Effect of Bio-Oss® on osseointegration of dental implants surrounded by circumferential bone defects of different dimensions: an experimental study in the dog. Clin Oral Implants Res 2007;18:304–10.
[28] Artzi Z, Weinreb M, Carmeli G, Lev-Dor R, Dard M, Nemcovsky CE. Histomorphometric assessment of bone formation in sinus augmentation utilizing a combination of autogenous and hydroxyapatite/biphasic tricalcium phosphate graft materials: at 6 and 9 months in humans. Clin Oral Implants Res 2008;19:686–92.
[29] Covani U, Orlando B, Giacomelli L, Cornelini R, Barone A. Implant survival after sinus elevation with Straumann® BoneCeramic in clinical practice: ad-interim results of a prospective study at a 15-month follow-up. Clin Oral Implants Res 2011;22:481–4.
[30] Giuliani A, Manescu A, Larsson E, Tromba G, Luongo G, Piattelli A, et al. In vivo regenerative properties of coralline-derived (biocoral) scaffold grafts in human maxillary defects: demonstrative and comparative study with Beta-tricalcium phosphate and biphasic calcium phosphate by synchrotron radiation x-ray microtomography. Clin Implant Dent Relat Res 2014;16:736–50.
[31] Wikesjo UM, Lim WH, Razi SS, Sigurdsson TJ, Tatakis DN, Hardwick WR. Periodontal repair in dogs: a bioabsorbable calcium carbonate coral implant enhances space provision for alveolar bone regeneration in conjunction with guided tissue regeneration. J Periodontol 2003;74:957–64.
[32] Demers C, Hamdy CR, Corsi K, Chellat F, Tabriziam M, Yahia L. Natural coral exoskeleton as a bone graft substitute: a review. Biomed Mater Eng 2002;12:15–35.
[33] Geim AK, Novoselov KS. The rise of graphene. Nat Mater 2007;6:183–1291.
[34] Zhang Y, Zhang L, Zhou C. Review of chemical vapor deposition of graphene and related applications. Acc Chem Res 2013;46:2329–39.
[35] Balan A, Kamar R, Boukhicha M, Beyssac O, Bouillard JC, Taverna D, et al. Anodic bonded graphene. J Phys D Appl Phys 2010;43:374013.
[36] Rollings E, Gweon GH, Zhou SY, Mun BS, McChesney JL, Hussain BS, et al. Synthesis and characterization of atomically-thin graphite films on a silicon carbide substrate. J Phys Chem Solids 2006;67:2172–7.
[37] Lippert G, Dabrowski J, Yamamoto Y, Herziger F, Maultzsch J, Baringhaus J, et al. Molecular beam epitaxy of graphene on mica. Phys Status Solidi B 2012;249:2507–10.
[38] Kosynkin DV, Higginbotham AL, Sinitskii A, Lomeda JR, Dimiev A, Price K, et al. Longitudinal unzipping of carbon nanotubes to form graphene nanoribbons. Nature 2009; 458:872–6.
[39] Zhang W, Cui J, Tao C, Wu Y, Li Z, Ma L, et al. A strategy for producing pure single-layer graphene sheets based on a confined self-assembly approach. Angew Chem 2009;48:5864–8.
[40] Yang X, Dou X, Rouhanipour A, Zhi L, Räder HJ, Müller K. Two dimensional graphene nanoribbons. J Am Chem Soc 2008;130:4216–7.
[41] Coleman JN. Liquid exfoliation of defect-free graphene. Acc Chem Res 2013;46:14–22.
[42] Kalbacova M, Broz A, Kong J, Kalbac M. Graphene substrates promote adherence of human osteoblasts and mesenchymal stromal cells. Carbon 2010;48:4323–9.
[43] Talukdar Y, Rashkow JT, Lalwani G, Kanakia S, Sitharaman B. The effects of graphene nanostructures on mesenchymal stem cells. Biomaterials 2014;35:4863–77.
[44] Fan HL, Wang LL, Zhao KK, Li N, Shi Z, Ge Z, et al. Fabrication, mechanical properties, and biocompatibility of graphene-reinforced chitosan composites. Biomacromolecules 2010;11:2345–51.

[45] Nayak TR, Andersen H, Makam VS, Khaw C, Bae S, Xu X, et al. Graphene for controlled and accelerated osteogenic differentiation of human mesenchymal stem cells. ACS Nano 2011;5:4670–8.
[46] Shen H, Zhang L, Liu M, Zhang Z. Biomedical applications of graphene. Theranostics 2012;2:283–94.
[47] La WG, Park S, Yoon HH, Jeong GJ, Lee TJ, Bhang SH, et al. Delivery of a therapeutic protein for bone regeneration from a substrate coated with graphene oxide. Small 2013;9: 4051–60.
[48] La WG, Jin M, Park S, Yoon HH, Jeong GJ, Bhang SH, et al. Delivery of bone morphogenetic protein-2 and substance P using graphene oxide for bone regeneration. Int J Nanomedicine 2014;9(Suppl. 1):107–16.
[49] Chen GY, Pang DW, Hwang SM, Tuan HY, Hu YC. A graphene-based platform for induced pluripotent stem cells culture and differentiation. Biomaterials 2012;33:418–27.
[50] Oyefusi A, Olanipekun O, Neelgund GM, Peterson D, Stone JM, Williams E, et al. Hydroxyapatite grafted carbon nanotubes and graphene nanosheets: promising bone implant materials. Spectrochim Acta A Mol Biomol Spectrosc 2014;132:410–6.
[51] Ettorre V, De Marco P, Zara S, Perrotti V, Scarano A, Di Crescenzo A, et al. In vitro and in vivo characterization of graphene oxide coated porcine bone granules. Carbon 2016; 103:291–8.

Mechanical modification of dental implants to control bone retention

2

H. Alexander[1], J. Ricci[2]
[1]Orthogen LLC, Springfield, NJ, United States; [2]New York University College of Dentistry, New York, NY, United States

2.1 Introduction

Over a number of decades, researchers and clinicians have empirically observed the effects of surface roughness (or lack of it) on soft and hard tissue response [1]. Rough and smooth surfaces affect osseointegration. However, there has been little understanding of the mechanisms involved.

Empirically, device manufacturers have, for many years, been using surface roughening techniques to enhance bone apposition to implants. The final outer finish of a dental implant is believed to play an important role in the ability of the bone to grow on the implant surface. There are, indeed, a great variety of finishes presently in use throughout the dental implant industry. For example, machined, acid etched, laser machined, blasted, and alloys coated with materials that induce bone activity are currently in use. Combinations of these techniques are often used to optimize implant fixation. For example, Szmukler-Moncler et al. [2] have shown that sandblasting with large grit followed by acid etching increases bone growth on the surface by 50% after 10 weeks of healing.

Conversely, smooth surfaces are often used to ensure a fibrous tissue barrier with the bone. A machined finish creates grooves on the order of 0.5−1 μm. Once a machined finish is polished, the surface of the implant is smooth to the nanometer level. On the cellular level, neither a machined finish nor a polished finish provides a surface with a texture promoting osseointegration. For example, fracture fixation devices have smooth polished surfaces because they are designed to be easily removed when no longer functional. This chapter discusses what is known of the mechanisms that allow cells to respond to surface topography. Reliance will be mainly on the cell biology and tissue engineering literature. This rich literature has provided often-overlooked clues to how cells respond to surfaces. The ways in which this information can be used to tissue engineer surfaces and examples of surfaces that have been engineered for cell response will be described.

Bone Response to Dental Implant Materials. http://dx.doi.org/10.1016/B978-0-08-100287-2.00002-1

2.2 The implant as extracellular matrix

The most accurate way to view cell response to surfaces is to look at any surface that interfaces with cells as one would view extracellular matrix (ECM). Normally, we view ECM as the tissue matrix where the cells reside within. Similarly, the implant surfaces should also be considered as a form of ECM. Cells never interact directly with any synthetic surface (in vivo or in vitro) as long as there are proteins present. In surgical sites, implants immediately come in contact with blood proteins and many of these proteins adhere to these surfaces because virtually all tissue-integrated implant surfaces are relatively hydrophilic and bind proteins immediately upon contact. In addition, over time, as cell–surface interfaces mature, the nature of the protein interface changes as the proteins change and cells change their attachment proteins [3]. Thus, proteins always mediate the interface between cells and surfaces. So the interface between cells and artificial surfaces is analogous to that of cells and ECM. When cells and either ECM or implant surfaces are discussed, it should be assumed that there is a proteinaceous interface between them.

2.3 Cell attachment

Cells form direct attachments to both ECM and implant surfaces. The first cells that reach the surface after implantation are macrophages and polymorphonuclear leukocytes (PMNs). These are immune system cells, and although they play an important role in the healing process, they are mostly transient at the interface. The cells that produce tissue at the interface (in the case of dental implants) are mostly fibroblasts, osteoblasts, and epithelial cells.

Attachments formed by cells are discontinuous and are analogous to "spot welds" between the cells and the surface. These attachments, which are collections of cell attachment proteins, are referred to as cell attachment plaques, or hemidesmosomes, in the case of epithelial cells attached to dental implants and teeth. These collections of proteins are cell-signaling molecules (ligands) that interact with clusters of integrins, which are transmembrane molecules that internalize the cell attachment signal into the cellular machinery, including the cell cytoskeleton and its associated cellular structures [4,5].

The combination of cell attachment plaques, integrins, and the cell cytoskeleton represents the mechanism by which the cell internalizes information from the ECM or implant surface. It is the three-dimensional arrangement of these cell attachments that determines how the cell responds to ECM and implant surfaces. Mechanotransduction and cell response to surface micro- and nanostructure are closely related. Mechanotransduction is simply the process by which mechanical forces cause changes in ECM configuration, which results in changes in the way cells respond to ECM. Ingber has authored an excellent summary of the mechanisms involved with mechanotransduction [6]. A further exposition on macro-mechanotransduction explaining the effects of mechanical stress on the bone can be found in Section 2.8.

2.4 Cell behavior on smooth surfaces

To determine how cells respond to topography, it is best to examine how cells behave when there is a lack of significant topography. Because researchers have been growing cells on flat culture plates for a very long time, there is extensive literature on this type of behavior. For instance, it is known that in media containing significant amounts of protein a typical mammalian cell such as a fibroblast will attach, spread extensively, form stress fibers, which are organized collections of cytoskeleton components, and proliferate at very high rates until the cells reach monolayer (confluence) conditions. There is also considerable historical evidence that there is an inverse relationship between proliferation and ECM production, suggesting that extensive proliferation causes dedifferentiation [7].

It is now clear that proliferation is partly based on extensive cell spreading and cell attachment plaque formation, as this has been shown to have a stimulatory effect on cell proliferation [5]. Early landmark studies of cell attachment showed that, if surfaces were modified to limit cell spreading, cell proliferation is also limited [8]. A significant determinant of this behavior, in vitro, is probably based on the three-dimensional configuration of the cell attachment plaques on the flat surface. Because these cell attachments are arranged in a planar array they internalize this information and control the arrangement of the cytoskeleton accordingly. Because these cells live in the normal ECM, which almost never exists as a perfectly flat surface in vivo, this flat arrangement of cell attachments is an unusual arrangement for these cells, and the cells respond by spreading extensively, proliferating at abnormally high rates, and dedifferentiating.

2.5 Cell behavior on three-dimensional and roughened surfaces

Cells behave much differently in ECM, roughened surfaces, and tissue-engineered surfaces compared to flat surfaces. This is based on a concept called contact guidance. Contact guidance refers to the way in which cells respond to surface micro- and nanostructure. Ross G. Harrison, a pioneer in cell culture techniques and the first to grow neurons in culture [9], was supposedly the first to observe this phenomenon in 1907, although the referenced paper does not specifically mention this. He supposedly noted the way in which growing neurons followed structural defects in glass culture plates. Harrison mentored Paul Weiss in the 1930s, and Weiss coined the term "contact guidance," and studied this phenomenon extensively. Weiss and Garber published a landmark paper in 1952 [10] that examined the morphology of cells cultured in three-dimensional fibrin clots of different concentrations and orientations. They found that cells in disorganized fibrin were more stellate in appearance and lacked significant orientation, whereas cells in organized fibrin became organized parallel to the fibrin and more spindle shaped. This was the first publication that demonstrated how organized ECM caused cells to orient and change shape. It is widely recognized as the first tissue engineering publication that examined cell response to three-dimensional scaffolds and defined the ways in which cells respond to changes in ECM organization by changing their cellular morphology. Although the mechanisms of contact guidance were unknown at the time, we now know that contact guidance is based on the way cells extend filopodia to explore ECM and then form cell attachment plaques with the ECM. The three-dimensional arrangement of these cell attachment plaques is the key to the cell response to ECM.

On complex surfaces, the arrangement of cell attachment plaques follows the three-dimensional arrangement of the surface, with cell attachment plaques forming on micro- and nanostructural peaks rather than in the valleys. Cell attachments do not form in the small valleys of these surfaces because of the dynamics of the cell cytoskeleton, and so the actual amount of available surface area for cell attachment on these surfaces is limited relative to flat surfaces. Cell attachment processes contain cytoskeleton elements, which are tensile and compressive in nature and form linear arrays. Thus, they cannot form effectively around sharp corners. This makes them incapable of conforming to small nano- and microindentations, and so they attach to the crests of the structures rather than the depressions [11]. In effect, this means that cell processes are not capable of "reaching" around sharp corners and conforming to extremely complex surfaces. Stem cells have been shown to respond to roughened surfaces by changing differentiation, which is partially mediated by RhoA (Ras homolog gene family member A protein) [12].

In addition, because the surfaces are three-dimensionally complex, the arrangement of cell attachments is also three-dimensionally complex as determined by the surface. This suggests that this change in attachment configuration results in (1) smaller numbers or lesser area of cell attachment, resulting in less signaling for proliferation, and (2) a three-dimensional cytoskeletal arrangement more like the one that is normally seen in the ECM, resulting in changes in cell differentiation.

2.6 Mechanisms involved with translation of cell configuration to differentiation

There is an extremely large body of literature that addresses the mechanisms involved with translation of cell attachment configuration with cell differentiation. As with most biologic processes, there are multiple pathways and significant redundancy built into the system. One particular system is very well documented and seems to be involved with mechanotransduction as well as cell response to surfaces. This system can be summarized as follows:

1. The signals from the cell attachments, mediated by integrin transmembrane proteins, are internalized into the cellular machinery including the cytoskeleton.
2. The configuration of the cytoskeleton controls many cellular signaling events, including cellular response to growth and differentiation factors [5].
3. This process is at least partially controlled by a system of small GTPase (guanosine triphosphate hydrolase enzyme) proteins such as Ras family proteins [13], Rho family proteins and subfamily proteins such as Rac and Rac1, and proteins such as ROCK1 (Rho associated

protein kinase 1), which is a downstream effector of RhoA [14]. These signaling molecules make up one of the systems that control cell spreading, proliferation, and differentiation. Knocking out the Ras signaling system has been shown to stop cell migration and proliferation, effectively paralyzing the cell [13]. Supplemental data from this publication, in the form of time-lapse videos of cell migration and proliferation dramatically, show the effect on cells when these Ras proteins are knocked out. This effectively stops cell response to surfaces by interrupting cell cytoskeleton function.

4. In the case of mechanotransduction, changes in the GTPase protein system are more dynamic and based on changes in the ECM configuration. However, the mechanisms behind this process are probably similar to the cell response to ECM in general.

Signaling molecules such as these GTPases have been shown to be the major pathways by which the signals from cell attachments and their three-dimensional patterns are translated into changes in the cell cytoskeleton and modulation of cell function and gene expression [5]. The effects of these signaling molecules are complex and it is not entirely clear how they are related as they respond differently to different surfaces and in different cells. A detailed study of this system is beyond the scope of this chapter. It is, however, important to note that these molecules represent an important and well-documented intermediate signaling system between the ECM, cell attachment plaques, the cell cytoskeleton, and overall cell function (migration, proliferation, differentiation, and apoptosis).

2.7 Using controlled surface configuration to control cell function—tissue engineering surfaces

It is only recently that controlled surfaces have begun to be used to control cell function. This has been done most successfully using two different methods: control of surface chemistry (protein and surface chemistry patterning) and control of surface micro- and nanogeometry. Both will be elaborated upon in this section.

Protein and surface chemistry patterning usually employs controlled microstructure "stamps" that are produced using soft lithography and then used to apply cell attachment proteins to surfaces (such as stamping ink on paper) in very controlled patterns where cell attachment is desired. Other surface chemistries are also used in conjunction with these methods to produce hydrophobic surfaces to prevent cell attachment where it is not wanted. Some of the best examples of the effects of the use of micro- and nanofabricated surfaces to control cell spreading, growth, and migration have been produced using these methods [15,16]. In fact, supplemental data from the article by Doyle et al. [16], which is in the form of time-lapse videos of cell migration, show exactly how controlling cell attachment can control cell spreading and migration. The videos by Doyle et al. show how cells respond when they are confined to channels, respond to flat surfaces, and respond to cross-hatched surfaces (a similar concept to roughening). These methods have worked well in vitro, where the presence of other proteins in the environment can be controlled. However, in vivo, these protein-patterned surfaces face interference from additional attached proteins and have not been found to be effective.

Most current roughened surfaces are randomly roughened meaning that they consist of a wide variety of surface structures depending on the method of processing. This has been shown empirically to work well for osseointegration and to strongly influence cell spreading and shape [17], but optimization of these surfaces has been elusive as their structure is not controlled. Consequently, many investigators in the tissue-engineering field have developed controlled micro- and nanotextured surfaces that demonstrate how specific surface configurations can be used to control cell function in vitro [18–20]. An excellent example of the use of controlled surface effects on cell and tissue formation, in vitro, can be found in the work of Guilemette et al. [21], where cell culture substrates containing cell-sized microgrooves were used to organize cells and the ECM produced by these cells. This was done to engineer multilayered tissue in vitro. Their results indicated that layers of cells and ECM, when cultured on these controlled surfaces, self-assembled into organized tissues. Multiple cell types were examined and in many cases, when multiple layers of cells and ECM were used, additional layers aligned based on the initial layers on the controlled surfaces. In a publication examining the response of bone cells to oriented surfaces [22], it was found that the cellular response was mediated at least in part by the RhoA/ROCK pathway.

Ricci et al. [18] have worked with similar microgrooved surfaces for a different purpose. Based on the previously noted data on the effects of cell spreading on proliferation, it was hypothesized that microgrooved surfaces, if produced in the proper sizes relative to cell size, could be used to inhibit cell spreading and thus their proliferation. A systematic study of microgroove dimensions was performed, ranging from 2 to 12 μm (ridge and groove dimension as well as depth), and their effects on both fibroblasts and bone marrow-derived osteoblast-like cells were evaluated. These surfaces, which were produced using silicon wafer technology similar to that used in the microelectronics industry, had profound effects on cell cytoskeleton configuration, cell orientation, spreading, and proliferation [19,20]. Microgrooves and ridges in the range of 6–12 μm (12–24 μm repeat spacing), and with similar depths, were shown to reduce cell proliferation up to 50% while causing orientation and migration of the cells parallel to the microgrooves, and preventing orientation and migration perpendicular to the microgrooves.

A method was then developed for producing similar microgroove patterns on titanium alloy surfaces using ultraviolet laser micromachining. These surfaces were characterized using specialized software and scanning electron microscopy (SEM) and compared with machined surfaces and a successful and widely used random roughened surface known as the resorbable blast textured surface (Figs. 2.1–2.3). The results indicated that the machined surface had Sa (roughness height) and Rc (profilometry feature height) values of 0.459 and 0.802 μm, respectively, and an Sdr (developed surface area or area percent in excess of a flat surface) of 13.09%. The roughened surface had Sa, Rc, and Sdr values of 3.07, 7.80 μm, and 30.51%, respectively, and the laser microchanneled (8 μm microchannel) surfaces had Sa, Rc, and Sdr values of 2.94, 7.93 μm, and 66.74%, respectively. In addition, the Rsm (spacing between major features) of the laser microchanneled surface was 16.18 μm. The Rc and Rsm values were precisely at specification for the 8 μm microchanneled surface, demonstrating the precision of manufacturing and reproducibility of this surface. Other

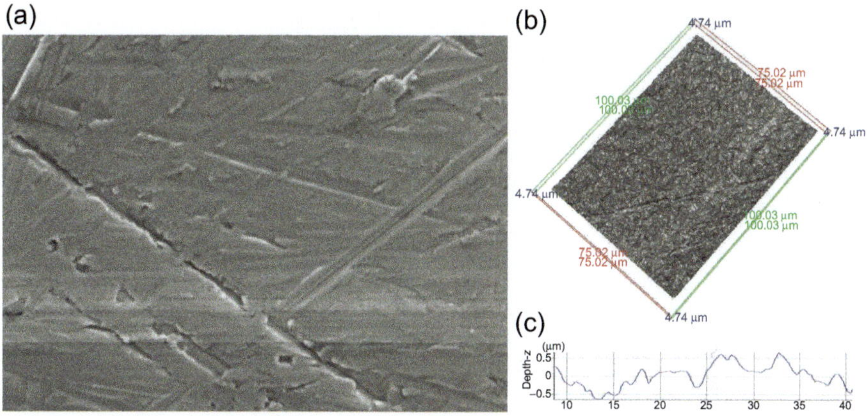

Figure 2.1 Scanning electron micrograph (a), three-dimensional reconstruction (b), and surface profilometry tracing (c) of a titanium alloy machined surface. Bar = 15 μm.
Reproduced from Int J Periodontics Restorative Dent 2016;36(suppl.):s39−46 with permission from Quintessence Publishing Co., Inc.

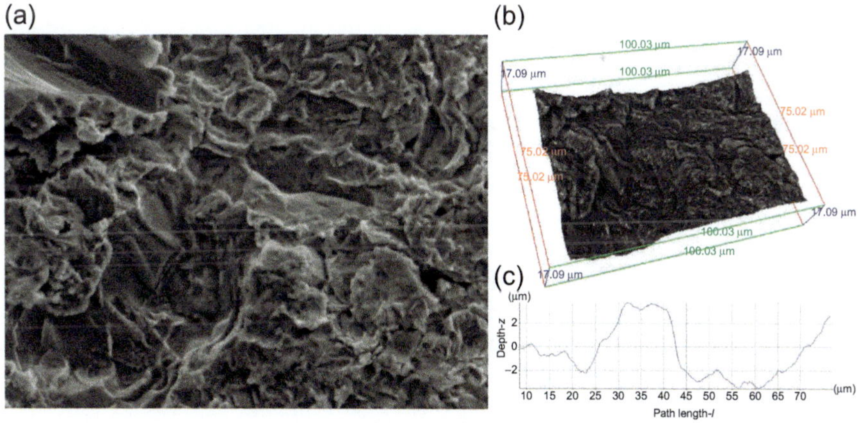

Figure 2.2 Scanning electron micrograph (a), three-dimensional reconstruction (b), and surface profilometry tracing (c) of a roughened titanium alloy surface. Bar = 15 μm.
Reproduced from Int J Periodontics Restorative Dent 2016;36(suppl.):s39−46 with permission from Quintessence Publishing Co., Inc.

than the organization of this surface, the significant increase in the Sdr value of this surface may also be one of the reasons for its success. Figs. 2.1−2.3 show the SEM images, three-dimensional reconstructions, and profilometry tracings of these surfaces.

Surfaces with 8 and 12 μm microchannels (16 and 24 μm repeat spacing), with similar depths, were initially tested in an implantable chamber model placed in the canine femur [23,24]. The results indicated that these surfaces developed more extensive bone ingrowth and contact than either machined surfaces or roughened surfaces

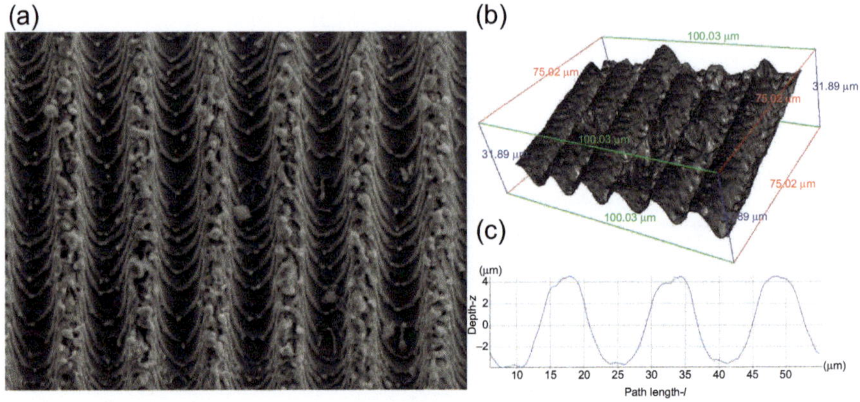

Figure 2.3 Scanning electron micrograph (a), three-dimensional reconstruction (b), and surface profilometry tracing (c) of a laser microchanneled titanium alloy surface (8 µm groove and ridge size). Bar = 15 µm.
Reproduced from Int J Periodontics Restorative Dent 2016;36(suppl.):s39–46 with permission from Quintessence Publishing Co., Inc.

made of the same alloy and that in the case of the microchannel surfaces, the bone organized parallel to the microchannels. Mechanical tensile testing of the interface between new tissue and these surfaces indicated significant bone adhesion to the microchannels. Areas of fibrous tissue interface, such as those seen in marrow spaces, also showed attachment to these laser micromachined surfaces.

These 8 and 12 µm surfaces were then produced on the collars of dental implants and tissue response was examined in a canine, functionally loaded study [25]. When these microchanneled implant collars were placed in the bone, the bone was observed to attach and remain at crestal levels, and in a significant number of cases, grow slightly up the collars (referred to as the bone upgrowth). When portions of the collars were left supracrestal, it was observed that the microchannels inhibited epithelial downgrowth, and these surfaces developed significant areas of fibrous tissue attachment. Perhaps the most significant observation, and one that was not fully appreciated at the time, was that the orientation of fibrous tissue in these areas was not the parallel (to the implant surface) collagen orientation that we usually observe at machined and random roughened surfaces (Figs. 2.4 and 2.5), but was oriented tangentially to the surface (Fig. 2.6). Fibrous tissue cells were also observed to be oriented within the microchannels (Fig. 2.7). This was an unexpected result, but extremely significant, as these fibers, while not Sharpey's fibers (there is no cementum observed), could be interpreted to function like the supracrestal fibers that are part of biologic width around the natural teeth. These results were equivalent using either the 8 or 12 µm surfaces. Human histological studies have confirmed these results [26], and these studies, as well as observations of microchanneled abutments retrieved from human patients, have shown that the epithelial and fibrous attachments to these surfaces is extremely robust (Fig. 2.8). In human and animal studies of microchanneled implants and abutments [26,27] and in retrieved specimens, when mechanical

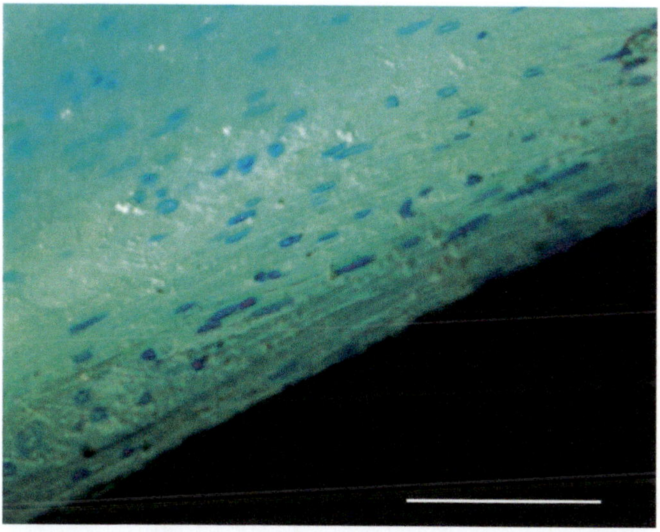

Figure 2.4 Interference transmitted light photomicrograph of soft tissue adjacent to a machined dental implant collar in a mechanically loaded canine model at 6 months. The collagenous tissue and fibroblasts are organized parallel to the implant surface. Bar = 200 μm; toluidine blue staining.

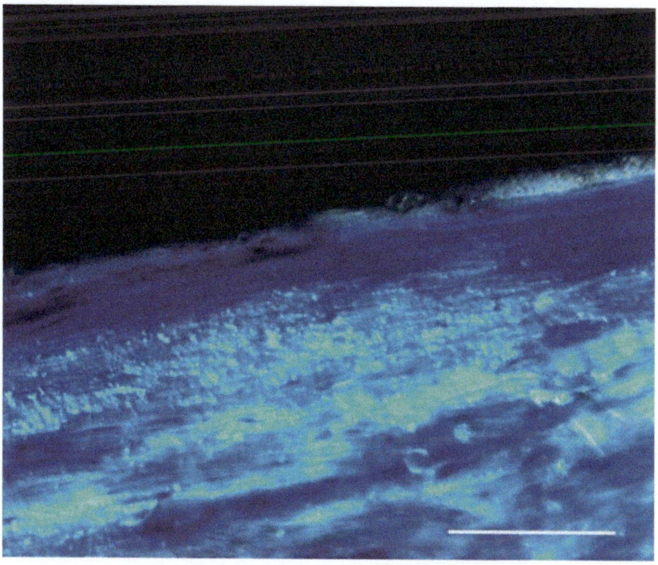

Figure 2.5 Transmitted light photomicrograph of the soft tissues adjacent to a roughened dental implant collar in a mechanically loaded canine model at 6 months. The collagenous tissue and fibroblasts are organized parallel to the implant surface. Bar=500 μm; toluidine blue staining.

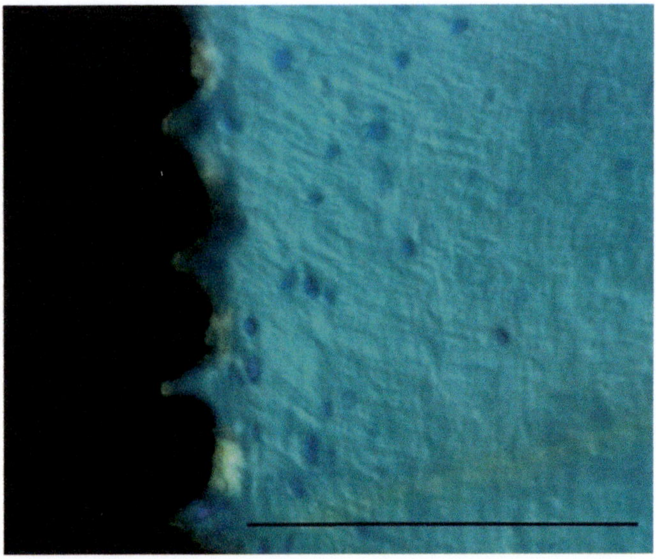

Figure 2.6 Interference transmitted light photomicrograph of soft tissues adjacent to a laser microchanneled (12 μm ridge and groove) dental implant collar in a mechanically loaded canine model at 6 months. The plane of section is perpendicular to the microchannels. The collagenous tissue is organized tangentially relative to the implant surface. Bar = 50 μm; toluidine blue staining.

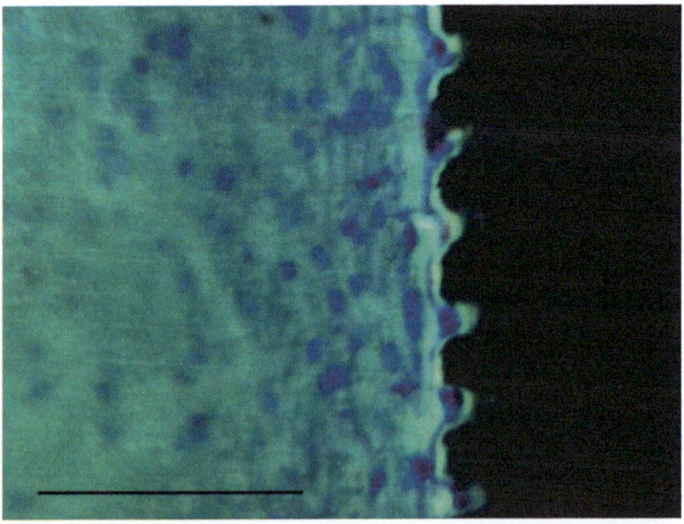

Figure 2.7 Transmitted light photomicrograph of soft tissues adjacent to a laser microchanneled (12 μm ridge and groove) dental implant collar in a mechanically loaded canine model at 6 months. The plane of section is perpendicular to the microchannels. Many of the dark blue-stained fibroblasts at the implant interface can be seen within the microchannels and appear to be oriented perpendicular to the plane of section. Bar = 50 μm; toluidine blue staining.

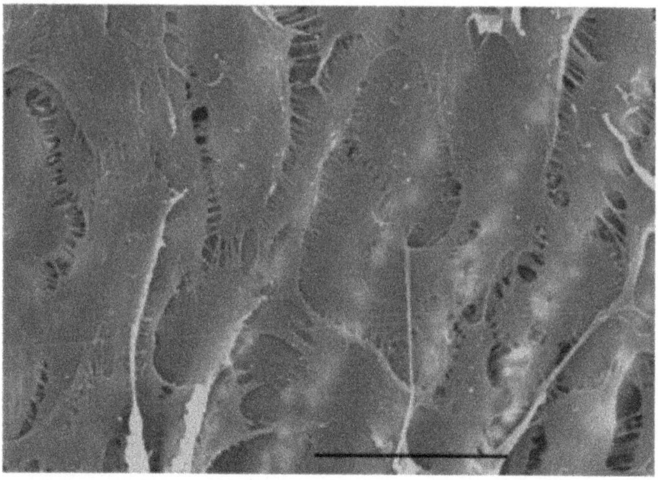

Figure 2.8 Scanning electron micrograph of an 8 μm laser microchanneled abutment that had been removed from a human patient after 2 months. No attempt was made to preserve the tissue attachment upon removal, and the only attached tissue was observed on the microchannels. The rows of cells in and on the microchannels appear to be gingival epithelial cells. In other areas of this abutment (not shown), there were areas of fibrous tissue attachment. Bar = 30 μm.

separation of the soft tissue from the surface is attempted, layers of epithelial cells, fibrous tissue, or both were observed to remain attached to the microchanneled surfaces and failure is observed to occur within the soft tissue rather than at the tissue–implant interface. This suggests that the soft tissue attachment to these surfaces is stronger than the tissue itself.

2.8 Mechanical basis for bone retention around dental implants

In an effort to try to understand the mechanical basis for the bone retention around implants that attach better to the adjacent tissue, Alexander et al. [28] performed an analytical study, through finite element analysis, to predict the minimization of crestal bone stress resulting from implant collar surface treatment. Axial and side loading were studied for two different collar–bone interfaces (nonbonded and bonded, to simulate smooth and microchanneled surfaces, respectively).

Dental implants are designed to bear the loads caused by the teeth during mastication. The goal is to have the maximum amount of bone engaged with the body of the implant and thus provide the most stability. In the past, it was well documented throughout the literature that crestal bone loss averages more than 1 mm in the first year, and at least 0.10 mm each the following year [29]. Accumulation of crestal bone loss over the lifetime of an implant affects the load-bearing capability of the implant and leads to cosmetic problems or implant failure. Crestal bone loss results from bone response to biological factors present at the bone–implant interface and bone response to mechanical factors of loading. As a result, the crestal bone around the implant often takes a saucer-like shape, which continues to become more pronounced as time progresses.

Dental implants are loaded in multiple ways. Teeth are subject to axial loads, bending and twisting moments, shear forces, and a combination of any or all of these loading mechanisms. The transfer of loads from the implant to the bone, along with the stress ranges created by the loads, is assumed to affect the osseointegration and bone remodeling around the implant. Mechanosensing theory, evidence supporting the concept, and how it applies to the levels of loading along the bone–implant interface have been the subjects of many research efforts.

There certainly is evidence in animal evolution that the bone has a mechanism of performing mechanosensory functions. It is, however, not absolutely established whether the mechanosensitivity mechanism is governed by the local stress, the local strain, or the frequency of the loading phenomenon, or a combination thereof. The work of Moseley and Lanyon [30] seems to argue for a strain rate response for bone remodeling. There is also evidence that bone responds to local strain [31] or to stress [32,33] but, is it total stress that governs or a component, deviatoric or dilatational?

Burger and Klein-Nulend [34,35] proposed that there is a bone cell network that links the bone cell signal caused by strain to a cellular signal, which causes bone resorption or bone formation. Mechanotransduction in the bone is described by them through the following mechanism: bone loading > matrix strain > mechanosensing of bone cells > bone formation by osteoblasts or bone resorption by osteoclasts. Within the bone lies a complex three-dimensional network of lacunae and canaliculi. These micropores are filled with the interstitial fluid that supply the bone cells with nutrients and, it is proposed, provide a means for the bone cells to sense mechanical changes. As the bone is stressed, the interstitial fluid flow causes mechanical shear stress and strain-generated potentials. By measuring the production of anabolic factors, nitric oxide, and prostaglandins, it has been experimentally shown that osteocytes have the ability to sense fluid flow and communicate intracellularly. Furthermore, the presence of nitric oxide and prostaglandins during bone loading has been correlated with other cellular reactions, i.e., endothelial cells in blood vessels, which require intracellular communication. The recruited bone cells are transferred through the lacuno-canalicular porosity to the necessary area of the bone. A combination of the anabolic messages and cell transfer brings either osteoclasts to remove the bone or osteoblasts to form the bone.

Ingber's excellent summary of the mechanisms of mechanotransduction [6], discussed in Section 2.3, although more related to soft tissue cells, probably also relates to Burger's theory [34,35] because squeeze flow most likely triggers flow receptors on the cell surface. Ingber described that at the molecular level the flow receptors connect to the same or similar systems through integrins or the cytoskeleton. Therefore, Ingber's theory may, on a cytoskeleton and molecular level, explain Burger's "squeeze flow" hypothesis.

The mechanotransduction mechanism as described by Burger [34] can be used to explain the cellular activity involved with bone remodeling under various load conditions. It is proposed, that under normal load conditions, bone has just enough mechanical stimulation to provide osteocytes with nutrients and waste removal. Disuse of bone leads to extremely low mechanical stimulation and nearly zero fluid flow. A low level of fluid shear does not create the necessary flow needed for nutrient supply and waste removal. As a result, disuse causes osteocyte death. Recruitment of osteoclasts causes the elimination of bone until the cell supporting fluid shear returns to normal and re-establishes osteocyte activity [34]. Damage to the network from overstress (beyond the yield stress) also leads to osteocyte death and the consequent recruitment of osteoclasts and bone destruction. The von Mises criterion, also known as the octahedral shearing stress theory, predicts failure by yielding when the octahedral shearing stress at a point achieves one-half the maximum principle stress at yielding [36]. Alexander, Ricci, and Hrico [28] used the von Mises stress to assess the bone–implant interface using the finite element method. Crestal bone response with and without a bone-attaching collar was evaluated. It was determined that with exposure to an 80 N side load, the maximum crestal bone stress was more than four times higher in the bone adjacent to an unattached collar as opposed to an attached collar. They hypothesized that the high relative motion from distortional stress overload can result in the loss of crestal bone and fibrous tissue formation.

Earlier, it was believed that fibrous encapsulation was optimal, and, therefore, the loading timeline was not a concern. Fibrous tissue formation is believed to occur via the following mechanism. During early bone healing, micromotion damages the tissue and vascular structure. Micromotion probably interferes with the development of adequate early scaffolding from a fibrin clot, and disrupts the reestablishment of a new vasculature to the healing tissue, which in turn interferes with the arrival of regenerative cells. Eventually, the healing process is re-routed into repair by collagenous scar tissue instead of regeneration of bone [37]. The resulting encapsulation is significantly inferior to adequate bone response at the bone–implant interface.

As understanding evolved, it was realized that the longevity of implants depends on the quality of bone fixation. As a result, implants were placed and given a long period of time, 3–6 months, under low stress to allow for sufficient osseointegration. In the 1970s, the concept of micromotion affecting bone response at the implant interface was introduced. In the years leading up to the present, many expansions on the concept of micromotion have been made. Furthermore, it is now known that there is a threshold for excessive micromotion between 50 and 150 μm, above which the bone formation turns to fibrous encapsulation [38]. It also appears that the threshold value for micromotion is a function of the implant design and surface characteristics. Pilliar et al. [39] also utilized finite element analysis to investigate the crestal bone stress state around porous-surfaced implants versus machined threaded implants. They concluded that the observed greater retention of crestal bone next to porous-surfaced implants was attributable to lower peak stresses developed in the crestal peri-implant bone.

Similarly, aggressively attaching bone to the microchanneled collar of an implant is predicted to diminish crestal bone stress, and, therefore, this fibrous tissue formation

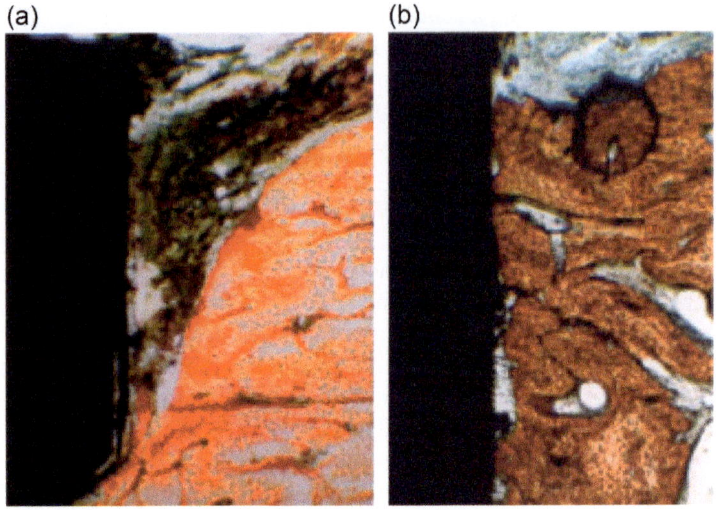

Figure 2.9 Tissue response to machined and microchanneled collars at 9 months postimplantation in a canine model. (a) Machined histology. (b) Microchanneled histology. Bar = 500 μm. SVG stain (Stevenel's blue and counterstained with van Gieson's picro fuchsin).
Reproduced from Weiner S, Simon J, Ehrenberg DS, Zweig B, Ricci J. Advanced surface microtexturing techniques to enhance bone and soft tissue response to dental implants. Implant Dent 2008;17(2):217–28, with permission from Lippincott Williams and Wilkins.

effect. This may be the explanation for crestal bone retention. Canine implantation study results reported by Weiner et al. [25] appear to bear out this proposition. Fig. 2.9 demonstrates the difference in the crestal bone response between two different implant collars (C is "as machined" and LL is "microchanneled"). Because canines use their teeth to shear food rather than grind it, the comparison with the side loading state analyzed in Alexander et al. [28] would appear to be appropriate. The higher stresses predicted with the unattached collar should result in bone loss. This is born out by the histology shown in Fig. 2.9(a). The low stress predicted with the attached collar should be crestal bone protective. This is born out by the histology shown in Fig. 2.9(b).

Clinical testing was performed in a prospective, controlled 37-month study by Pecora et al. [40]. Each patient received two single tooth implants of the same design with either machined or microchanneled collars. The study was performed with a total of 15 patients who received 20 sets of implants. The crestal bone loss data are the most dramatic result of this study. The differences between the LL (microchanneled) and C (machined) implants were tested at each study visit by a paired t-test resulting in p-values $<.005$ for all time periods after 5 months post-op.

As is shown in Fig. 2.10, the microchanneled collar bone loss is limited to the 0.6 mm range, whereas the machined collar demonstrated up to almost 2 mm of bone loss.

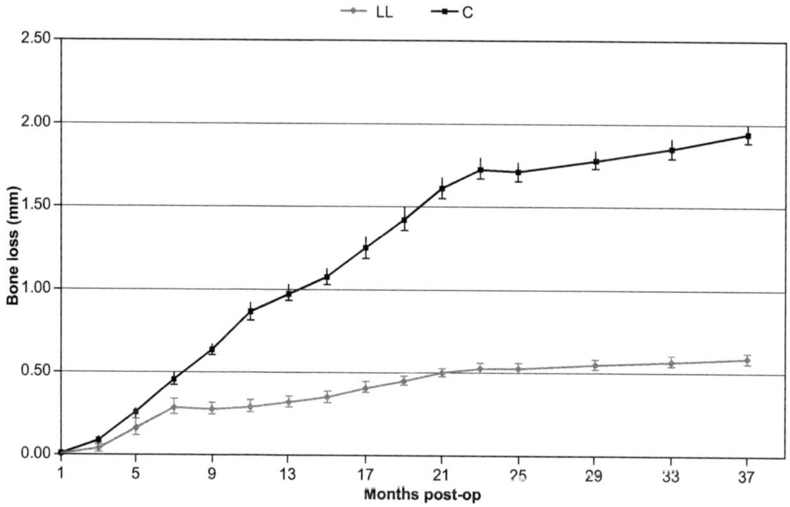

Figure 2.10 Crestal bone loss microchanneled versus machined control in a 3-year prospective, controlled clinical study. Error bars = standard error: $p < .005$ after month 5.
Reproduced from Pecora GE, Ceccarelli R, Bonelli M, Alexander H, Ricci J. Clinical evaluation of laser microtexturing for soft tissue and bone attachment to dental implants. Impl Dent 2009; 18(1):57–66, with permission from Lippincott Williams and Wilkins.

These surfaces are now used on the BioHorizons Laser-Lok implants (BioHorizons Inc., Birmingham, AL, USA), and a significant body of literature has described their efficacy. A review of this literature has been prepared by Ketabi and Deporter [41].

2.9 Conclusion

Cell and tissue response to surfaces can be controlled through chemical modification, microgeometric modification, or both. However, the chemical modification approach, while effective in vitro, has not shown such impressive results in vivo; probably because of interference by adsorbed proteins from body fluids and other cellular processes at the interface. Microgeometric modification, however, shows every indication of being a long-term solution in vivo and a clear idea of the mechanisms involved now exists. The results of the in vitro and in vivo studies noted earlier have established a direct link between the three-dimensional organization of cell attachments to ECM and implant surfaces, their influence on the organization of the cell cytoskeleton, the resultant effects on the GTPase signaling system, and ultimately the effects on cell differentiation and cell function. There is no longer a knowledge gap between how cells attach to surfaces and the related mechanisms that significantly control cell function.

Understanding the cellular response to surfaces has resulted in the utilization of high surface area, organized microtextures to encourage the bone integration.

With tissue attachment shown to decrease local tissue stresses, further loss of bony tissue is diminished. This provides a further mechanical explanation for the superiority of such surfaces in retaining the bone in the critical crestal area of a dental implant.

Indeed, in a significant article on tissue engineering from 2009, Bettinger et al. suggested that the way to control cell response is through the use of micro and nanotextured surfaces [42]. This approach is now being used to tissue engineer implant surfaces to mimic the effects of ECM, and, as is documented above, the first generation of these surfaces has been very successful. Hopefully, this is only the beginning of tissue-engineered surfaces that will revolutionize tissue response to all types of implantable medical devices.

References

[1] Ricci JL, Spivak JM, Blumenthal NC, Alexander H. Modulation of bone ingrowth by surface chemistry and roughness. In: Davies JE, editor. The bone−biomaterial interface. University of Toronto Press; 1991. p. 334−49.

[2] Shmukler-Moncler S, Perrin D, Ahossi V, Magnin G, Bernard J-P. Biological properties of acid etched titanium implants: effect of sandblasting on bone anchorage. J Biomed Mater Res B 2004;68:149−59.

[3] Kasemo B, Lausmaa J. Biomaterial and implant surfaces: a surface science approach. Int J Oral Maxillofac Implants 1988;3(4):247−59.

[4] Baetscher M, Pumplin DW, Block RJ. Vitronectin at sites of cell-substrate contact in cultures of rat myotubes. J Cell Biol 1986;103:369−78.

[5] Lee JW, Juliano R. Mitogenic signal transduction by integrin and growth factor receptor-mediated pathways. Mol Cells 2004;17(2):188−202.

[6] Ingber DE. Cellular mechanotransduction: putting all the pieces together again. FASEB 2006;20:812−27.

[7] Schwarz RI, Farson DA, Bissell MJ. Requirements for maintaining the embryonic state of avian tendon cells in culture. In Vitro 1979;15(12):941−8.

[8] Folkman J, Moscona A. Role of cell shape in growth control. Nature 1978;273(5661):345−9.

[9] Harrison RG. Observations of the living developing nerve fiber. Pro Soc Exper Biol Med 1907;4:140−3.

[10] Weiss P, Garber B. Shape and movement of mesenchymal cells as functions of the physical structure of the medium. Contributions to a quantitative morphology. Proc Nat Acad Sci 1952;38(3):264−80.

[11] Ghibaudo M, Trichet L, Le Digabel J, Richert A, Hersen P, Ladoux B. Substrate topography induces a crossover from 2D to 3D behavior in fibroblast migration. Biophys J 2009;97:357−68.

[12] Ongino Y, Liang R, Mendonca DBS, Mendonca G, Nagasawa M, Koyano K, et al. RhoA-mediated functions in C3H10Ti/2 osteoprogenetors are substrate topography dependent. J Cell Physiol 2015. http://dx.doi.org/10.1002/jcp.25100.

[13] Drosten M, Dhawahir A, Sum E, Urosevic J, lechuga C, Esteban L, et al. Genetic analysis of Ras signaling pathways in cell proliferation, migration and survival. EMBO J 2010;29(6):1091−104.

[14] Mammoto A, Huang S, Moore K, Oh P, Ingber DE. Role of RhoA, mDia, and ROCK in cell shape-dependent control of the Skp2-p27kip1 pathway and the G1/S transition. J Biol Chem 2004;279(25):26323–30.

[15] Thomas CH, Collier JH, Sfeir CS, Healy KE. Engineering gene expression and protein synthesis by modulation of nuclear shape. PNAS 2002;99(4):1972–7.

[16] Doyle AD, Wang FW, Matsumoto K, Yamada KM. One-dimensional topography underlies three-dimensional fibrillar cell migration. J Cell Biol 2009;184(4):481–90.

[17] Kunzler TP, Drobek T, Schuler M, Spencer ND. Systematic study of osteoblast and fibroblast response to roughness by means of surface-morphology gradients. Biomaterials 2007;28:2175–82.

[18] Ricci JL, Charvet J, Chang R, Alexander H. Influence of surface microgeometry on in vitro cell growth and migration. In: Sudarshan TS, editor. Surface modification techniques, VII. London: Institute of Materials; 1994. p. 491–508.

[19] Ricci JL, Grew JC, Alexander H. Connective-tissue responses to defined biomaterial surfaces: Part I. Growth of rat fibroblast and bone marrow cell colonies on microgrooved substrates. J Biomed Mater Res 2008;85A:313–25.

[20] Grew JC, Ricci JL, Alexander H. Connective-tissue responses to defined biomaterial surfaces: Part II. Behavior of rat and mouse fibroblasts cultured on microgrooved substrates. J Biomed Mater Res 2008;85A:326–35.

[21] Guillemette MD, Cui B, Roy E, Gauvin R, Giasson CJ, Esch MB, et al. Surface topography induces 3D self-orientation of cells and extracellular matrix resulting in improved tissue function. Integr Biol 2009;1:196–204.

[22] Calzado-Martin A, Mendez-Vilas A, Multigner M, Saldana L, Gonzalez-Carrasco JL, Gonzalez-Martin ML, et al. On the role of RhoA/ROCK signaling in contact guidance of bone-forming cells on anisotropic Ti6Al4V surfaces. Acta Biomater 2011;7:1890–901.

[23] Ricci JL, Charvet J, Frenkel SR, Chang R, Nadkarni P, Turner J, et al. Bone response to laser microtextured surfaces. In: Davies JE, editor. Bone engineering. Toronto: EM2 Inc.; 2000. p. 282–94.

[24] Frenkel SR, Simon J, Alexander H, Dennis M, Ricci JL. Osseointegration on metallic implant surfaces: effects of microgeometry and growth factor treatment. J Biomed Mater Res Appl Biomater 2002;63(6):706–13.

[25] Weiner S, Simon J, Ehrenberg DS, Zweig B, Ricci J. Advanced surface microtexturing techniques to enhance bone and soft tissue response to dental implants. Implant Dent 2008; 17(2):217–28.

[26] Nevins M, Nevins ML, Camelo M, Boyeson JL, Kim DM. Human histologic evidence of a connective tissue attachment to a dental implant. Int J Periodontics Restor Dent 2008;28: 111–21.

[27] Nevins M, Kim DM, Jun SH, Guze K, Schupbach P, Nevins ML. Histologic evidence of a connective tissue attachment to laser microgrooved abutments: a canine study. Int J Periodontics Restor Dent 2010;30:245–55.

[28] Alexander H, Ricci J, Hrico J. Mechanical basis for bone retention around dental implants. J Biomed Mater Res Part B 2007;88B:306–11.

[29] Small PN, Tarnow DP. Gingival recession around implants: a one year longitudinal prospective study. Int J Oral Maxillofac Implants 2000;15:527–32.

[30] Moseley JR, Lanyon LE. Strain rate as a controlling influence on adaptive modeling. Bone 1998;23:313–8.

[31] Prendergast PJ, Taylor G. Prediction of bone adaptation using damage accumulation. J Biomech 1994;27:1067–76.

[32] Cowin SC. Bone stress adaptation models. J Biomech Eng B 1993;115:528–33.

[33] Cowin SC, Moss ML. Mechanosensory mechanisms in bone. In: Cowin SC, editor. Bone mechanics handbook. Boca Raton: CRC Press; 2001. 29(1–17).
[34] Burger EH. Experiments on cell mechanosensitivity; Bone cells as mechanical engineers. In: Cowin SC, editor. Bone mechanics handbook. Boca Raton: CRC Press LLC; 2001. 28(1–16).
[35] Burger EH, Klein-Nulend J. Mechanotransduction in bone – role of the lacuno-canalicular network. FASEB J 1999;13(Suppl.):S101–12.
[36] Ugural AC, Fenster SK. Advanced strength and applied elasticity. New York: Elsevier; 1975. p. 105–6.
[37] Brunski JB. In vivo bone response to biomechanical loading at the bone/dental-implant interface. Adv Den Res 1999;13:99–119.
[38] Szmukler-Moncler S, Salama H, Reingewirtz Y, Dubruille JH. Timing of loading and effect of micromotion on bone-dental implant interface; Review of experimental literature. J Biomed Mater Res B 1998;43:192–203.
[39] Pilliar RM, Sagals G, Meguid SA, Oyonarte R, Deporter DA. Threaded versus porous-surfaced implants as anchorage units for orthodontic treatment: three-dimensional finite element analysis of peri-implant bone tissue stresses. Int J Oral Maxillofac Implants 2006; 21:879–89.
[40] Pecora GE, Ceccarelli R, Bonelli M, Alexander H, Ricci J. Clinical evaluation of laser microtexturing for soft tissue and bone attachment to dental implants. Impl Dent 2009; 18(1):57–66.
[41] Ketabi M, Deporter D. The effects of laser microgrooves on hard and soft tissue attachment to implant collar surfaces: a literature review and interpretation. Int J Periodontics Restor Dent 2013;33(6):145–52.
[42] Bettinger CJ, Langer R, Borenstein JT. Engineering substrate micro- and nano-topography to control cell function. Angew Chem Int Ed Engl 2009;48(30):5406–15.

Surface modification of dental biomaterials for controlling bone response

3

I.-S. Yeo
Seoul National University, Seoul, Korea

Dental implants made of titanium (Ti), especially commercially pure Ti, have become a well-established treatment modality for the replacement of missing teeth and are state of the art in the field of dental restoration. Since it was first described by Brånemark, osseointegration, which refers to close contact between bone and Ti and its alloys at the light microscope level, has advanced substantially in clinical application. Successful long-term clinical results, i.e., those over 10 years, have been well documented [1]. The six factors that are key to the long-term success of implants include the following [1]:

1. Biocompatibility
2. Implant design
3. Surface characteristics
4. Host factors
5. Surgical technique
6. Loading condition

Biologic responses at the interface between the implant surface and bone play a vital role in the longevity of implant osseointegration and the function of implant-supported prostheses. In vivo findings have supported this by showing that changes in implant surface design have immense effects on bone response to the surface [2–4].

Originally, the principles established by the Göteborgs group required a latency period of several months for bone healing and hard tissue attachment to the surface of a commercially pure Ti implant, which is now called a turned Ti implant [5]. Turned Ti implants inserted into patients' jawbones were not placed under intraoral functional load during the healing period until the implants underwent osseointegration. Clinically, this meant that patients underwent long edentulous periods before implants were loaded or before the implant-supported prostheses were installed in patients' mouths. Thus, there was a need for improved techniques that would allow for earlier loaded implants and, therefore, shortened edentulous periods. Also, as more patients received implants, there was a greater demand for improvements in clinical utility, such as use in areas with poor bone quantity or quality or in the setting of negative local or systemic influences.

Titanium is a biologically stable metal that is used because it is inert, remains unchanged, and does not provoke foreign body reactions or activate biocompatible

Bone Response to Dental Implant Materials. http://dx.doi.org/10.1016/B978-0-08-100287-2.00003-3

responses when introduced into human bodies [6,7]. To improve the speed and strength of bone formation and to thereby allow more rapid loading of the implant, researchers have investigated the effects of modifying implant surfaces. They have demonstrated that several types of surface treatment may enhance surface biocompatibility and bone response around the implant, resulting in rapid osseointegration and early loading [6,8−14]. The surface modification is considered to start from the topographical change of the surface or increasing the roughness of the Ti surface. Surface scientists found that a rougher Ti surface increases surface free energy, which promotes the adhesion and differentiation of osteogenic cells [7]. Various surface treatment methods have been introduced to modify the Ti implant surface for enhanced affinity to the biological environment: (1) changing the surface topography using physical and/or chemical methods; (2) transforming surface properties by coating with a highly biocompatible material, such as calcium phosphate and functional peptide; and (3) performing the above changes in combination.

This chapter first describes the bone healing process around implant surfaces. Then, it introduces several modified surfaces and their effects on the biological response. It focuses on modifications of Ti surfaces specifically because Ti and Ti alloys remain one of the most widely used implant materials for biomedical applications [15]. Implants made of zirconia have been recently investigated. However, zirconia implants have not yet been used clinically, and the modification methods for zirconia implants are similar to those for Ti. An additional consideration is that, in reality, surface modifications change both the topography and chemical properties, even if the method is described and classified here as primarily belonging to one of these two categories. For example, calcium phosphate coating on the Ti surface changes the morphological structure of the surface as well as the surface characteristics from Ti oxide to calcium phosphate.

3.1 Bone responses to implant surfaces

When holes are drilled with dental implant drills and the implants are inserted, bleeding and hemostasis occur in the bone from the surgical trauma, lasting from minutes to hours. The bone debris and matrix generated from the surgical procedure of implant drilling may release various growth and differentiation factors and bone matrix proteins, including bone morphogenetic proteins, which are activated by the bone trauma. Bleeding and damaged endothelium from injured blood vessels form platelet plugs, and simultaneously provoke the coagulation cascade of the tissue factor pathway (the extrinsic pathway) and the contact activation pathway (the intrinsic pathway), leading to fibrin formation for hemostasis. When an implant is placed into the bone, the implant surface is thought to first make contact with water molecules and ions. The surface polarity changes, and the major plasma proteins such as albumin bind to the surface. Slowly, extracellular matrix proteins including vitronectin, which plays a role in cell adhesion, replace the major plasma proteins (Fig. 3.1). The hydrophilic Ti surface appears to allow the initial processes to occur more easily than the hydrophobic surface, because the first contact material with the surface is water and hydrophilicity is advantageous in preserving the conformation (and therefore function)

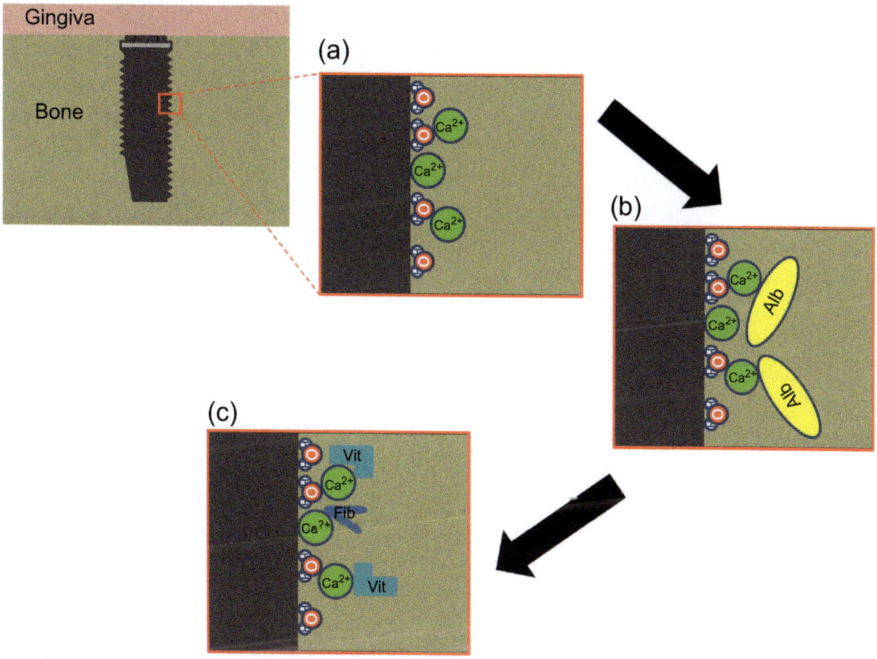

Figure 3.1 Schematic diagrams of the molecular events around the implant surface during hemostasis are shown. First, water (H_2O) and ions (here, calcium ions, Ca^{2+}) adhere to the surface (a). Note that the positive side (hydrogen) of a water molecule has the direct contact with the surface, which is known to be negative. Calcium ions are known to play a bridge role in that the plasma proteins (b) and the subsequently exchanged extracellular ones (c) attach to the Ti implant surface. *Alb*, albumin; *Vit*, vitronectin; *Fib*, fibronectin.

of the adsorbed proteins [16]. Cells begin to adhere to the Ti surface by binding to the coating of vitronectin, fibronectin, and other extracellular matrix proteins.

Activated platelets from the platelet plugs release stored granules, which contain various growth factors and cytokines. Platelet degranulation results in vasodilation and an inflammatory reaction, beginning after about 10 min and lasting for some days after surgery [16]. Polymorphonuclear leucocytes, macrophages, and the complement system are responsible for the initial immune response to bacterial insult. Immune cells arrive at the site of surgical injury through the process of diapedesis and chemotaxis. The period of early inflammation (i.e., the first 3 h) is critical because it dictates the course of the subsequent reaction: either enhanced and prolonged inflammation or subsided inflammation and progressive healing. Therefore, clean surgical technique is very important for a desirable bone response to the implant surface. Macrophages have Janus kinase activity and continually secrete proinflammatory molecules, prolonging the inflammation as long as bacteria are present. However, they secrete angiogenic and fibrogenic molecules, stopping inflammation and preparing bone healing if they can remove tissue debris and bacteria from the site of surgery.

Granulation tissue is formed by new extracellular matrix and angiogenesis. This newly formed tissue is established during the "proliferative phase," which lasts for a few days to a few weeks [16]. Fibroblasts are a key component in the formation of this granulation tissue as they produce collagens and other extracellular matrix proteins after arriving at the wound site. They also break down the blood clot with metalloproteinases and attach to the arginine–glycine–aspartate (RGD) sequence of fibronectin via their transmembrane receptors, integrins. Additionally, angiogenesis by endothelial cells occurs simultaneously; endothelial cells are stimulated and attracted by angiogenic molecules secreted by macrophages, primarily vascular endothelial growth factor. New bone can be formed from the blood vessels made from this angiogenesis. After osteoprogenitor cells adhere to the implant surfaces where the extracellular matrix proteins are adsorbed, they differentiate into osteoblasts. Osteoblasts also maintain adhesion to fibronectin through integrins binding to the RGD motif. Other motifs—for example, those derived from laminins—are also thought to contribute to cell adhesion via integrins or syndecans [17–19]. In fact, this cell attachment at the bone–implant interface is the most critical biological step in the clinical healing phase of a dental implant [20]. In the case of bone trauma, such as implant drilling, bone morphogenetic proteins, which are stored in the bone matrix, are released and activated. Likewise, other cytokines and growth factors participate in the new bone formation. Newly formed bone makes contact with the implant surface after 1 week of implant insertion [21]. The first bone at the bone healing site is woven bone, which begins with the secretion of collagen matrices by osteoblasts, followed by hydroxyapatite mineralization.

Woven bone is replaced by lamellar bone through a process of bone remodeling. Osteoclasts are the major contributors to this process and function by providing space for the lamellar or compact bone. Bone remodeling can continue for years depending on the load distribution around the implant and the bone [16]. Actually, bone resorption by osteoclasts is balanced with the bone formation by osteoblasts. Differentiated osteoblasts forming the bone detach from the surface of the formed bone using collagenases. Migrating osteoclast precursors are then attracted by the newly exposed bone surface. These precursors adhere to the surface, differentiate into osteoclasts, and osteoclasts form a resorption apparatus, which is called Howship's lacuna and ruffled borders, absorbing the bone. Osteoblastic precursor cells can detect the texture of the bone surface in the Howship's lacuna with pseudopodia, gaining information of the bone quantity necessary to fill the lacuna [22]. This feature appears to be involved in the enhanced bone formation activity of osteoblasts detecting the irregularities of topographically modified Ti surfaces [23]. The Haversian system, the fundamental functional unit of the new lamellar bone, is produced to effectively bear the load transferred via the inserted implant.

3.2 Roughening the surface

3.2.1 Surface characteristics

Surface topography is defined by three characteristics: lay, waviness, and surface roughness. Lay indicates the direction of the principal surface configuration such as the horizontal pattern of machining grooves created during the milling process to make a Ti implant. Waviness is a measure of surface irregularities that are usually larger than those of surface roughness, which indicates the fine deviations of a surface. Implant surface can be classified by its surface roughness, specifically one of the surface parameters, S_a: the arithmetic mean height of a surface. This chapter mainly focuses on microroughness that ranges from about 1 to 5 μm of S_a. Macroroughness, including implant geometry and threads, and nanoroughness less than 100 nm of S_a are partially described in this chapter. The classification of microroughness is here based on the system of Albrektsson and Wennerberg [6], wherein smooth surfaces have less than 0.5 μm of S_a, minimally rough surfaces have an S_a of 0.5–1.0 μm, moderately rough surfaces have an S_a of 1.0–2.0 μm, which is considered to be optimal in bone responses, and rough surfaces have more than 2.0 μm of S_a.

The turned Ti surface is without any modification process of the surface. Surface machining by computer numerical control (CNC) milling produces the features of this surface, a smooth surface with some machining grooves (Fig. 3.2). The surface roughness is generally less than 0.5 μm of S_a, which is classified as "smooth." As mentioned above, this type of surface has shown long-term clinical success in restoring the missing teeth, although it requires a long period for osseointegration before loading. Therefore, the turned Ti surface has served as a control in many studies evaluating the quality of modified surfaces.

Physically blasting (or grit blasting) the Ti surface with certain particles, called blast media, modifies the surface mainly topographically. Frequently used blast media include aluminum oxide (Al_2O_3), titanium oxide (TiO_2), or calcium phosphorus

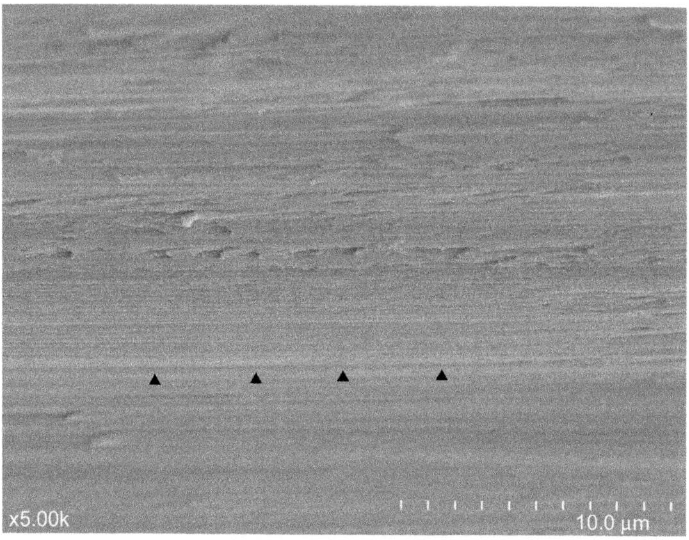

Figure 3.2 The scanning electron microscopic image of a turned Ti surface is shown (Deep Implant System, Inc., Seongnam, South Korea). The grooves (*black arrowheads*) are made during the process of machining by CNC milling (×5000 magnification).

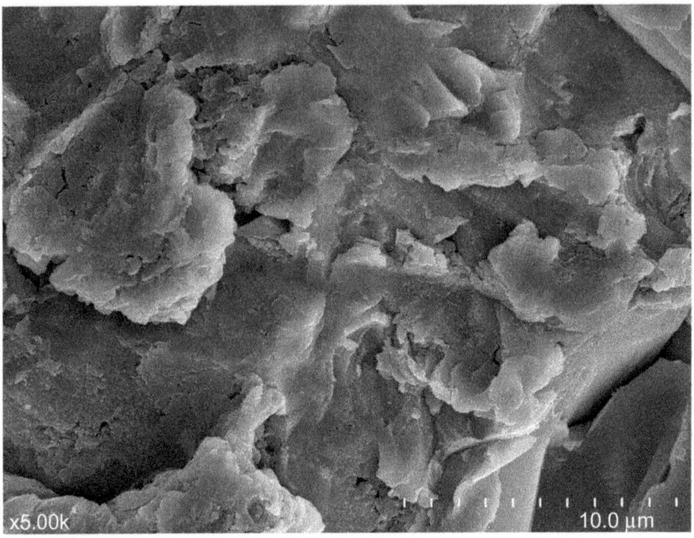

Figure 3.3 The scanning electron microscopic image of a blasted Ti surface (Deep Implant System, Inc., Seongnam, South Korea) shows many irregularities that are formed during the process of blasting. The diameter of the blast media (here, about 50 μm), type of the media (here, Al_2O_3), and blasting pressure influence the surface morphology. Usually, the sizes of the irregularities are larger than those formed by etching (×5000 magnification).

(CaP) particles in the field of dental implantology (Fig. 3.3). Particle size, blasting time and pressure, and distance from the particle nozzle to the surface all influence the resulting roughness. The optimal roughness of the blasted surface that shows the best removal torque and bone-to-implant contact data is a moderately rough surface with about 1.5 μm of S_a [12].

Although Ti itself is resistant to corrosion by acid, acids can erode and form pits on the surface of Ti implants when the implants are immersed in acidic solutions because commercially pure Ti has trace impurities that are acid labile. The diameter of the produced pits is approximately 0.5–2 μm (Fig. 3.4). Hydrochloric acid, sulfuric acid, and hydrofluoric acid are largely applied to the Ti surface for modification of the dental implant. The microstructure of the etched surface depends on the type, concentration and temperature of the acidic solution, and the time of etching. The S_a value of this etched surface has been evaluated to be less than 1.0 μm. Thus, the roughness may be "smooth" or "minimally rough."

The Ti surface can be sandblasted with large-grit particles, which are generally 250–500 μm in size, and then immersed into acidic solutions for etching, resulting in the sandblasted, large-grit, and acid-etched (SLA) surface (Fig. 3.5). This combined surface is one of the most widely used and with a long history of clinical use in the market of dental implants, although the topography is different from surface to surface based on the combination of conditions used for blasting and etching. The SLA surface has an S_a value that is "moderately rough" in most studies. Additionally, it has shown

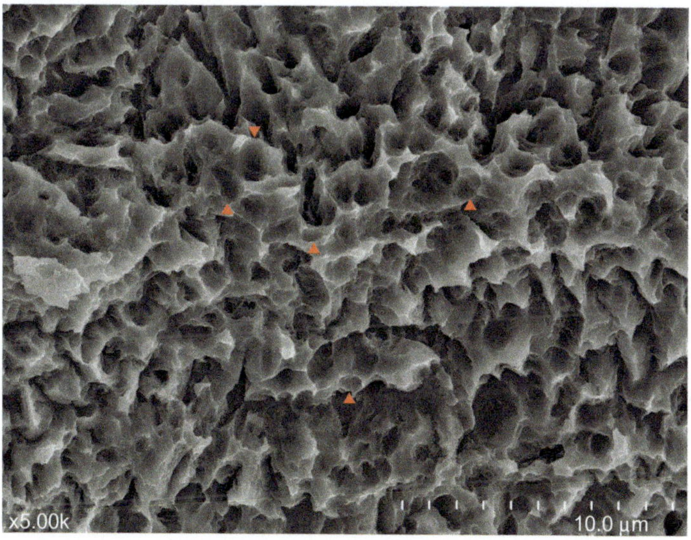

Figure 3.4 Smaller honeycomb-shaped irregularities (*red arrowheads*) are found on the entire Ti surface modified by acid etching (Deep Implant System, Inc., Seongnam, South Korea) (scanning electron microscopic, ×5000 magnification).

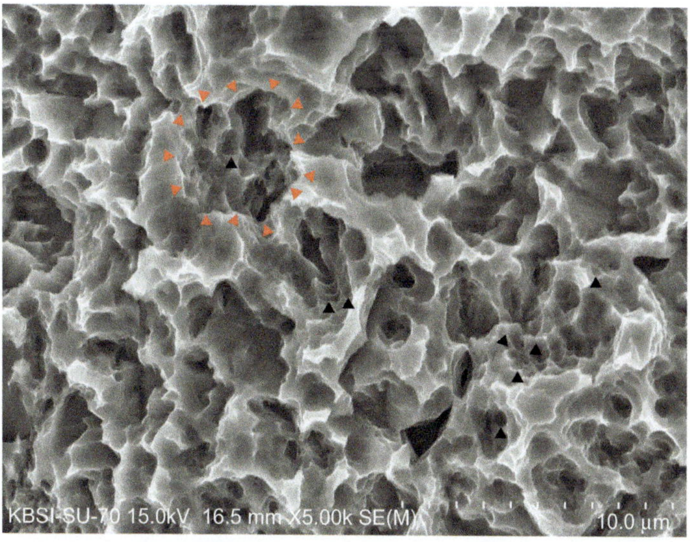

Figure 3.5 The Ti surface sandblasted with large particles, followed by acid etching, shows characteristic irregularities (Deep Implant System, Inc., Seongnam, South Korea) (scanning electron microscopic, ×5000 magnification). The irregularities consist of large crater-like structures, resulting from the blasting procedure (*red arrowheads*), and small honeycomb-shaped micropits (*black arrowheads*), which are formed by the application of acids to the surface.

higher biocompatibility compared to surfaces that were blasted only or etched only. Therefore, the SLA surface is considered an adequate positive control in comparison studies evaluating a new modified surface.

The SLA surface with additional hydrophilic properties has been developed and is being used in the market of clinical dentistry. This type of surface is called hydrophilic SLA or modified SLA (modSLA) surface. The existing SLA without the additional hydrophilicity is sometimes called standard or hydrophobic SLA for clarity. Rinsing the standard SLA surface in water under nitrogen protection and storing the surface in isotonic NaCl solution without atmospheric contact is known to make the SLA surface water friendly [24]. The hydrophilic SLA surface has topographical features similar to those of the standard SLA surface (Fig. 3.6), i.e., it is "moderately rough." However, there have been some studies showing an S_a higher than 2.0 μm in the modSLA surface, which would be classified as "rough" [25,26].

A Ti oxide layer is naturally formed on the Ti surface upon exposure to oxygen in air. The oxide layer can be thickened by placing the Ti surface as an anode in a galvanic cell and applying voltage to the electrolyte solution. Scanning electron microscopy shows many micropores with different diameters on the oxidized Ti oxide surface (Fig. 3.7). The surface roughness used in dental Ti implants is often minimally rough, and the surface characteristics can be changed depending on the applied voltage, the contents of electrolytes, and the time of electric current (oxidation time). Furthermore, Ti oxide—not Ti itself—is biocompatible. Therefore, anodic oxidation procedures are considered to provide this surface with higher biocompatibility by increasing the thickness of the Ti oxide layer and by changing the surface topographically.

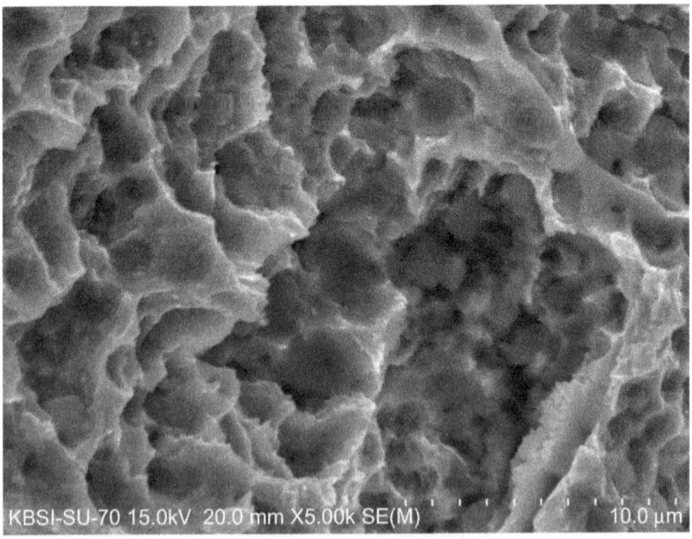

Figure 3.6 The scanning electron microscopic (SEM) image of a hydrophilic SLA surface is shown (SLActive, Institute Straumann AG, Basel, Switzerland). Actually, there is no specific SEM feature differentiating between the hydrophilic and standard SLA surfaces (×5000 magnification).

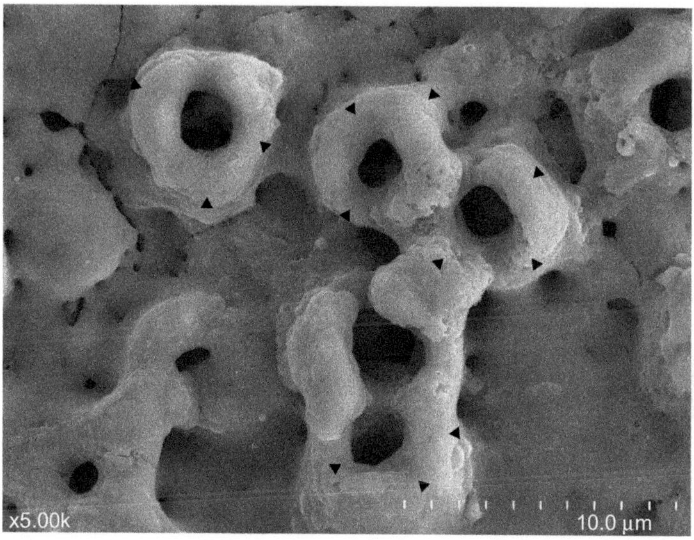

Figure 3.7 This scanning electron microscopic image shows typical surface characteristics of an anodically oxidized Ti surface, which include protruded open pores (*black arrowheads*) (×5000 magnification).

Extremely rough surfaces are developed by a method, called direct metal laser sintering (DMLS). This method is one of the additive manufacturing (publicly, 3D printing) techniques, in which thermal energy by laser fuses Ti alloy powder (here, 90% Ti, 6% aluminum, 4% vanadium, or Ti-6Al-4V) by melting as the powder deposits to an implant shape instead of milling a Ti alloy block with a CNC machine (Fig. 3.8). Very rough surfaces are made through this procedure. R_a (two-dimensional version of S_a) value is shown to be about 60 μm, not optimal, but to be similar in biocompatibility to the sandblasted and etched surface [27–29]. This surface is still under investigation, not marketed yet, although some human cases have been reported [30,31].

3.2.2 The effect of surface topography on bone healing

There has been rapid development in the field of Ti dental implant surface modifications. Various novel surfaces known to be biocompatible have been clinically introduced and tested. Generally, the hierarchical approach is accepted for evaluating biologic responses to modified surfaces [32]. Surfaces are first tested in vitro on cells, and properties such as cell adhesion, spreading, and expression of some important marker genes are evaluated. Second, in vivo animal research including histomorphometric evaluations is performed. Third, retrospective and/or prospective clinical investigations follow. As mentioned above, modified surfaces have been evaluated in many laboratory and clinical studies using the turned Ti surface as a control.

Blasted surfaces have been shown to have better histomorphometry compared to turned surfaces [33]. Specifically, blasted surfaces exhibit better bone-to-implant

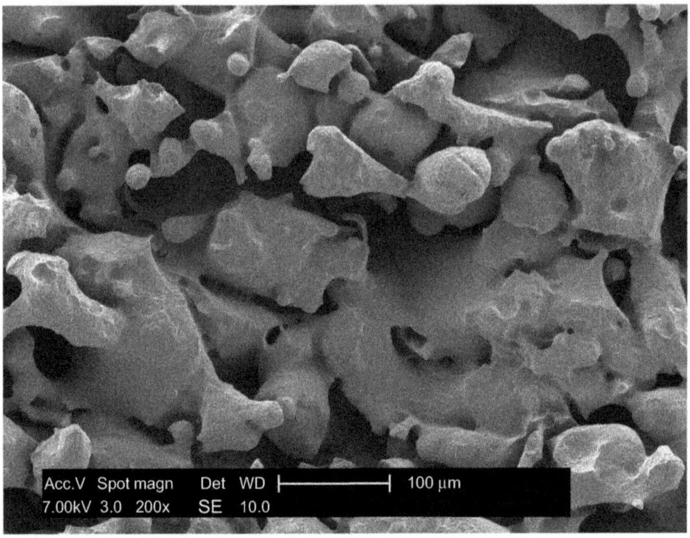

Figure 3.8 The surface made by DMLS is very rough and porous (×200 magnification). Notice the low magnification for this image (×200), compared to much higher magnification for other scanning electron microscopic images in this chapter (×5000). The additive manufacturing technique melts and fuses Ti alloy powder to produce such an extremely irregular surface morphology with ridge-like and globular protrusions, interspersed by intercommunicating pores and narrow crevices.
Courtesy of Dr. Adriano Piattelli.

contact (BIC), which is defined as the ratio of the direct bone–implant contact length along a defined implant length at a light microscopic level, and larger bone area, which is defined as the ratio of the newly formed bone to a defined area around the implant. Previous studies indicate a positive correlation between increased roughness and blasting and osseointegration [34,35]. In comparison studies with the turned surface, by conducting experiments on animals, it has been found that the etched surface also has been found to achieve faster and stronger osseointegration [36,37]. Many studies have also shown better results in both in vitro and in vivo experiments when the SLA, hydrophilic SLA, or oxidized surface is compared to the turned surface [14]. Some studies have also found that hydrophilic SLA surfaces show more bone formation and more potentiated osteogenic effects than standard SLA [9,24]. Those topographically modified implants have been reported to have high success on survival rates in clinical trials.

However, many studies have failed to find any significant differences in bone responses when modified surfaces are compared with one another. Although the hydrophilic SLA surface in the previous study showed better results in comparison with the standard SLA, another study reported similar data between the hydrophilic SLA and oxidized surfaces [38]. Another previous study found no significant in vitro or in vivo differences between the standard SLA and oxidized surfaces [3]. Many researchers believe that topographical features other than roughness may impact the biological response to the implant surfaces, but how these characteristics affect the response remains unknown. For example, we do not yet know which of the surface morphologies is more biocompatible in bone formation, the honeycomb shape of the SLA surface (Fig. 3.5) or the volcano-like micropore of the oxidized surface (Fig. 3.7).

Overall, the topographical changes on the Ti implant surface by various modification methods induce faster bone healing and osseointegration around the implant compared to the turned surface. At the cellular level, modified surfaces with higher S_a than the turned surface stimulate attachment, spreading, and activation of bone cells. Ti implants with topographically modified surfaces may be advantageous in faster bone healing at the animal level. Clinically, such implants are considered to be more adequate in early loading, when compared to the turned implants, although both the turned and topographically modified implants have been successful in clinical trials with the conventional loading protocol. The important thing is that, however, the exact roles of the changed roughness and the other topographical features (including chemical features), resulting from the surface treatments, are still poorly understood.

3.3 Application of inorganic elements to implant surfaces

3.3.1 Calcium phosphorus

CaP coating on the Ti surface is thought to make the implant surface bioactive. The surface is highly osteoconductive to the surrounding bone and it can even be osteoinductive when used with bone morphogenetic proteins. This biocompatibility stems from the fact that calcium and phosphorus are the main components of the human bone. Traditionally, the CaP-coated surface is made using the plasma-spraying method, which is still widely used for CaP coating on the Ti implant surface (Fig. 3.9). Briefly, hydroxyapatite particles are injected into a plasma flame at a high temperature of about 15,000–20,000K, and these heated particles are projected onto the Ti surface [39]. Thus, a CaP coating layer, which is approximately 50–100 μm thick, is formed on the surface. The bone response to the CaP coating is influenced by the uniformity and crystallinity of the coating layer, as well as by the calcium/phosphorus atomic ratio (coating composition). Alteration of this ratio can control the rate of dissolution and degradation of the coating layer in the biological environment.

Clinically, CaP-coated implants have been shown to be successful and functional in patients' mouths over long-term service periods [40,41]. In vivo biomechanical removal torque and histomorphometrical BIC of the CaP-coated implants have been reported to be higher than those of the turned and blasted implants, indicating earlier and more rapid bone formation and osseointegration [42]. However, many concerns have been raised about this method, including possible delamination and cohesive failure of the CaP-coating layer. In particular, CaP coating by plasma spraying has been documented to obstruct bone apposition at the dissolving area and attract inflammatory cells such as macrophages and multinucleated cells [43,44]. These findings have made

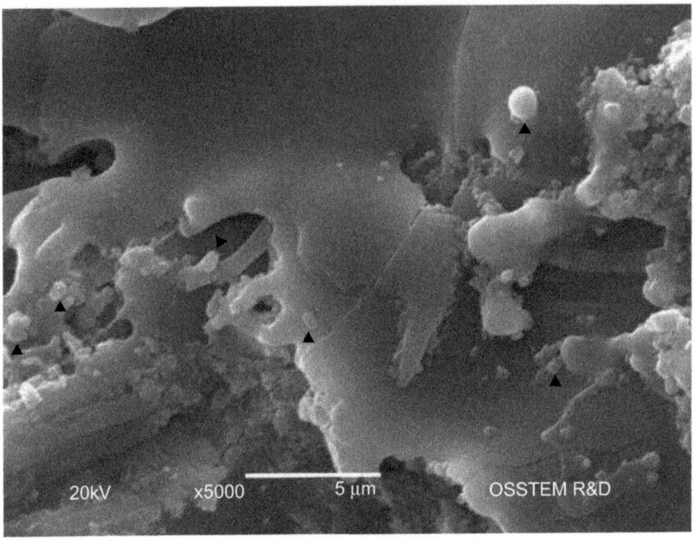

Figure 3.9 Many hydroxyapatite particles (*black arrowheads*) are observed on the plasma sprayed, hydroxyapatite coated surface (Osstem Implant, Busan, South Korea) in scanning electron microscopic (×5000 magnification).

dental practitioners hesitate to use CaP-coated implants, leading to an investigation into a coating method that resolves the problems associated with plasma spraying.

The higher osteoconductive property of the CaP-coating layer and stronger osseointegration behavior of the surrounding hard tissue remain attractive when treating patients with dental implants, who have limited bone quantity and quality. Thin coating of the CaP layer has been developed through various processes including sol–gel deposition and ion sputtering (Fig. 3.10). These methods not only decrease the film

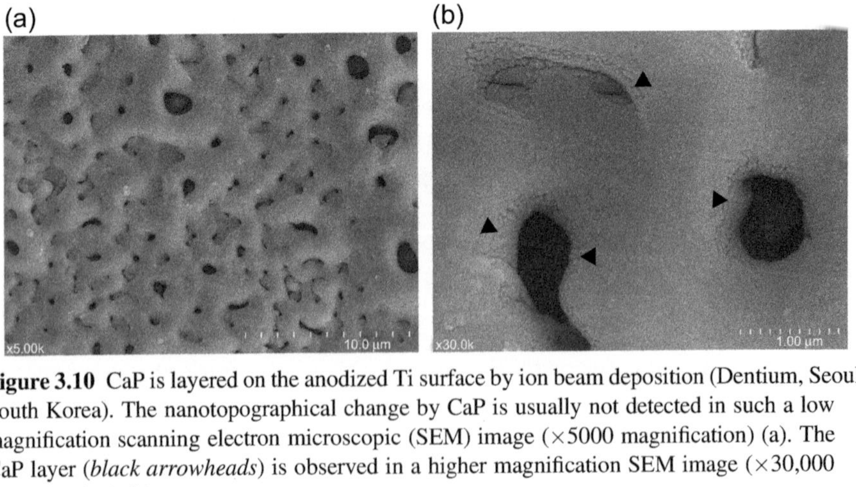

Figure 3.10 CaP is layered on the anodized Ti surface by ion beam deposition (Dentium, Seoul, South Korea). The nanotopographical change by CaP is usually not detected in such a low magnification scanning electron microscopic (SEM) image (×5000 magnification) (a). The CaP layer (*black arrowheads*) is observed in a higher magnification SEM image (×30,000 magnification) (b).

thickness of the CaP layer but also change the surface topography at the nanoscale level. Typically, the thickness ranges from 1 to 5 μm. The size of the coated materials has been reported to be 20–100 nm in some previous studies [45,46]. The CaP-coated surface modified at the nanometer level has shown better osseointegration, higher bioactivity, and superior histomorphometric results, when compared with uncoated surfaces [32,45,47,48]. A dental implant modified by CaP nanocoating on a minimally rough etched Ti surface (NanoTite, Biomet 3i, Palm Beach Gardens, FL, USA) is commercially available.

Modified surface topographies at the nanoscale level are expected to promote protein adsorption and enhance the adhesion of bone forming cells in the early bone response. However, the benefits and effects of these nanomodifications are not yet fully understood at the level of cells or tissues when compared to their counterparts at the microscale level. Also, the optimal size and distribution of the nanoparticles and their application in implant surfaces remain unclear. In addition, the limitations of surface modification at both the nanoscale and microscale should be noted. Even the bioactive coating such as CaP has demonstrated disastrous failure in clinical use when the material was coated on the surface of the cylinder-shaped Ti dental implant. After the geometry of the implant was changed from a cylinder shape to a screw shape at the macroscale, this bioactive coating was successful for long-term clinical use.

3.3.2 Fluoride treatment

Fluoride (F) has a specific attraction for calcium and phosphates, which are the major elements of the human bone. The Ti surface is reduced on a cathode, when the Ti surface is immersed into a hydrofluoric acid solution at a low concentration. The reduction reaction of the Ti surface allows the attraction of F ions on the Ti surface. This surface is called an F-modified surface. In the market of dental implants, only OsseoSpeed (Astra Tech, Dentsply, Waltham, MA, USA) uses an F-modified surface. Hydrogen fluoride at a low concentration is applied on Ti surface blasted with Ti dioxide particles. Such an F reduction results in the incorporation of F into Ti dioxide without the significant change of the blasted surface micro-structure. The roughness of OsseoSpeed surface is about 1.5 μm in S_a, which makes it moderately rough (Fig. 3.11). X-ray photoelectron spectroscopy detects trace amounts of F on the surface, whereas energy dispersive spectroscopy finds no F content on the surface [25,49].

Fluoride is thought to act primarily on osteoprogenitor cells and undifferentiated osteoblasts, but not on differentiated osteoblasts. It increases growth factor synthesis in these cells and facilitates their differentiation into osteoblasts [50–52]. The nucleation ability of calcium and phosphate ions is improved on the F-modified surface [53]. Thus, F may enhance the bone formation and accelerate early bone response to the modified implant surface. Several in vitro cell tests have shown that the messenger RNA expression levels of various osteogenic marker genes increase on F-modified Ti surfaces [53]. There have been in vivo animal experiments indicating accelerated bone formation and mineralization on the F-modified surface compared to its predecessor, the Ti dioxide-blasted surface without F modification [53–55].

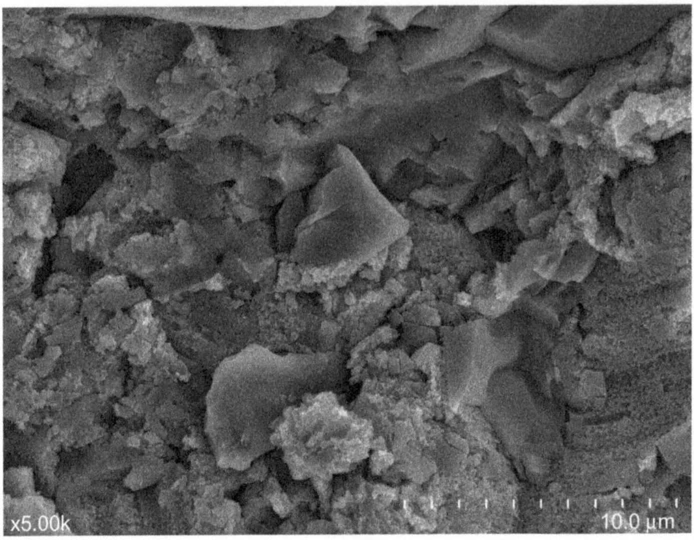

Figure 3.11 The F-treated surface is shown (OsseoSpeed, Astra Tech, Dentsply, Waltham, MA, USA). The surface is F treated after it is blasted with Ti dioxide particles. Therefore, the scanning electron microscopic image is similar to that of the Ti dioxide–blasted surface without further F modification (×5000 magnification).

Clinically, F-modified implants are successful, with 5-year survival rates higher than 95% in early loading [56,57].

The F-modified surface is considered to be bioactive because it, similar to a CaP-coated surface, has stronger interaction with the bone at the bone–implant interface than a topographically modified surface. The F-modified surface probably exhibits the compounding effects of modified topography and chemistry. The F-modified surface forms strong osseointegration that is very difficult to dismantle; cutting between the bone and implant sides is significantly harder than in the original surface without further F modification. However, it is interesting that the advanced quality observed between the newly developed surface and its predecessor is not easily found when this new surface is compared with other topographically modified surfaces. For example, some in vivo studies have found no significant differences in histomorphometry when the F-modified surface is compared with the oxidized Ti surface or with the SLA surface [49,58]. Likewise, a previous in vivo study concluded similar early bone responses between the CaP-coated and the blasted surfaces [33]. The chemical effects of these bioactive inorganic elements on bone responses should be further investigated.

3.4 Application of organic compounds to implant surfaces

Extracellular matrix proteins adsorb to the implant surface during hemostasis when the implant is inserted into the bone. Some of the extracellular matrix proteins are involved in the adhesion of bone forming cells. Osteoblasts have transmembrane proteins that recognize the adhesion molecules such as fibronectin, vitronectin, and laminin. In particular, one of these transmembrane proteins, integrin, is well studied. The binding of integrin to an extracellular matrix protein is known to be an important mechanism by which osteoblasts interact with the extracellular matrix, and this interaction controls cell morphology, proliferation, and differentiation [59]. Cell adhesion and subsequent cell signaling and interaction for bone healing occur through those transmembrane proteins. The bone response is accelerated if the adhesion proteins are coated on the implant surface because bone healing begins with the attachment of osteogenic cells on the surface. Another idea that has been explored is using the small binding units—functional peptides—for coating on the implant surface, if the amino acid sequences of the peptides are known. This is preferable to using whole proteins as the proteins are large and multifunctional, which can provoke undesirable immune responses in the host and make cellular reactions difficult to control. These adhesion molecules on the implant surface bind to the receptors (transmembrane proteins) of osteoblasts and the intracellular events for cellular activation are triggered (Fig. 3.12).

Functionalized Ti surfaces coated with the RGD peptides show higher histomorphometric values, indicating accelerated osteogenesis when compared with uncoated Ti surfaces [60,61]. Recently, two functional peptides contributing to cell adhesion

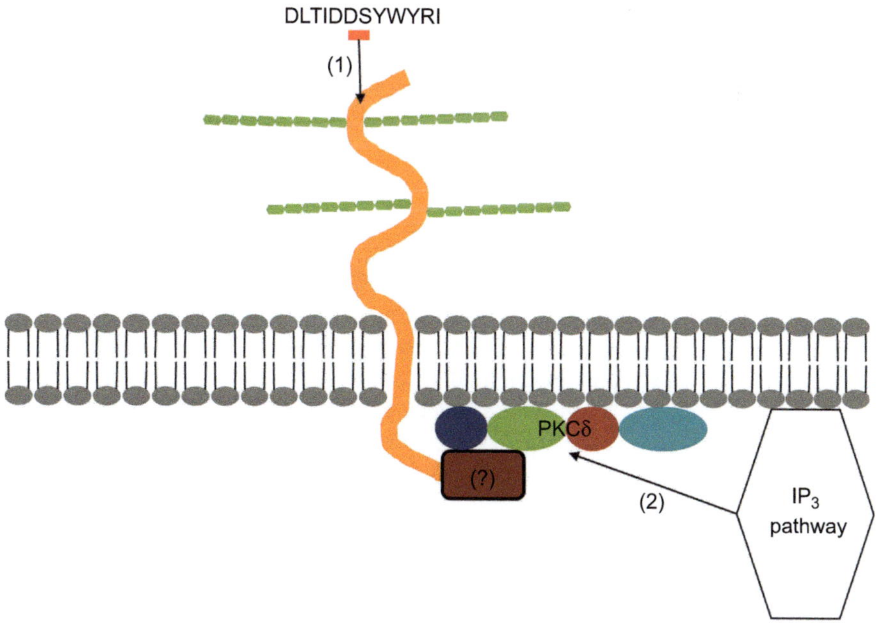

Figure 3.12 A proposed mechanism about the intracellular triggering for cell adhesion by the functional peptide, DLTIDDSYWYRI. This functional peptide binds to the syndecan-1, a transmembrane proteoglycan (1). Then, the PKCδ-mediated inositol triphosphate pathway (2) promotes the cell attachment. The protein designated with question mark (?) remains unknown at present. *PKCδ*, protein kinase Cδ; *IP_3*, inositol triphosphate.

have been found from human laminin [18,19]; one is a dodecamer (12-amino acid sequence; DLTIDDSYWYRI) and the other is a nonamer (nine-amino acid sequence; PPFEGCIWN). These peptides also actively bind to bone forming cells and the mechanism by which these peptides trigger intracellular cascades has been hypothesized (Fig. 3.13). The dodecamer has been found to overwhelm the topography and chemistry of the underlying Ti surface in the activity of bone cell attachment, although both the implant surface structure and the coating organic compounds are known to affect cellular and tissue responses [18,53].

Cytokines, especially growth factors, are another category of biomolecules that can enhance the bone formation. One candidate that is clinically available in dental implantology is the bone morphogenetic protein (BMP) family. Human recombinant BMP-2 (rhBMP-2) is currently used clinically. Some studies have found that rhBMP-2–coated implants accelerate the bone formation in vivo [62–64]. However, a cytokine is not an adhesion molecule and a BMP cannot be effective in its coated form because its bone healing effect is a result of its free floating action in the tissue microenvironment. A previous study reported that BMP-2 directly applied to osteoblastic cells was sufficient to promote cellular adhesion to Ti surfaces by increasing the expression of adhesion molecules [65]. BMPs are temporal signals and have complicated biological effects, depending on their concentration and the condition of surrounding tissues. Some studies have reported conflicting results about BMP-2 that indicated osteolysis or negative effects on osteogenesis around BMP-2–treated implants [64,66,67]. Another consideration is that BMP-2 is not easy to directly coat onto Ti surface. Some studies have used BMP-2 as a free form [66,68], whereas others have evaluated coated BMP-2 after the base Ti surface was modified by CaP coating, anodic oxidation, or applications of other growth factors, where the effects on bone responses were mixed [62,63,67].

To provide the bone healing site with more biomimetic environment, a growth factor can be combined with an adhesion molecule-coated Ti surface. One study proposed that the bone induction effects of an adhesion molecule are possible in the presence of BMPs [69]. A Ti surface functionalized with adhesion molecules and nanocarriers has also been considered, wherein nanocarriers contain growth factors, releasing them as free forms after implant insertion. In this method, the initial bone responses and the subsequent bone remodeling phase can be manipulated by controlling the time of release of the bioactive molecules. Although these biologically modified Ti surfaces have not yet been introduced clinically, they are expected to be in the near future.

3.5 Concluding remarks

Sometimes, it is said that the research of surface modification for dental implantology is no longer necessary because existing implants have shown long-term success rates over 90–95%, which are very high compared to those of other grafting surgeries. However, humans have 28 permanent teeth, which should not be overlooked. Imagine that a dental clinician has 10 patients, each of whom has been treated with 10 implants

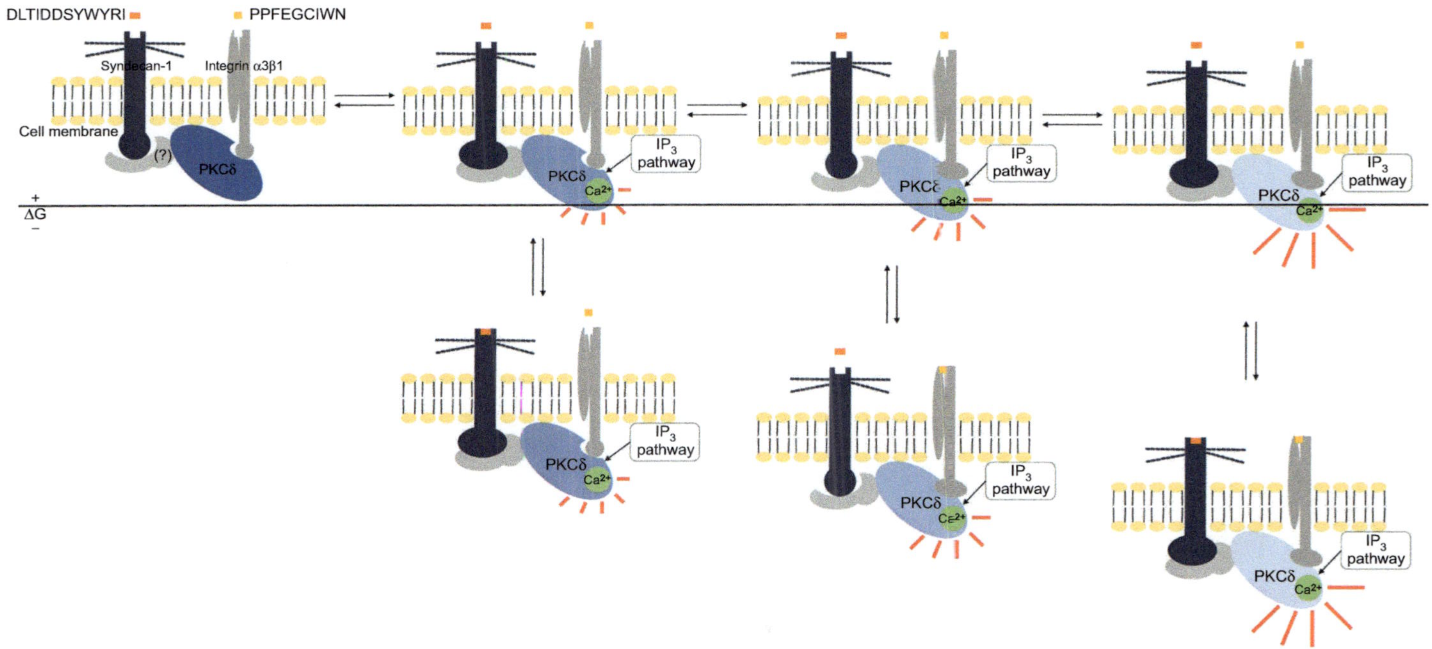

Figure 3.13 This hypothetical mechanism for the two laminin-derived bioactive peptides is based on a probabilistic interpretation of allostery. The *black horizontal line* means that the Gibbs-free conformational energy difference (ΔG) is zero. The lower, the more stable energy state is below the line. The brightness and the shining degree (*red lines*) of protein kinase Cδ (PKCδ) indicate how much this enzyme is activated. Various conformational energy states are assumed when the functional peptides bind to the transmembrane proteins that have tunable sensitivity for PKCδ phosphorylation. PKCδ can be reversibly activated even if the peptides do not bind to their receptors. That is, equilibrium is reached between the inactive (the most left state) and active states when neither of the peptides binds to transmembrane receptors. However, such activated states are probably very difficult to maintain because their free energy states are still high. When either PPFEGCIWN or DLTIDDSYWYRI or both bind to the receptors, circumstances become different. The bound forms stabilize the conformations significantly, increasing the probabilities of the active states. Finally, the increased number of the active states effectively trigger the intracellular events via the transmembrane proteins, promoting cell adhesion. IP_3, Inositol triphosphate; Ca^{2+}, calcium ion; *(?)*, unknown protein.

for his/her missing teeth, assuming that the implant has a 10% failure rate. In total, 100 implants have been inserted and 10 implants will statistically fail. Therefore, all of the 10 patients will visit the dental office for one failed implant of each patient in the worst case. This is a very embarrassing situation. Efforts to develop more biocompatible dental implants should be still made to increase long-term clinical success rates.

There are a number of surface modifications for Ti dental implants. This chapter has explored some representative modified surfaces. It is clear that those modified surfaces demonstrate faster and stronger osteogenic responses than the original commercially pure Ti turned surfaces. It is unclear, however, that one modified surface is more biocompatible for bone healing in comparison with another modified surface, although the topographical and chemical features of the surface influence the biologic responses to the surface. This chapter describes the bone healing process, including hemostasis, inflammation, proliferative phase, remodeling, and their substeps. The key information about which step is the most critical for accelerated bone formation remains missing. There is now a growing field of research on osteoporotic patients and their therapies and our knowledge about bone physiology is expanding. It may be possible to find an effective modified surface through related research.

The surface modifications that this chapter describe focus mainly on microstructures. The microstructural modification changes cell behavior around the modified surface, but it has its own limits. For instance, such a modified surface cannot avoid implant failure resulting from shear force due to the occlusal load on the bone–implant interface. This type of failure can be bypassed by providing the implant macrodesign with threads, which convert shear force into compressive force that the bone–implant interface endures much better. Surface characteristic is just one of all the six key factors for the clinical success of a dental implant. Researchers should consider both the implant macro- and microstructure to better understand clinical bone response to the dental implant.

Recently, researchers have investigated the effects of nanolevel surface structure and chemistry on biologic responses to dental implantation. CaP nanocoating, modifications adding Ti dioxide nanotubes to the surface, and other strategies are being tested. At the molecular level, functional peptides, adhesion molecules, and growth factors are being applied on the Ti surface to control the bone response. Such control at the nanoscale level is expected not only to boost bone formation reactions around the modified surface, but also to manipulate the bone response at certain time points (early or late) of bone metabolism if those molecules are appropriately combined. However, the clinical use of novel materials as Ti surface modifiers requires supporting data from large, prospective clinical studies or clinical trials, which have not yet been performed.

References

[1] Albrektsson T, Branemark PI, Hansson HA, Lindstrom J. Osseointegrated titanium implants. Requirements for ensuring a long-lasting, direct bone-to-implant anchorage in man. Acta Orthop Scand 1981;52:155–70.

[2] Buser D, Schenk RK, Steinemann S, Fiorellini JP, Fox CH, Stich H. Influence of surface characteristics on bone integration of titanium implants. A histomorphometric study in miniature pigs. J Biomed Mater Res 1991;25:889–902.

[3] Koh JW, Kim YS, Yang JH, Yeo IS. Effects of a calcium phosphate-coated and anodized titanium surface on early bone response. Int J Oral Maxillofac Implants 2013;28:790–7.

[4] Trisi P, Lazzara R, Rebaudi A, Rao W, Testori T, Porter SS. Bone-implant contact on machined and dual acid-etched surfaces after 2 months of healing in the human maxilla. J Periodontol 2003;74:945–56.

[5] Branemark PI, Adell R, Breine U, Hansson BO, Lindstrom J, Ohlsson A. Intra-osseous anchorage of dental prostheses. I. Experimental studies. Scand J Plast Reconstr Surg 1969;3:81–100.

[6] Albrektsson T, Wennerberg A. Oral implant surfaces: Part 1—review focusing on topographic and chemical properties of different surfaces and in vivo responses to them. Int J Prosthodont 2004;17:536–43.

[7] Kulkarni M, Mazare A, Gongadze E, Perutkova S, Kralj-Iglic V, Milosev I, et al. Titanium nanostructures for biomedical applications. Nanotechnology 2015;26:062002.

[8] Albrektsson T, Wennerberg A. Oral implant surfaces: Part 2—review focusing on clinical knowledge of different surfaces. Int J Prosthodont 2004;17:544–64.

[9] Buser D, Broggini N, Wieland M, Schenk RK, Denzer AJ, Cochran DL, et al. Enhanced bone apposition to a chemically modified SLA titanium surface. J Dent Res 2004;83:529–33.

[10] Ivanovski S. Osseointegration—the influence of implant surface. Ann R Australas Coll Dent Surg 2010;20:82–5.

[11] Lemons JE. Biomaterials, biomechanics, tissue healing, and immediate-function dental implants. J Oral Implantol 2004;30:318–24.

[12] Wennerberg A, Albrektsson T. Effects of titanium surface topography on bone integration: a systematic review. Clin Oral Implants Res 2009;20(Suppl. 4):172–84.

[13] Wennerberg A, Albrektsson T. On implant surfaces: a review of current knowledge and opinions. Int J Oral Maxillofac Implants 2010;25:63–74.

[14] Yeo IS. Reality of dental implant surface modification: a short literature review. Open Biomed Eng J 2014;8:114–9.

[15] Roy P, Berger S, Schmuki P. TiO_2 nanotubes: synthesis and applications. Angew Chem Int Ed Engl 2011;50:2904–39.

[16] Terheyden H, Lang NP, Bierbaum S, Stadlinger B. Osseointegration—communication of cells. Clin Oral Implants Res 2012;23:1127–35.

[17] Jung SY, Kim JM, Kang HK, Jang Da H, Min BM. A biologically active sequence of the laminin alpha2 large globular 1 domain promotes cell adhesion through syndecan-1 by inducing phosphorylation and membrane localization of protein kinase Cdelta. J Biol Chem 2009;284:31764–75.

[18] Kang HK, Kim OB, Min SK, Jung SY, Jang Da H, Kwon TK, et al. The effect of the DLTIDDSYWYRI motif of the human laminin alpha2 chain on implant osseointegration. Biomaterials 2013;34:4027–37.

[19] Yeo IS, Min SK, Kang HK, Kwon TK, Jung SY, Min BM. Identification of a bioactive core sequence from human laminin and its applicability to tissue engineering. Biomaterials 2015;73:96–109.

[20] Ogle OE. Implant surface material, design, and osseointegration. Dent Clin North Am 2015;59:505–20.

[21] Berglundh T, Abrahamsson I, Lang NP, Lindhe J. De novo alveolar bone formation adjacent to endosseous implants. Clin Oral Implants Res 2003;14:251–62.

[22] Sims NA, Gooi JH. Bone remodeling: multiple cellular interactions required for coupling of bone formation and resorption. Semin Cell Dev Biol 2008;19:444–51.
[23] Gray C, Boyde A, Jones SJ. Topographically induced bone formation in vitro: implications for bone implants and bone grafts. Bone 1996;18:115–23.
[24] Wall I, Donos N, Carlqvist K, Jones F, Brett P. Modified titanium surfaces promote accelerated osteogenic differentiation of mesenchymal stromal cells in vitro. Bone 2009; 45:17–26.
[25] Hong YS, Kim MJ, Han JS, Yeo IS. Effects of hydrophilicity and fluoride surface modifications to titanium dental implants on early osseointegration: an in vivo study. Implant Dent 2014;23:529–33.
[26] Park JW, Kwon TG, Suh JY. The relative effect of surface strontium chemistry and superhydrophilicity on the early osseointegration of moderately rough titanium surface in the rabbit femur. Clin Oral Implants Res 2013;24:706–9.
[27] Mangano C, Raspanti M, Traini T, Piattelli A, Sammons R. Stereo imaging and cytocompatibility of a model dental implant surface formed by direct laser fabrication. J Biomed Mater Res A 2009;88:823–31.
[28] Stubinger S, Mosch I, Robotti P, Sidler M, Klein K, Ferguson SJ, et al. Histological and biomechanical analysis of porous additive manufactured implants made by direct metal laser sintering: a pilot study in sheep. J Biomed Mater Res B Appl Biomater 2013;101: 1154–63.
[29] Traini T, Mangano C, Sammons RL, Mangano F, Macchi A, Piattelli A. Direct laser metal sintering as a new approach to fabrication of an isoelastic functionally graded material for manufacture of porous titanium dental implants. Dent Mater 2008;24:1525–33.
[30] Mangano C, Piattelli A, D'avila S, Iezzi G, Mangano F, Onuma T, et al. Early human bone response to laser metal sintering surface topography: a histologic report. J Oral Implantol 2010;36:91–6.
[31] Mangano C, Piattelli A, Raspanti M, Mangano F, Cassoni A, Iezzi G, et al. Scanning electron microscopy (SEM) and X-ray dispersive spectrometry evaluation of direct laser metal sintering surface and human bone interface: a case series. Lasers Med Sci 2011;26: 133–8.
[32] Coelho PG, Granjeiro JM, Romanos GE, Suzuki M, Silva NR, Cardaropoli G, et al. Basic research methods and current trends of dental implant surfaces. J Biomed Mater Res B Appl Biomater 2009;88:579–96.
[33] Yeo IS, Han JS, Yang JH. Biomechanical and histomorphometric study of dental implants with different surface characteristics. J Biomed Mater Res B Appl Biomater 2008;87: 303–11.
[34] Ivanoff CJ, Hallgren C, Widmark G, Sennerby L, Wennerberg A. Histologic evaluation of the bone integration of TiO(2) blasted and turned titanium microimplants in humans. Clin Oral Implants Res 2001;12:128–34.
[35] Piattelli A, Manzon L, Scarano A, Paolantonio M, Piattelli M. Histologic and histomorphometric analysis of the bone response to machined and sandblasted titanium implants: an experimental study in rabbits. Int J Oral Maxillofac Implants 1998;13:805–10.
[36] Abrahamsson I, Zitzmann NU, Berglundh T, Wennerberg A, Lindhe J. Bone and soft tissue integration to titanium implants with different surface topography: an experimental study in the dog. Int J Oral Maxillofac Implants 2001;16:323–32.
[37] Klokkevold PR, Nishimura RD, Adachi M, Caputo A. Osseointegration enhanced by chemical etching of the titanium surface. A torque removal study in the rabbit. Clin Oral Implants Res 1997;8:442–7.

[38] Bonfante EA, Janal MN, Granato R, Marin C, Suzuki M, Tovar N, et al. Buccal and lingual bone level alterations after immediate implantation of four implant surfaces: a study in dogs. Clin Oral Implants Res 2013;24:1375−80.
[39] Gupta A, Dhanraj M, Sivagami G. Status of surface treatment in endosseous implant: a literary overview. Indian J Dent Res 2010;21:433−8.
[40] Lee JJ, Rouhfar L, Beirne OR. Survival of hydroxyapatite-coated implants: a meta-analytic review. J Oral Maxillofac Surg 2000;58:1372−9. discussion 1379−80.
[41] Van Oirschot BA, Bronkhorst EM, Van Den Beucken JJ, Meijer GJ, Jansen JA, Junker R. Long-term survival of calcium phosphate-coated dental implants: a meta-analytical approach to the clinical literature. Clin Oral Implants Res 2013;24:355−62.
[42] Gotfredsen K, Wennerberg A, Johansson C, Skovgaard LT, Hjorting-Hansen E. Anchorage of TiO_2-blasted, HA-coated, and machined implants: an experimental study with rabbits. J Biomed Mater Res 1995;29:1223−31.
[43] Bauer TW. Severe osteolysis after third-body wear due to hydroxyapatite particles from acetabular cup coating. J Bone Joint Surg Br 1998;80:745.
[44] Karabuda C, Sandalli P, Yalcin S, Steflik DE, Parr GR. Histologic and histomorphometric comparison of immediately placed hydroxyapatite-coated and titanium plasma-sprayed implants: a pilot study in dogs. Int J Oral Maxillofac Implants 1999;14:510−5.
[45] Meirelles L, Arvidsson A, Andersson M, Kjellin P, Albrektsson T, Wennerberg A. Nano hydroxyapatite structures influence early bone formation. J Biomed Mater Res A 2008;87: 299−307.
[46] Mendes VC, Moineddin R, Davies JE. Discrete calcium phosphate nanocrystalline deposition enhances osteoconduction on titanium-based implant surfaces. J Biomed Mater Res A 2009;90:577−85.
[47] Gan L, Wang J, Tache A, Valiquette N, Deporter D, Pilliar R. Calcium phosphate sol-gel-derived thin films on porous-surfaced implants for enhanced osteoconductivity. Part II: short-term in vivo studies. Biomaterials 2004;25:5313−21.
[48] Novaes Jr AB, De Souza SL, De Barros RR, Pereira KK, Iezzi G, Piattelli A. Influence of implant surfaces on osseointegration. Braz Dent J 2010;21:471−81.
[49] Choi JY, Lee HJ, Jang JU, Yeo IS. Comparison between bioactive fluoride modified and bioinert anodically oxidized implant surfaces in early bone response using rabbit tibia model. Implant Dent 2012;21:124−8.
[50] Bellows CG, Heersche JN, Aubin JE. The effects of fluoride on osteoblast progenitors in vitro. J Bone Miner Res 1990;5(Suppl. 1):S101−5.
[51] Kassem M, Mosekilde L, Eriksen EF. 1,25-dihydroxyvitamin D3 potentiates fluoride-stimulated collagen type I production in cultures of human bone marrow stromal osteoblast-like cells. J Bone Min Res 1993;8:1453−8.
[52] Kassem M, Mosekilde L, Eriksen EF. Effects of fluoride on human bone cells in vitro: differences in responsiveness between stromal osteoblast precursors and mature osteoblasts. Eur J Endocrinol 1994;130:381−6.
[53] Ellingsen JE, Thomsen P, Lyngstadaas SP. Advances in dental implant materials and tissue regeneration. Periodontol 2006;2000(41):136−56.
[54] Cooper LF, Zhou Y, Takebe J, Guo J, Abron A, Holmen A, et al. Fluoride modification effects on osteoblast behavior and bone formation at TiO_2 grit-blasted c.p. titanium endosseous implants. Biomaterials 2006;27:926−36.
[55] Taxt-Lamolle SF, Rubert M, Haugen HJ, Lyngstadaas SP, Ellingsen JE, Monjo M. Controlled electro-implementation of fluoride in titanium implant surfaces enhances cortical bone formation and mineralization. Acta Biomater 2010;6:1025−32.

[56] Mertens C, Steveling HG. Early and immediate loading of titanium implants with fluoride-modified surfaces: results of 5-year prospective study. Clin Oral Implants Res 2011;22: 1354–60.

[57] Oxby G, Oxby F, Oxby J, Saltvik T, Nilsson P. Early loading of fluoridated implants placed in fresh extraction sockets and healed bone: a 3- to 5-year clinical and radiographic follow-up study of 39 consecutive patients. Clin Implant Dent Relat Res 2015;17: 898–907.

[58] Jimbo R, Anchieta R, Baldassarri M, Granato R, Marin C, Teixeira HS, et al. Histomorphometry and bone mechanical property evolution around different implant systems at early healing stages: an experimental study in dogs. Implant Dent 2013;22:596–603.

[59] Stephansson SN, Byers BA, Garcia AJ. Enhanced expression of the osteoblastic phenotype on substrates that modulate fibronectin conformation and integrin receptor binding. Biomaterials 2002;23:2527–34.

[60] Germanier Y, Tosatti S, Broggini N, Textor M, Buser D. Enhanced bone apposition around biofunctionalized sandblasted and acid-etched titanium implant surfaces. A histomorphometric study in miniature pigs. Clin Oral Implants Res 2006;17:251–7.

[61] Ryu JJ, Park K, Kim HS, Jeong CM, Huh JB. Effects of anodized titanium with Arg-Gly-Asp (RGD) peptide immobilized via chemical grafting or physical adsorption on bone cell adhesion and differentiation. Int J Oral Maxillofac Implants 2013;28:963–72.

[62] Kim JE, Kang SS, Choi KH, Shim JS, Jeong CM, Shin SW, et al. The effect of anodized implants coated with combined rhBMP-2 and recombinant human vascular endothelial growth factors on vertical bone regeneration in the marginal portion of the peri-implant. Oral Surg Oral Med Oral Pathol Oral Radiol 2013;115:e24–31.

[63] Liu Y, Hunziker EB, Layrolle P, De Bruijn JD, De Groot K. Bone morphogenetic protein 2 incorporated into biomimetic coatings retains its biological activity. Tissue Eng 2004;10: 101–8.

[64] Wikesjo UM, Qahash M, Polimeni G, Susin C, Shanaman RH, Rohrer MD, et al. Alveolar ridge augmentation using implants coated with recombinant human bone morphogenetic protein-2: histologic observations. J Clin Periodontol 2008;35:1001–10.

[65] Shah AK, Lazatin J, Sinha RK, Lennox T, Hickok NJ, Tuan RS. Mechanism of BMP-2 stimulated adhesion of osteoblastic cells to titanium alloy. Biol Cell 1999;91:131–42.

[66] Kang JD. Another complication associated with rhBMP-2? Spine J 2011;11:517–9.

[67] Liu Y, Enggist L, Kuffer AF, Buser D, Hunziker EB. The influence of BMP-2 and its mode of delivery on the osteoconductivity of implant surfaces during the early phase of osseointegration. Biomaterials 2007;28:2677–86.

[68] Lee BC, Yeo IS, Kim DJ, Lee JB, Kim SH, Han JS. Bone formation around zirconia implants combined with rhBMP-2 gel in the canine mandible. Clin Oral Implants Res 2013;24:1332–8.

[69] Ebara S, Nakayama K. Mechanism for the action of bone morphogenetic proteins and regulation of their activity. Spine (Phila Pa 1976) 2002;27:S10–5.

Bone response to calcium phosphate coatings for dental implants

4

S. Anil[1], *J. Venkatesan*[2], *M.S. Shim*[2], *E.P. Chalisserry*[3], *S.-K. Kim*[3]
[1]Prince Sattam Bin Abdulaziz University, AlKharj, Saudi Arabia; [2]Incheon National University, Incheon, Republic of Korea; [3]Pukyong National University, Busan, Korea

4.1 Introduction

The success of dental implant depends, in part, on the quality of the material used to make the implant, its manufacturing routes, mechanical properties, biological stabilization, and biocompatible surface coating. Biocompatibility of the implant with body and bone tissue is essential to allow adequate new bone adaptation to the implant surface. Titanium and its alloys have arisen as adequate materials that fulfill those requirements, that is, good mechanical strength and bioinertness when implanted. Geometry and surface topography are crucial for the short- and long-term success of dental implants. Implant surfaces have been developed in the last decade in a concentrated effort to provide bone in a faster and improved osseointegration process [1]. Dental implant quality depends on the chemical, physical, mechanical, and topographic characteristics of the surface. These different properties interact and determine the activity of the attached cells that are close against the dental implant surface. Dental implants have been designed to provide textures and shapes that may enhance cellular activity and direct bone apposition. Osteogenesis at the implant surface is influenced by several mechanisms. A series of coordinated events, including cell proliferation, transformation of osteoblasts, and bone tissue formation might be affected by different surface topographies. Moreover, their surface can be modified to improve fixation by direct bonding with bone [2].

Chemical methods have been applied to induce the formation of bioactive apatite nucleation points on the titanium surface [3], but the most extended method clinically used to enhance the adhesion of implants is the application of bioactive ceramic coatings on their surface [4]. These coatings provide the interface to which leaving tissues can attach, avoiding the formation of a fibrous capsule that can cause failure of the implant. The ceramic coating of metallic implants functions as a transition layer between the bone tissue and the metal surface, enhancing the contact and conducting bone growth along the surface of the implant. Calcium phosphate (CaP) ceramics, particularly hydroxyapatite (HA) and tricalcium phosphate (TCP), have received much attention as implant coating materials and are widely used in dentistry due to their excellent biocompatibility properties. Techniques, such as sputtering [5,6], enameling [7,8], electrophoretic deposition (EPD) [9,10], or solgel [11,12], have been used

Bone Response to Dental Implant Materials. http://dx.doi.org/10.1016/B978-0-08-100287-2.00004-5

to produce bioactive coatings. Among them, pulsed laser deposition (PLD) of bioactive glass has arisen as a very interesting alternative to coat metallic substrates for implantation [13] due to the high adhesion of the coatings to the metallic substrates and absence of contamination and porosity [14]. Reports showed that nanometer-sized HA coatings on electropolished surfaces can result in approximately 300% more bone-to-implant contact when compared to noncoated electropolished surfaces [15].

4.2 The bone implant interface

A systematic review concluded that there was a positive correlation between surface roughness and bone-to-implant contact [16]. As a consequence, over the last 30 years, various surface modification techniques have been introduced, including blasting, etching, oxidizing, titanium (Ti) plasma spraying, and incorporation of HA or other forms of CaP [17]. CaP has been investigated extensively because of its biocompatibility and mineral chemistry, which resembles those of the human bone [18]. As a coating material, CaP has been widely applied to titanium implants. HA-coated implants showed faster healing and bone attachment compared to noncoated implants [19,20]. CaP-coated implants also showed excellent clinical outcome when implanted in fresh extraction sites, grafted maxillary sinuses, and areas with poor bone quality [21,22].

The quality of the bone implant interface is determined by the quantity of the implant surface in intimate contact with the mineralized bone tissue as well as the mechanical quality of the bone tissue around the interface. Two interfaces contribute to mechanical implant fixation: the *implant-coating interface* and the *coating-bone interface.* Regarding the *implant-coating interface,* the mechanical properties of the coating and the bonding strength to the metal substrate are important. The bond strength of the implant-coating interface could be reduced due to the disintegration of the coating [23]. Recrystallization of the amorphous phase in CaP coatings also might result in stress accumulation leading to reduced strength [24]. The rate of resorption of the coating also influences the bond strength between bone and implant [25].

The coated surface of the titanium implant plays a crucial role in determining the biological response of the bone [26]. The CaP coating generally alters the surface properties, including morphology, physicochemical composition, and surface energy [27]. Although the surface alterations, such as the roughness, have improved the outcome of osseointegration, the exact mechanism is poorly understood [19]. This could be due to the topographical alterations, fabrication-related changes in surface composition, or changes in the wettability characteristics [28]. It is well established that the CaP-based coating of titanium favors the bone response compared with the uncoated titanium [25,29,30].

The adsorption of biomolecules and the subsequent interactions of cells on an implant surface determine the fate of the implant. The rough topography generally increases the surface area of the implant adjacent to the bone and improves the cell adhesion to the surface, thereby enhancing the bone-to-implant contact and biomechanical integrity. The CaP-based surfaces bind more attachment proteins, such as fibronectin and vitronectin, for the integrin-mediated binding action of osteoprogenitors compared with titanium surfaces [31].

CaP-based coatings on titanium implants are now accepted as suitable for enhancing the bone formation around implants and thus improving the clinical success at an early stage after implantation. The biological interface reactions can be summarized as follows [32].

1. Dissolution of CaP-based coatings,
2. Reprecipitation of apatite,
3. Ion exchange accompanied by absorption and incorporation of biological molecules,
4. Cell attachment, proliferation, and differentiation,
5. Extracellular matrix formation and mineralization.

The dissolution of HA coating is a key step to induce the precipitation of bone-like apatite on the implant surface.

4.3 Methods of calcium phosphate coating

The addition of calcium- and phosphorous-based materials as coatings has received significant attention because these elements are the same as the basic components of the natural bone and coatings can be applied along the implant surfaces by various industrial processing methods [33]. The osseointegration of the dental implant with plasma-sprayed HA is faster than uncoated implants. In vivo studies on rabbit femoral condyles have demonstrated a higher level of osseointegration for the HA-coated samples compared to the uncoated ones. Bone maturation was reported to be more significant at the bone−implant interface and coating of titanium with HA led to improve maturation of the newly formed bone tissue [34]. These observations were attributed to the presence of porous HA in the coated samples. Due to the high biocompatibility and osteoconduction of CaP materials, they have been widely used for different hard tissue applications such as HA-coated metallic implants and bone substitute materials.

CaP coating may undergo extensive dissolution in tissue fluids and demonstrate rapid breakdown around the implant surface [35]. Various coating methods have been tried to achieve optimal quality of the bone implant interface (Fig. 4.1). Each of the techniques has its own technical limitations, and so far, an optimal method for producing a bioactive coating with high bonding strength on an implant remains to be developed.

Several techniques have been used to create the HA coating on metallic implants, such as plasma spraying process, thermal spraying, sputter coating, pulsed laser ablation, dynamic mixing, dip coating, solgel, EPD, biomimetic coating, ion-beam-assisted deposition (IBAD), and hot isostatic pressing.

4.3.1 *Plasma sprayed coatings*

Plasma-sprayed HA coatings were introduced in the 1980s and are the most frequently used method for clinical application of CaP coatings [26]. The implant surface is

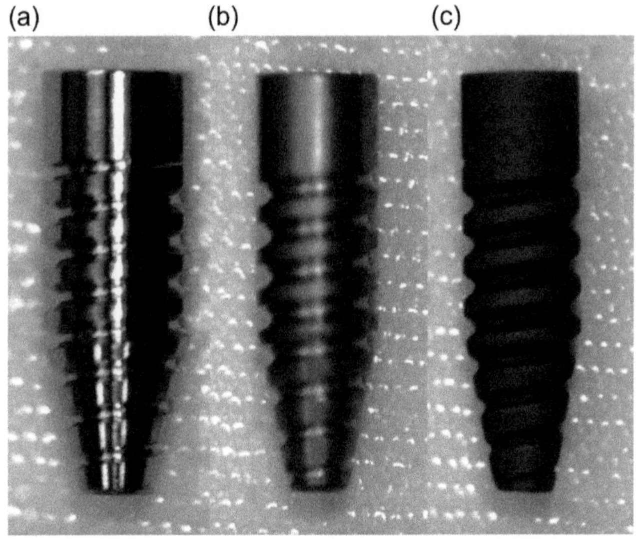

Figure 4.1 Titanium implant without any surface modification (a). An anodized titanium implant (b) and a CaP-coated titanium implant (c).

roughened by grit-blasting, shot peening, or etching before plasma spraying. The plasma spraying process is very critical for the coating quality and several parameters have to be controlled, including the purity and the crystallinity of the HA used [36]. The coating crystallinity depends on the particle temperature in the plasma flame, particle position within the flame, the flame velocity, residence time in the flame, and particle size. It also changes with the distance between spray gun and substrate. The stability of the melted powder in the plasma is determined by its chemical composition. The heat treatment has shown to improve bonding strength by further diffusion of the coating into the substrate surface [37]. Other plasma spraying methods such as vacuum plasma spraying and high velocity flame sprayed coatings produced coatings with good adhesion strength and fewer pores [38,39]. Even though these methods produce coatings with good adhesion strength and fewer pores, they might overheat the metal substrate, thereby changing its mechanical properties.

4.3.2 Thermal spray coating technique

Thermal spray technology is a coating process that provides functional surfaces to protect or improve the performance of a substrate or component. Thermal spraying of CaP on the implant devices can be compared with plasma spray-coating technique, having the advantage of high deposition rate and low cost [40]. Thermal spray technique has the ability to produce HA layer with thickness from 30 to 200 μm depending on the coating condition However, films deposited by thermal spraying suffer from poor coating–substrate adherence and nonuniform crystallinity, which reduce the lifetime of implants [23, 41]. The thermal spray coating requires high sintering temperature, which may result in crack propagation on the surface of the coating [41].

4.3.3 Solgel coating

The solgel method represents a simple and low-cost procedure to deposit thin coatings, with homogenous chemical composition onto substrates with large dimensions and complex design. The high mechanical strength and toughness of titanium alloys are the most important advantages over bioactive HA ceramics. A system that joins both materials has the mechanical advantage of the underlying (metallic) substrate and biological affinity of the HA. Coating of metallic implants with bioactive materials, such as HA, may accelerate bone formation during initial stages of osseointegration, improving implant fixation [42]. Thin HA film on titanium substrates can be prepared using solgel [11] or electrophoresis techniques [43]. The solgel and electrophoresis methods are capable of improving chemical homogeneity in the resulting HA coating to a significant extent when compared to conventional methods, such as solid state reactions, wet precipitation, and hydrothermal synthesis [44]. These methods are also simple and less expensive than the plasma-spraying method that is widely used for biomedical applications. In vivo bone tissue evaluations of surfaces modified using the solgel method have shown better osseointegration, with no adverse reaction [12,45]. However, the behavior of solgel modifications of loaded osseointegrated implants in the long term remains unknown.

4.3.4 Sputter deposition

This technique involves the vaporization of atoms or molecules from a solid surface by momentum transfer from bombarding energetic atomic-sized particles. These particles are ions of a gaseous material accelerated in an electric field. Physical sputtering can be divided into a number of methods, including radiofrequency (RF) magnetron sputtering and high-energy ionic scattering. A common drawback inherent in all these methods is that the deposition rate is very low and the process itself is very slow [46]. The deposition rate is improved by using a magnetically enhanced variant of diode sputtering, known as radio frequency magnetron sputtering.

Magnetron sputtering: Magnetron sputtering is a viable thin-film technique as it allows the mechanical properties of titanium to be preserved while maintaining the bioactivity of the coated HA. Films were deposited in a custom-built sputter deposition chamber at room temperature. This technique shows strong HA titanium bonding associated with outward diffusion of titanium into the HA layer, forming TiO_2 at the interface [47].

RF sputtering: RF magnetron sputtering is largely used to deposit thin films of CaP coatings on titanium implants. RF magnetron sputtering is a very suitable technique to deposit standardized CaP coatings on titanium substrates. The advantage of this technique is that the coating shows strong adhesion to the titanium and the CaP ratio and crystallinity of the deposited coating can be varied easily. Studies in animals have shown higher BIC percentages with sputter-coated implants [48,49]. Studies have shown that these coatings were more retentive, with the chemical structure being precisely controlled [50].

4.3.5 Pulsed laser deposition

PLD technique has evolved as an alternative and added advantage of preservation of stoichiometry of target phase. PLD is very promising for coatings of bioactive glass on implant metals. The PLD technique involves three main steps: ablation of the target material, formation of a highly energetic plume, and the growth of the film on the substrate. PLD technique also possesses the ability to form desired film thickness, morphology, and composition by varying the deposition parameters. This method additionally provides deposition of different target materials of unique physicochemical and biological properties over single substrate for functionally graded coatings [51,52]. The process ensures the titanium surface with increased hardness, corrosion resistance, and a high degree of purity with a standard roughness and thicker oxide layer [53,54]. Biological studies evaluating the role of titanium ablation topography and chemical properties showed the potential of the grooved surface to orientate osteoblast cells attachment and control the direction of ingrowth [55].

4.3.6 Dip-coating technique

HA can be homogenously coated onto metal substrates to obtain coating thickness in the range of 0.05−0.5 mm. The technique allows uniform coating of HA on the metal surface. In addition, the processing time for dip coating is short and can be used for substrate with complex shapes. The coating layer is deposited on the surface of the substrate without decomposition or reaction with the metal substrate [56]. A highly porous surface with bonding strengths of more than 30 MPa can be obtained with this technique [57].

4.3.7 Ion beam assisted deposition of CaP

IBAD method is used in CaP coating. With this method, the dissolution rate of the CaP coating has decreased remarkably, whereas the bonding strength between the layer and Ti substrate has increased [58]. An atomic intermixing layer is formed between the HA coating and Ti substrate during the IBAD method and this chemical bonding may enhance the interfacial adhesive bonding strength [59]. Studies have shown that implants coated with CaP by the IBAD method showed a higher bone-to-implant contact ratio compared to blasted surface implants and machined surface implants [60]. Better biocompatibility and contact osteogenesis have also been reported [35]. Bone defects adjacent to implants coated with IBAD CaP showed better bone response in resolving them [35,61].

4.3.8 Electrophoretic deposition

EPD is a process in which particles in a suspension are coated onto an electrode under the effect of an electric field. A good degree of controlled coating can be achieved by regulating the deposition conditions and the ceramic powder size and shape for obtaining a coating thickness from 1 mm to more than 100 μm thick [62]. A uniform thin coating of HA on titanium with good mechanical strength can be obtained with EPD hydroxyapatite [63]. EPD of HA can be processed at room temperature or lower, which avoids problems related to formation of amorphous phases. One of the drawback is the development of porosities, which may later on lead to corrosion and delamination of the titanium caused by penetration of body fluids into the substrate. Even though post-treatment high temperature sintering can be utilized to minimize the porosity by increasing the coating density, chances of formation of cracks in the coating can occur due to the difference in the thermal expansion coefficients [64].

4.3.9 Hot isostatic pressing technique

Hot isostatic pressing (HIP) is a method of producing a HA coating on a Ti substrate using pressure to exert the required load at the desired temperature. The advantages of HIP are better temperature control as compared to uniaxial hot pressing, and a resultant homogeneous material structure and properties. The reduced sintering temperature enables control or even avoidance of grain growth and undesirable reactions. HIP technique is useful in reducing the porosity and improving the physical and mechanical properties of ceramic coatings [65].

4.3.10 Biomimetic precipitation

Biomimetic HA deposition is mimicking the natural process of remineralization of HA, but without involving the cellular and organic levels. Because the biomimetic HA coatings have a low degree of crystallinity and porous structure, their solubility is higher than the dense hydroxyapatite coatings deposited with other methods [66]. The crystallized titanium oxides induce bone-like HA on its surface, which can be hypothesized as an important early step for osseointegration. The deposition of biomimetic hydroxyapatite on titanium oxide surfaces, acting as a bonding layer to the bone, might improve the bone-bonding ability and enhance the biological responses to bone-anchored implants. The biological benefits of biomimetic HA and the possibilities to use them as coatings on titanium implants for improved response have been reported [67].

4.4 Surface coating and peri-implant wound healing process

Even though a high level of success has been achieved with dental implants, there is still scope for improving the osseointegration phenomenon through promoting osteoblast differentiation and proliferation as well as reducing the healing period. One approach to enhance osteoinductivity is to modify the implant surface to mimic the natural structure of tissue, namely, a biomimetic approach. Better communication between cells and extracellular matrix components is crucial for the maintenance and regeneration of relevant tissue (Fig. 4.2). The extracellular matrix governs

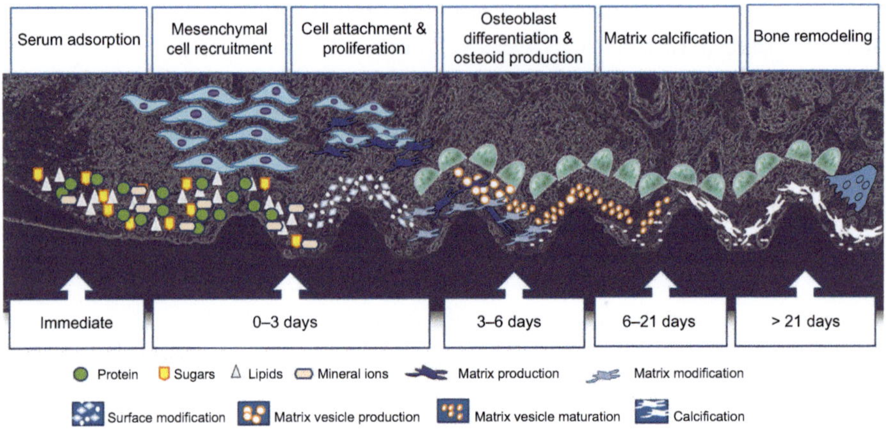

Figure 4.2 Illustration showing the cellular phenomena at the implant–bone interface during the healing of the implant.

various cellular events of osteoblasts, including cell adhesion, proliferation, and differentiation [68].

There are three major stages, which are involved in direct healing: woven bone formation, adaptation of bone mass to load, and adaptation of bone structure or bone remodeling [69]. Osteoconductivity and osteoinductivity are two key processes of the formation of the new bone. Osteoblasts and osteoclasts are the main cells involved in remodeling of bone, osteoblasts lay down bone matrix, whereas osteoclasts are involved in resorbing the bone tissue.

Osteogenic factors have been applied with success in the bone implant interface [70]. CaP, including HA, coatings have been proposed to enhance bone integration of metal implants [71]. Stimulation of new bone formation around CaP-coated implants is based on dissolution of the coating soon after implantation followed by formation of a bone-inductive carbonated CaP layer (Fig. 4.3). The biological advantages of these coatings include the enhancement of bone formation and accelerated bonding between the implant surface and the surrounding bone (Fig. 4.4) [72,73].

CaP coatings have osteoconductive properties, which enhance the bone formation at the implant–bone interface. A carbonated apatite layer is generated at the surface between the coated implant and bone. The formation of this layer is by the local degradation of the CaP surface followed by secondary crystal growth between the artificial HA and the bone. Moreover, reprecipitation might occur leading to a physicochemical bonding mechanism [74,75]. It has been hypothesized that bone formation on CaP coatings is due to selective adsorption of serum protein to the surface, which might be responsible for enhanced osteoblast adhesion [76]. The cascade of events has been suggested, which involves early formation of an afibrillar globular calcified layer on the implant surface produced by osteoblasts, to be crucial for bonding of the bone to the implant surface. This layer fuses to form a homogenous line analogous with cement lines or lamina limitans with which collagen fibers become incorporated. Formation of carbonate-containing apatite crystals has been observed in both the bone and

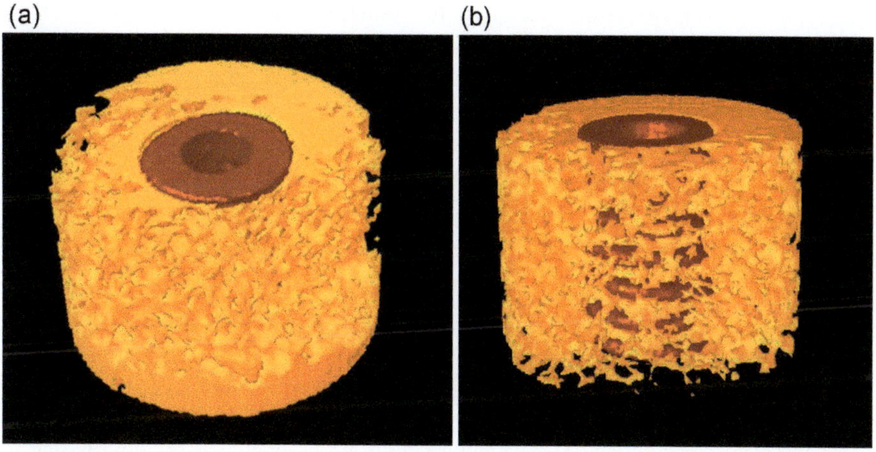

Figure 4.3 Microcomputed tomography (CT) images showing the bone implant contact around HA-coated (a) and noncoated titanium implants (b) installed (8 weeks healing) in the tibia of beagle dog. Three-dimensional images were generated from micro-CT data for both titanium implants and HA-coated implants.

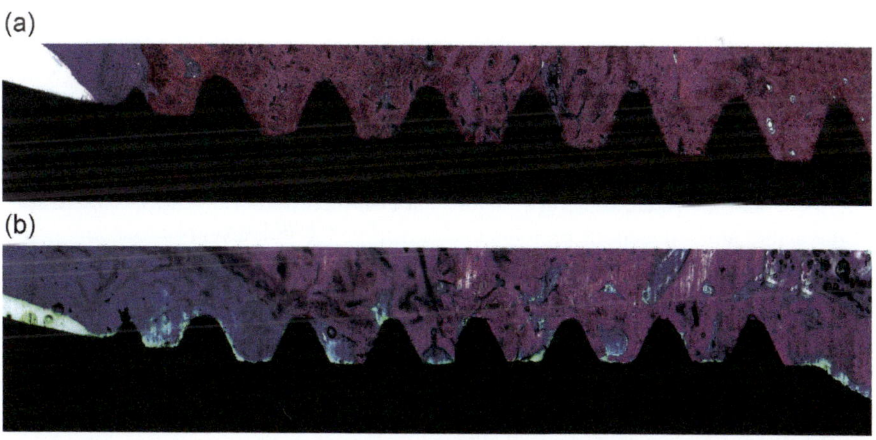

Figure 4.4 Histological section of the HA-coated titanium implant (a) and noncoated titanium implant (b) installed in the mandible of dog. Note the dense bone HA coated around the implant (hematoxylin and eosin and basic fuchsin stained, magnification objective ×10).

extraskeletally, whereas the true bone formation as characterized histologically has only been demonstrated in bony sites.

A comparative study of the HA-coated and uncoated implants in the femoral condyles of dogs showed that the coated implants were able to help in bridging a gap of 1–2 mm [77]. Several other studies also showed significantly higher bone formation than uncoated implants [72,78]. The biomimetic-coating deposition aids in producing a homogeneous coating and because the CaP is deposited under physiological temperatures it is possible to incorporate functional biological agents, such as growth factors. The CaP ratio and coating thickness can be varied, and the structure of the formed crystals is more akin to the bone mineral than that produced in conventional ways [79,80].

4.5 Factors influencing the coated implant bone interface

Biomechanical and biochemical anchorage mechanisms are involved in the bone–implant interface bonding. Biomechanical binding is when the bone ingrowth occurs into micrometer-sized surface irregularities. Biochemical bonding occurs with certain bioactive materials showing primarily a chemical bonding, with possible supplemental biomechanical interlocking. The advantage with the biochemical bonding is that the anchorage is accomplished within a relatively short period of time, whereas biomechanical anchorage takes weeks to develop [81]. CaPs are widely used osteoconductive materials in coating implant surface. Coating of titanium implants with CaP increases the surface area, biocompatibility, and osteoconductive effect that favors cellular activity, thereby enhancing osseointegration.

The bioinorganics can modulate angiogenesis to accelerate healing, induce osteogenic differentiation, stimulate osteoblast proliferation, and control the resorptive activity of osteoclasts. Calcium induces platelet activation and release of their intragranular content. At calcium-modified implant surfaces, these platelet-derived factors may create a concentration gradient of chemoattractants for mesenchymal and osteoprogenitor cells and stimulate their activity [82,83]. Calcium is present abundantly at the implant–bone interface, not only in the mineral structure but also incorporated to the anionic residues of the acidic noncollagenous proteins that constitute the first layers of osseointegration [84]. The calcium on titanium surfaces alters the electrical characteristics of the surface and thereby the composition of the adsorbed biofilm [85].

The integration of bone-to-implant interface in a coated implant is influenced by the following factors:

- Surface morphology
- The chemical composition and CaP ratio
- Phase composition and structure

4.5.1 Surface morphology/surface topography

Surface topography plays a crucial role in osseointegration. By modifying the characteristics of the Ti surface, biocompatibility can be improved, faster osseointegration can be provoked [86]. The dynamics of cell populations and of the biomolecules that drive to regeneration around implants are strongly influenced by the implant surface roughness [87]. Commonly, implant surface roughness is divided, depending on the dimension of the measured surface features, into macro-, micro-, and nanoroughness. Typically, these different roughness features are related to distinct effects during wound healing and osseointegration (Fig. 4.5). A moderately roughened surface (1.0–2.0 μm) results in a stronger bone response than smoother or rougher surfaces. Microrough surfaces have been generally interpreted as biocompatible with limited ability to directly affect the initial fate of surrounding tissues, that is, the ability to enhance the bone formation or to prevent bone resorption [88]. Several methods have been developed to create surface roughness, such as titanium plasma-spraying, blasting with ceramic particles, acid etching, and anodization. Creation of nanoscale topographies plays an important role in the adsorption of proteins, adhesion of osteoblastic cells, and thus the rate of osseointegration [89]. However, reproducible surface roughness in the nanometer range is difficult to produce with chemical treatments. The optimal surface nanotopography

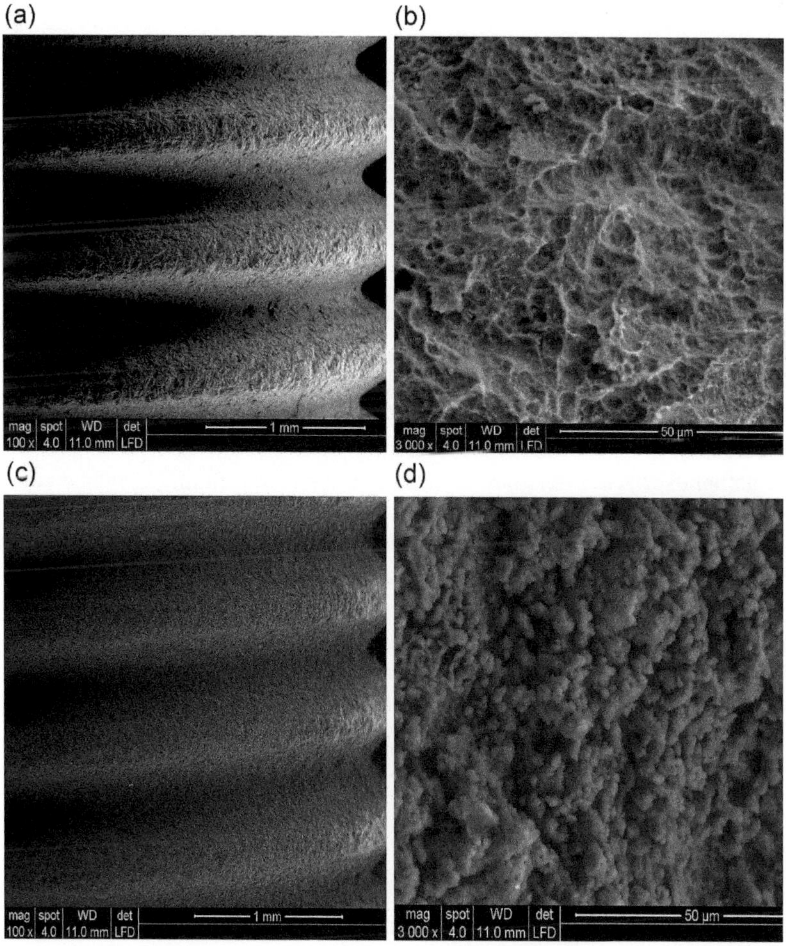

Figure 4.5 Micrographs showing the appearance of the titanium implant (a), implant having PLD deposited HA (c), scanning electron microscope (SEM) image (×3000) of bare titanium surface before coating (b), SEM image (×3000) of titanium implant with HA (d).

helps in the selective adsorption of proteins leading to the adhesion of osteoblastic cells and rapid bone apposition [88].

CaP-derived coatings, have been widely documented, and several experimental studies have suggested that bone integration may occur faster around an implant coated with CaP [25]. Calcium induces platelet activation and release of their intragranular contents. These platelet-derived factors may create a concentration gradient of chemoattractants for mesenchymal and osteoprogenitor cells at the coated surface and stimulate their activity [83,90]. The platelet activation and subsequent clot formation provide the biochemical cues and the mechanical structure for the recruitment of osteogenic cells and the generation of an osteoconductive microenvironment. The calcium is present at the implant–bone interface in the mineral structure and incorporated to the anionic residues of the acidic noncollagenous proteins constituting the first layers of osseointegration [84]. The presence of calcium on titanium surfaces alters the electrical characteristics of the surface and thereby the composition of the adsorbed biofilm [85]. Clinically, an implant that has a thin $CaPO_4$ coating on the acid-etched surface yielded a stronger bone response than the etched surface alone [91].

4.5.2 The chemical composition and CaP ratio

CaPs can exist in different phases depending on temperature, impurities, and the presence of water. All CaPs do not have similar bioactivity and degradation behavior, which generally depend on the CaP ratio, crystallinity, and phase purity. Among the various CaPs, HA and β-TCP are the most commonly used phases because of their osteogenic property and the ability to form strong bonds with host bone tissues. Solubility of β-TCP is much higher than HA, and thus β-TCP is termed a bioresorbable ceramic [92,93]. The degradation process of CaP can be controlled by the development of biphasic CaP–based biomaterials consisting of HA and β-TCP [94].

The implant surface differs based on the surface treatment, the chemical composition, and the charges on the implant surface. The chemical composition of a surface layer might influence different in vivo reactions such as reactive bond formations. Protein adsorption occurs immediately upon implant contact with the biological environment and surface properties, such as surface energy and wettability, which are pivotal parameters determining the final composition of this adsorbate [95]. The binding of proteins to the implant surface and the subsequent cell reactions could be influenced by the continuous exchange of water and various ions [96]. The composition and charges are critical for protein adsorption and cell attachment. Highly hydrophilic surfaces seem to be more desirable than hydrophobic ones because of their interactions with biological fluids, cells, and tissues [97–99].

4.5.3 Phase composition and structure

Melting of the hydroxyapatite occurs within the plasma stream, and when the particles impact on the cooler metallic substrate, a range of disordered CaP phases are formed possessing differing biologic dissolution kinetics, which favor both short- and long-term osseointegration. These phases include predominately amorphous CaP, β-TCP, and HA. The reported relative biological solubility of these compounds varies with the composition. The dissolution rate of various forms is not only related to crystal chemistry, but also affected by physical parameters such as the size of melted splats, the amount of porosity within the coating, the presence of thermally induced cracks, pits or other defects, and the coating's crystallinity [100]. An enhanced level of bone growth occurs when the coating contains a higher percentage of the amorphous phase.

4.5.4 Coating dissolution of HA

The success of a coated implant depends on the stability of the coating. Stability of the coating is controlled by its physical and mechanical properties such as crystallinity, phase composition, dissolution characteristics, coating thickness, and coating strength [101]. Chemical resorption and dissolution of the coating are two non−cell-mediated processes that contribute to the overall loss of the HA coating during service. CaP coating may undergo dissolution in tissue fluids and demonstrate breakdown around the implant surface [102,103]. The resorption of HA coating in clinical scenario happens mainly due to the dissolution at neutral pH, and osteoclastic resorption of the coating as part of normal bone remodeling [35,104]. Even though partial dissolution of the HA coating is essential to trigger bone growth, rapid dissolution leads to poor bone bonding and coating disintegration [105]. The bioactive property of a CaP coating is a direct consequence of the dissolution and reprecipitation process, which occurs in vivo. The formation of biological apatite resulting from surface reactions is believed to lead to the chemical bonding between the implant and bone.

Dissolution of the coating occurs due to the presence of extracellular fluid and the rate of dissolution is influenced by the presence of cracks and voids in the coating. A study showed that the resorption rate of HA coatings in the human trabecular bone is approximately 20% of the coating thickness per year [106]. The extracellular fluid in contact with the coated implant could generate progressive crystallization of amorphous phases, resulting in stress accumulation within the coating. This stress accumulation at the implant-coating interface results in instability of the coating and subsequent delamination [24]. The composition of the coating also influences the chemical resorption. The amorphous form of HA or TCP phases has a greater chance of dissolution compared to the crystalline HA phases [107].

With substitution and doping of elements to the CaP coating as well as application of current coating methods, the dissolution and resorption issues can be resolved. Further research is underway to optimize the process for creating the ideal bioactive coating over the titanium surface [26].

4.6 CaP coating as drug delivery system

Biomimetics is a potential way to prepare surfaces that provide a favorable bone tissue response, thus enhancing the fixation between the bone and implants. The biological performance of CaP coating can be enhanced by ionic substitution/doping or substitution of strontium (Sr), silicon (Si), and silver (Ag). These ion substitutions not only change the composition, solubility, and crystallinity of HA but also are important in cell proliferation, collagen synthesis, nuclei acid synthesis, and bone development. They also have pharmaceutical effects on the bone regeneration. CaPs have been used successfully in various drug delivery applications in the form of nanoscale (particulate systems), microscale (coating), and macroscale (calcium phosphate cement and scaffold) for local delivery and targeted delivery.

Composite coatings composed of collagen and CaP minerals could combine the benefits of the mineral phase and the collagenous matrix to affect cellular adhesion, subsequent proliferation, and differentiation phases [108]. The CaP—collagen composite coatings also showed an improved retention of CaP crystals onto implant surfaces [109]. Also factors such as bone morphogenetic protein 2 (BMP-2), BMP-7, growth factor 2, fibroblast, platelet-derived growth factor, and insulin-like growth factors have been codeposited with CaP or collagen coatings onto implant surfaces. In fact, growth factors (GF's) immobilized on titanium implants precoated with collagen, showed increased osteogenic properties compared to GFs bound to untreated titanium surfaces [110]. This may be due to a sustained delivery profile or a higher stability of the growth factor [111,112].

4.6.1 Silicon

Silicon (Si), although not labeled an essential trace element for human health, has showed beneficial effect bone formation, maintenance, and wound healing [113]. Substitution of silicate ions for phosphate ions at ultratrace levels will enhance the bioactivity of HA either through its effect on surface chemistry or through controlled local bioavailable Si release. During the early stages of the biomineralization process, silicon can be found at active calcification sites and the later stages of calcification. Silicon plays a direct role in mineralization by inducing the precipitation of HA from electrolyte solutions [114]. Studies have shown that silicon-substituted CaP showed better performance [18,115,116].

4.6.2 Strontium

Strontium (Sr) has bone-seeking behavior and has been shown to enhance bone regeneration when incorporated into synthetic bone grafts. Essentially, because it is very similar in size and charge to Ca, it is thought to displace Ca ions in osteoblast-mediated processes. The divalent strontium ions enhance the replication of preosteoblastic cells and bone matrix synthesis by binding to the calcium receptor and stimulation of local growth factor and osteoprotegerin (OPG) production [117,118]. Because strontium is chemically closely related to calcium, it is easily introduced as a natural substitute for calcium in HA [119]. Sr could not only enhance the positive effect of HA coatings on osseointegration and bone regeneration, but it also prevents undesirable bone resorption [120]. Research has shown that strontium probably stimulates the bone formation by a dual mode of action [121]. First, it activates the calcium sensing receptor in osteoblasts, which simultaneously increases OPG production and decreases receptor activator of nuclear factor kappa beta ligand expression [122]. Strontium-doped CaP material was found to increase endothelial cellular proliferation and tubule formation, both characteristics of angiogenic abilities. Strontium-doped material also showed between 5% and 10% increased new bone growth in vivo over 16 weeks when compared to a similar material without strontium [123]. The addition of strontium to CaP cement leads to a faster osseointegration of the implant into the osteoporotic bone [124].

4.6.3 Silver

Adherence and colonization of bacteria on the surface of the implant can lead to infections and peri-implantitis [125,126]. Silver-polysaccharide nanocomposite coatings were effective in killing both Gram-positive and Gram-negative bacterial strains [127,128]. The antibacterial effect of Ag is reported with plasma-sprayed, RF magnetron sputter–deposited, IBAD-deposited, and PLD-deposited Ag-HA coatings [129,130].

4.6.4 Bisphosphonate

Bisphosphonates are a class of agents that may have the potential to improve osseointegration of the implants. They potently inhibit the osteoclast differentiation, reduce their activity, and induce the osteoclast apoptosis [131,132]. Incorporation of bisphosphonates with HA coatings showed better bone–implant contact. A study showed that HA–zoledronate composite coating enhanced the peri-implant bone quality and implant stability in rats with aseptic loosening [133]. The bisphosphonates have a high affinity for bone minerals and bind strongly to HA resulting in selective uptake to the target organ and high local concentration in bone, particularly at the sites of active bone remodeling. The nitrogen-containing bisphosphonates bind to and inhibit farnesyl pyrophosphate synthase, a key enzyme of the mevalonate pathway, thereby preventing the prenylation and activation of small Guanosine-5′-triphosphate-ases (GTPases) that are essential for the bone resorption activity and survival of osteoclasts [134].

4.6.5 Proteins

CaP ceramic has been chosen as one of the most suitable carriers of proteins because of its wide clinical acceptance in many areas of orthopedics and dentistry based on its biocompatible and osteoconductive behavior. The incorporation of a protein into a CaP coating can modify its three-dimensional structure [135]. Due to the slow but definite degradation CaP they may be very suitable to serve as protein carriers, indeed the loaded proteins are gradually releasing during CaP dissolution. Reports have shown that bovine serum albumin can be used along with CaP coating as a source for releasing of biologically active proteins [136].

4.7 CaP coating and peri-implantitis

Bacterial colonization of dental implants can lead to inflammatory reactions, which prevent or result in the loss of osseointegration. Peri-implantitis is defined as "an inflammatory process affecting the soft and hard tissues surrounding an osseointegrated implant, resulting in the rapid loss of the supporting bone, bleeding, and suppuration." The implant surfaces and design play a role in peri-implant disease development. Rough surfaces on superstructures and abutments are reported to accumulate and retain more bacterial plaque than smooth surfaces and are more frequently surrounded by inflamed tissues [137,138]. The rough surfaces provide niches that protect bacteria from host defenses and routine oral hygiene treatments. HA coatings increase the surface roughness of implants. These coatings have also been reported to be at a higher risk for failure, due to peri-implant diseases, when compared with noncoated implants [139,140].

4.8 Conclusion

The implant surface plays an important role in enhancing osseointegration and achieving rapid secondary stability. Altering the implant surface through surface treatments may promote osteogenesis by increasing the surface area, enhancing cellular activity, and ultimately increasing bone attachment. CaP has been studied extensively because of its biocompatibility and mineral chemistry that resemble the bone. It is extensively used as a coating material over metallic implants. The HA-coated implants produce rapid healing responses, promote faster bone attachment, and show a high clinical survival rate when compared to noncoated implants. One of the major drawback is its dissolution in tissue fluids, demonstrating rapid breakdown around the implant surface. To overcome these drawbacks, alteration in the composition as well as newer method of CaP deposition has been tried during the recent past. Research in this field should focus on the effect of coatings' crystallinity, chemical composition/surface topography on the cell differentiation, and therapeutic capabilities of the coating. Further studies are mandatory to assess the long-term in vivo clinical trials to optimize coating properties and continue the preclinical research to provide additional understanding of the bone responses to the coated implant surfaces of different properties.

References

[1] Elias CN, Meirelles L. Improving osseointegration of dental implants. Expert Rev Med Dev 2010;7:241–56.

[2] Guo Z, Zhou L, Rong M, Zhu A, Geng H. Bone response to a pure titanium implant surface modified by laser etching and microarc oxidation. Int J Oral Maxillofac Implants 2010;25:130–6.

[3] Nishiguchi S, Kato H, Neo M, Oka M, Kim HM, Kokubo T, et al. Alkali-and heat-treated porous titanium for orthopedic implants. J Biomed Mater Res 2001;54:198–208.
[4] Dumbleton J, Manley MT. Hydroxyapatite-coated prostheses in total hip and knee arthroplasty. J Bone Joint Surg Am 2004;86-A:2526–40.
[5] Wang CX, Chen ZQ, Wang M. Fabrication and characterization of bioactive glass coatings produced by the ion beam sputter deposition technique. J Mater Sci Mater Med 2002;13:247–51.
[6] Yang Y, Kim K-H, Ong JL. A review on calcium phosphate coatings produced using a sputtering process—an alternative to plasma spraying. Biomaterials 2005;26:327–37.
[7] Kasuga T, Mizuno T, Watanabe M, Nogami M, Niinomi M. Calcium phosphate invert glass-ceramic coatings joined by self-development of compositionally gradient layers on a titanium alloy. Biomaterials 2001;22:577–82.
[8] Torricelli P, Verné E, Brovarone CV, Appendino P, Rustichelli F, Krajewski A, et al. Biological glass coating on ceramic materials: in vitro evaluation using primary osteoblast cultures from healthy and osteopenic rat bone. Biomaterials 2001;22:2535–43.
[9] Agata De Sena L, Calixto De Andrade M, Malta Rossi A, de Almeida Soares G. Hydroxyapatite deposition by electrophoresis on titanium sheets with different surface finishing. J Biomed Mater Res 2002;60:1–7.
[10] Han Y, Xu K, Lu J. Morphology and composition of hydroxyapatite coatings prepared by hydrothermal treatment on electrodeposited brushite coatings. J Mater Sci Mater Med 1999;10:243–8.
[11] Xu W, Hu W, Li M, Wen C. Sol-gel derived hydroxyapatite/titania biocoatings on titanium substrate. Mater Lett 2006;60:1575–8.
[12] Gan L, Wang J, Tache A, Valiquette N, Deporter D, Pilliar R. Calcium phosphate sol-gel-derived thin films on porous-surfaced implants for enhanced osteoconductivity. Part II: short-term in vivo studies. Biomaterials 2004;25:5313–21.
[13] Hamadouche M, Meunier A, Greenspan DC, Blanchat C, Zhong JP, La Torre GP, et al. Bioactivity of sol-gel bioactive glass coated alumina implants. J Biomed Mater Res 2000; 52:422–9.
[14] Teghil R, D'Alessio L, Ferro D, Barinov S. Hardness of bioactive glass film deposited on titanium alloy by pulsed laser ablation. J Mater Sci Lett 2002;21:379–82.
[15] Meirelles L, Arvidsson A, Andersson M, Kjellin P, Albrektsson T, Wennerberg A. Nano hydroxyapatite structures influence early bone formation. J Biomed Mater Res Part A 2008;87:299–307.
[16] Shalabi MM, Gortemaker A, Van't Hof MA, Jansen JA, Creugers NH. Implant surface roughness and bone healing: a systematic review. J Dent Res 2006;85:496–500.
[17] Wennerberg A, Albrektsson T. Effects of titanium surface topography on bone integration: a systematic review. Clin Oral Implants Res 2009;20(Suppl. 4):172–84.
[18] Preethanath RS, Rajesh P, Varma H, Anil S, Jansen JA, van den Beucken JJ. Combined treatment effects using bioactive-coated implants and ceramic granulate in a rabbit femoral condyle model. Clin Implant Dent Relat Res 2015.
[19] Alsayed A, Anil S, Jansen JA, van den Beucken JJ. Comparative evaluation of the combined application of titanium implants and calcium phosphate bone substitutes in a rabbit model. Clin Oral Implants Res 2015;26:1215–21.
[20] Lee SW, Hahn BD, Kang TY, Lee MJ, Choi JY, Kim MK, et al. Hydroxyapatite and collagen combination-coated dental implants display better bone formation in the peri-implant area than the same combination plus bone morphogenetic protein-2-coated implants, hydroxyapatite only coated implants, and uncoated implants. J Oral Maxillofac Surg 2014;72:53–60.

[21] Biesbrock AR, Edgerton M. Evaluation of the clinical predictability of hydroxyapatite-coated endosseous dental implants: a review of the literature. Int J Oral Maxillofac Implants 1995;10:712−20.

[22] McGlumphy EA, Peterson LJ, Larsen PE, Jeffcoat MK. Prospective study of 429 hydroxyapatite-coated cylindric omniloc implants placed in 121 patients. Int J oral Maxillofac Implants 2002;18:82−92.

[23] Mohseni E, Zalnezhad E, Bushroa A. Comparative investigation on the adhesion of hydroxyapatite coating on Ti−6Al 4V implant: a review paper. Int J Adhesion Adhesives 2014;48:238−57.

[24] Ogiso M, Yamashita Y, Matsumoto T. Microstructural changes in bone of HA-coated implants. J Biomed Mater Res 1998;39:23−31.

[25] Urquia Edreira ER, Wolke JG, Aldosari AA, Al-Johany SS, Anil S, Jansen JA, et al. Effects of calcium phosphate composition in sputter coatings on in vitro and in vivo performance. J Biomed Mater Res Part A 2015;103:300−10.

[26] Xuereb M, Camilleri J, Attard NJ. Systematic review of current dental implant coating materials and novel coating techniques. Int J Prosthodont 2015;28:51−9.

[27] Ong JL, Chan DC. Hydroxyapatite and their use as coatings in dental implants: a review. Crit Rev Biomed Eng 2000;28:667−707.

[28] Elias CN, Oshida Y, Lima JH, Muller CA. Relationship between surface properties (roughness, wettability and morphology) of titanium and dental implant removal torque. J Mech Behav Biomed Mater 2008;1:234−42.

[29] AlFarraj Aldosari A, Anil S, Alasqah M, Al Wazzan KA, Al Jetaily SA, Jansen JA. The influence of implant geometry and surface composition on bone response. Clin Oral Implants Res 2014;25:500−5.

[30] van Oirschot BA, Alghamdi HS, Narhi TO, Anil S, Al Farraj Aldosari A, van den Beucken JJ, et al. In vivo evaluation of bioactive glass-based coatings on dental implants in a dog implantation model. Clin Oral Implants Res 2014;25:21−8.

[31] Kilpadi KL, Chang PL, Bellis SL. Hydroxylapatite binds more serum proteins, purified integrins, and osteoblast precursor cells than titanium or steel. J Biomed Mater Res 2001; 57:258−67.

[32] Narayanan R, Seshadri SK, Kwon TY, Kim KH. Calcium phosphate-based coatings on titanium and its alloys. J Biomed Mater Res Part B, Appl Biomater 2008;85:279−99.

[33] Kirsch A. Plasma-sprayed titanium-I.M.Z. implant. J Oral Implantol 1986;12:494−7.

[34] Clark PA, Rodriguez A, Sumner DR, Hussain MA, Mao JJ. Modulation of bone ingrowth of rabbit femur titanium implants by in vivo axial micromechanical loading. J Appl Physiol 2005;98:1922−9.

[35] Hwang JW, Lee EU, Lee JS, Jung UW, Lee IS, Choi SH. Dissolution behavior and early bone apposition of calcium phosphate-coated machined implants. J Periodontal & Implant Sci 2013;43:291−300.

[36] de Groot K, Geesink R, Klein CP, Serekian P. Plasma sprayed coatings of hydroxylapatite. J Biomed Mater Res 1987;21:1375−81.

[37] Ji H, Marquis PM. Effect of heat treatment on the microstructure of plasma-sprayed hydroxyapatite coating. Biomaterials 1993;14:64−8.

[38] Hulshoff JE, Hayakawa T, van Dijk K, Leijdekkers-Govers AF, van der Waerden JP, Jansen JA. Mechanical and histologic evaluation of Ca-P plasma-spray and magnetron sputter-coated implants in trabecular bone of the goat. J Biomed Mater Res 1997;36:75−83.

[39] Yeung WK, Reilly GC, Matthews A, Yerokhin A. In vitro biological response of plasma electrolytically oxidized and plasma-sprayed hydroxyapatite coatings on Ti-6Al-4V alloy. J Biomed Mater Res Part B, Appl Biomater 2013;101:939−49.

[40] Bolelli G, Bellucci D, Cannillo V, Lusvarghi L, Sola A, Stiegler N, et al. Suspension thermal spraying of hydroxyapatite: microstructure and in vitro behaviour. Mater Sci Eng C 2014;34:287–303. Materials for biological applications.
[41] Hsiung J, Tzeng J, Kung K, Chen H. A study of thermal spray coating on artificial knee joints. Life Sci J 2013;10:236–41.
[42] Vidigal Jr GM, Aragones LC, Campos Jr A, Groisman M. Histomorphometric analyses of hydroxyapatite-coated and uncoated titanium dental implants in rabbit cortical bone. Implant Dent 1999;8:295–302.
[43] Wang C, Ma J, Cheng W, Zhang R. Thick hydroxyapatite coatings by electrophoretic deposition. Mater Lett 2002;57:99–105.
[44] Milev A, Kannangara G, Ben-Nissan B. Morphological stability of hydroxyapatite precursor. Mater Lett 2003;57:1960–5.
[45] Gil-Albarova J, Garrido-Lahiguera R, Salinas AJ, Roman J, Bueno-Lozano AL, Gil-Albarova R, et al. The in vivo performance of a sol-gel glass and a glass-ceramic in the treatment of limited bone defects. Biomaterials 2004;25:4639–45.
[46] Jansen JA, Wolke JG, Swann S, Van der Waerden JP, de Groot K. Application of magnetron sputtering for producing ceramic coatings on implant materials. Clin Oral Implants Res 1993;4:28–34.
[47] Wolke JG, van Dijk K, Schaeken HG, de Groot K, Jansen JA. Study of the surface characteristics of magnetron-sputter calcium phosphate coatings. J Biomed Mater Res 1994;28:1477–84.
[48] Vercaigne S, Wolke JG, Naert I, Jansen JA. A histological evaluation of TiO_2-gritblasted and Ca-P magnetron sputter coated implants placed into the trabecular bone of the goat: Part 2. Clin Oral Implants Res 2000;11:314–24.
[49] Vercaigne S, Wolke JG, Naert I, Jansen JA. A mechanical evaluation of TiO_2-gritblasted and Ca-P magnetron sputter coated implants placed into the trabecular bone of the goat: Part 1. Clin Oral Implants Res 2000;11:305–13.
[50] Ong JL, Bessho K, Cavin R, Carnes DL. Bone response to radio frequency sputtered calcium phosphate implants and titanium implants in vivo. J Biomed Mater Res 2002;59: 184–90.
[51] Garcia-Sanz FJ, Mayor MB, Arias JL, Pou J, Leon B, Perez-Amor M. Hydroxyapatite coatings: a comparative study between plasma-spray and pulsed laser deposition techniques. J Mater Sci Mater Med 1997;8:861–5.
[52] Rajesh P, Muraleedharan CV, Komath M, Varma H. Pulsed laser deposition of hydroxyapatite on titanium substrate with titania interlayer. J Mater Sci Mater Med 2011;22: 497–505.
[53] Gaggl A, Schultes G, Muller WD, Karcher H. Scanning electron microscopical analysis of laser-treated titanium implant surfaces—a comparative study. Biomaterials 2000;21: 1067–73.
[54] Hallgren C, Reimers H, Chakarov D, Gold J, Wennerberg A. An in vivo study of bone response to implants topographically modified by laser micromachining. Biomaterials 2003;24:701–10.
[55] Frenkel SR, Simon J, Alexander H, Dennis M, Ricci JL. Osseointegration on metallic implant surfaces: effects of microgeometry and growth factor treatment. J Biomed Mater Res 2002;63:706–13.
[56] Li T, Lee J, Kobayashi T, Aoki H. Hydroxyapatite coating by dipping method, and bone bonding strength. J Mater Sci Mater Med 1996;7:355–7.
[57] Mavis B, Taş AC. Dip coating of calcium hydroxyapatite on Ti-6Al-4V substrates. J Am Ceram Soc 2000;83:989–91.

[58] Choi JM, Kim HE, Lee IS. Ion-beam-assisted deposition (IBAD) of hydroxyapatite coating layer on Ti-based metal substrate. Biomaterials 2000;21:469–73.

[59] Liu JQ, Luo ZS, Cui FZ, Duan XF, Peng LM. High-resolution transmission electron microscopy investigations of a highly adhesive hydroxyapatite coating/titanium interface fabricated by ion-beam-assisted deposition. J Biomed Mater Res 2000;52: 115–8.

[60] Le IS, Kim DH, Kim HE, Jung YC, Han CH. Biological performance of calcium phosphate films formed on commercially pure Ti by electron-beam evaporation. Biomaterials 2002;23:609–15.

[61] Um Y-J, Song J-E, Chae G-J, Jung U-W, Chung S-M, Lee I-S, et al. The effect of post heat treatment of hydroxyapatite-coated implants on the healing of circumferential coronal defects in dogs. Thin Solid Films 2009;517:5375–9.

[62] Ma J, Liang CH, Kong LB, Wang C. Colloidal characterization and electrophoretic deposition of hydroxyapatite on titanium substrate. J Mater Sci Mater Med 2003;14: 797–801.

[63] Soares G, de Sena LÁ, Rossi AM, Pinto M, Muller CA, de Almeida Soares GD. Effect of electrophoretic apatite coating on osseointegration of titanium dental implants. In: Key engineering materials: trans tech publ; 2004. p. 729–32.

[64] Zhang Z, Dunn MF, Xiao T, Tomsia AP, Saiz E. Nanostructured hydroxyapatite coatings for improved adhesion and corrosion resistance for medical implants. In: Materials research society symposium proceedings. Cambridge Univ Press; 2002. p. 291–6.

[65] Hero H, Wie H, Jorgensen RB, Ruyter IE. Hydroxyapatite coatings on Ti produced by hot isostatic pressing. J Biomed Mater Res 1994;28:343–8.

[66] Lindgren M, Astrand M, Wiklund U, Engqvist H. Investigation of boundary conditions for biomimetic HA deposition on titanium oxide surfaces. J Mater Sci Mater Med 2009; 20:1401–8.

[67] Yang L, Perez-Amodio S, Barrere-de Groot FY, Everts V, van Blitterswijk CA, Habibovic P. The effects of inorganic additives to calcium phosphate on in vitro behavior of osteoblasts and osteoclasts. Biomaterials 2010;31:2976–89.

[68] Cooper LF, Deporter D, Wennerberg A, Hammerle C. What physical and/or biochemical characteristics of roughened endosseous implant surfaces particularly enhance their bone-implant contact capability? Int J Oral Maxillofac Implants 2005;20:307–12.

[69] Schenk RK, Buser D. Osseointegration: a reality. Periodontology 1998;2000(17):22–35.

[70] Kim TI, Jang JH, Kim HW, Knowles JC, Ku Y. Biomimetic approach to dental implants. Curr Pharm Des 2008;14:2201–11.

[71] Yu X, Wang L, Jiang X, Rowe D, Wei M. Biomimetic CaP coating incorporated with parathyroid hormone improves the osseointegration of titanium implant. J Mater Sci Mater Med 2012;23:2177–86.

[72] Barrere F, van der Valk CM, Meijer G, Dalmeijer RA, de Groot K, Layrolle P. Osteointegration of biomimetic apatite coating applied onto dense and porous metal implants in femurs of goats. J Biomed Mater Res Part B, Appl Biomater 2003;67: 655–65.

[73] Tsukeoka T, Suzuki M, Ohtsuki C, Tsuneizumi Y, Miyagi J, Sugino A, et al. Enhanced fixation of implants by bone ingrowth to titanium fiber mesh: effect of incorporation of hydroxyapatite powder. J Biomed Mater Res Part B, Appl Biomater 2005;75: 168–76.

[74] Daculsi G, LeGeros RZ, Deudon C. Scanning and transmission electron microscopy, and electron probe analysis of the interface between implants and host bone. Osseo-coalescence versus osseo-integration. Scanning Microsc 1990;4:309–14.

[75] Roy M, Bandyopadhyay A, Bose S. Induction plasma sprayed nano hydroxyapatite coatings on titanium for orthopaedic and dental implants. Surf Coatings Technol 2011; 205:2785−92.
[76] Yu X, Wei M. Cellular performance comparison of biomimetic calcium phosphate coating and alkaline-treated titanium surface. Biomed Res Int 2013;2013:832790.
[77] Soballe K. Hydroxyapatite ceramic coating for bone implant fixation. Mechanical and histological studies in dogs. Acta Orthop Scand Suppl 1993;255:1−58.
[78] Cook SD, Thomas KA, Dalton JE, Volkman TK, Whitecloud 3rd TS, Kay JF. Hydroxylapatite coating of porous implants improves bone ingrowth and interface attachment strength. J Biomed Mater Res 1992;26:989−1001.
[79] Biemond JE, Eufrasio TS, Hannink G, Verdonschot N, Buma P. Assessment of bone ingrowth potential of biomimetic hydroxyapatite and brushite coated porous E-beam structures. J Mater Sci-Mater Med 2011;22:917−25.
[80] Liu Y, Wu G, de Groot K. Biomimetic coatings for bone tissue engineering of critical-sized defects. J R Soc Interface/R Soc 2010;7(Suppl. 5):S631−47.
[81] Tejero R, Anitua E, Orive G. Toward the biomimetic implant surface: biopolymers on titanium-based implants for bone regeneration. Prog Polym Sci 2014;39:1406−47.
[82] Dvorak MM, Siddiqua A, Ward DT, Carter DH, Dallas SL, Nemeth EF, et al. Physiological changes in extracellular calcium concentration directly control osteoblast function in the absence of calciotropic hormones. Proc Natl Acad Sci USA 2004;101: 5140−5.
[83] Gruber R, Karreth F, Kandler B, Fuerst G, Rot A, Fischer MB, et al. Platelet-released supernatants increase migration and proliferation, and decrease osteogenic differentiation of bone marrow-derived mesenchymal progenitor cells under in vitro conditions. Platelets 2004;15:29−35.
[84] Puleo DA, Nanci A. Understanding and controlling the bone-implant interface. Biomaterials 1999;20:2311−21.
[85] Tejero R, Rossbach P, Keller B, Anitua E, Reviakine I. Time-of-flight secondary ion mass spectrometry with principal component analysis of titania-blood plasma interfaces. Langmuir ACS J Surf Colloids 2013;29:902−12.
[86] Wennerberg A, Albrektsson T. On implant surfaces: a review of current knowledge and opinions. Int J Oral Maxillofac Implants 2010;25:63−74.
[87] Le Guehennec L, Soueidan A, Layrolle P, Amouriq Y. Surface treatments of titanium dental implants for rapid osseointegration. Dent Mater Off Publ Acad Dent Mater 2007; 23:844−54.
[88] Mendonca G, Mendonca DB, Aragao FJ, Cooper LF. Advancing dental implant surface technology−from micron- to nanotopography. Biomaterials 2008;29:3822−35.
[89] Brett PM, Harle J, Salih V, Mihoc R, Olsen I, Jones FH, et al. Roughness response genes in osteoblasts. Bone 2004;35:124−33.
[90] Nakamura S, Matsumoto T, Sasaki J, Egusa H, Lee KY, Nakano T, et al. Effect of calcium ion concentrations on osteogenic differentiation and hematopoietic stem cell niche-related protein expression in osteoblasts. Tissue Eng Part A 2010;16:2467−73.
[91] Schopper C, Moser D, Goriwoda W, Ziya-Ghazvini F, Spassova E, Lagogiannis G, et al. The effect of three different calcium phosphate implant coatings on bone deposition and coating resorption: a long-term histological study in sheep. Clin Oral Implants Res 2005; 16:357−68.
[92] Matsushita N, Terai H, Okada T, Nozaki K, Inoue H, Miyamoto S, et al. A new bone-inducing biodegradable porous beta-tricalcium phosphate. J Biomed Mater Res Part A 2004;70:450−8.

[93] Li Y, Weng W, Tam KC. Novel highly biodegradable biphasic tricalcium phosphates composed of alpha-tricalcium phosphate and beta-tricalcium phosphate. Acta Biomater 2007;3:251−4.

[94] Arinzeh TL, Tran T, McAlary J, Daculsi G. A comparative study of biphasic calcium phosphate ceramics for human mesenchymal stem-cell-induced bone formation. Biomaterials 2005;26:3631−8.

[95] Vogler EA. Protein adsorption in three dimensions. Biomaterials 2012;33:1201−37.

[96] Koh JW, Kim YS, Yang JH, Yeo IS. Effects of a calcium phosphate-coated and anodized titanium surface on early bone response. Int J Oral Maxillofac Implants 2013;28:790−7.

[97] Buser D, Schenk RK, Steinemann S, Fiorellini JP, Fox CH, Stich H. Influence of surface characteristics on bone integration of titanium implants. A histomorphometric study in miniature pigs. J Biomed Mater Res 1991;25:889−902.

[98] Rupp F, Scheideler L, Olshanska N, de Wild M, Wieland M, Geis-Gerstorfer J. Enhancing surface free energy and hydrophilicity through chemical modification of microstructured titanium implant surfaces. J Biomed Mater Res Part A 2006;76:323−34.

[99] Zhao G, Schwartz Z, Wieland M, Rupp F, Geis-Gerstorfer J, Cochran DL, et al. High surface energy enhances cell response to titanium substrate microstructure. J Biomed Mater Res Part A 2005;74:49−58.

[100] Sun L, Berndt CC, Gross KA, Kucuk A. Material fundamentals and clinical performance of plasma-sprayed hydroxyapatite coatings: a review. J Biomed Mater Res 2001;58:570−92.

[101] Bose S, Tarafder S. Calcium phosphate ceramic systems in growth factor and drug delivery for bone tissue engineering: a review. Acta Biomater 2012;8:1401−21.

[102] Liao H, Fartash B, Li J. Stability of hydroxyapatite-coatings on titanium oral implants (IMZ). 2 retrieved cases. Clin Oral Implants Res 1997;8:68−72.

[103] Zeng H, Chittur KK, Lacefield WR. Dissolution/reprecipitation of calcium phosphate thin films produced by ion beam sputter deposition technique. Biomaterials 1999;20:443−51.

[104] Gross KA, Ray N, Rokkum M. The contribution of coating microstructure to degradation and particle release in hydroxyapatite coated prostheses. J Biomed Mater Res 2002;63:106−14.

[105] Wolke JG, van der Waerden JP, Schaeken HG, Jansen JA. In vivo dissolution behavior of various RF magnetron-sputtered Ca-P coatings on roughened titanium implants. Biomaterials 2003;24:2623−9.

[106] Overgaard S, Soballe K, Lind M, Bunger C. Resorption of hydroxyapatite and fluorapatite coatings in man. An experimental study in trabecular bone. J Bone Joint Surg Br 1997;79:654−9.

[107] Jinno T, Davy DT, Goldberg VM. Comparison of hydroxyapatite and hydroxyapatite tricalcium-phosphate coatings. J Arthroplasty 2002;17:902−9.

[108] Morra M, Cassinelli C, Cascardo G, Cahalan P, Cahalan L, Fini M, et al. Surface engineering of titanium by collagen immobilization. Surface characterization and in vitro and in vivo studies. Biomaterials 2003;24:4639−54.

[109] de Jonge LT, Leeuwenburgh SC, van den Beucken JJ, te Riet J, Daamen WF, Wolke JG, et al. The osteogenic effect of electrosprayed nanoscale collagen/calcium phosphate coatings on titanium. Biomaterials 2010;31:2461−9.

[110] Liu Y, Hunziker EB, Layrolle P, De Bruijn JD, De Groot K. Bone morphogenetic protein 2 incorporated into biomimetic coatings retains its biological activity. Tissue Eng 2004;10:101−8.

[111] Fischer U, Hempel U, Becker D, Bierbaum S, Scharnweber D, Worch H, et al. Transforming growth factor beta1 immobilized adsorptively on Ti6Al4V and collagen type I coated Ti6Al4V maintains its biological activity. Biomaterials 2003;24:2631−41.

[112] Uludag H, Gao T, Porter TJ, Friess W, Wozney JM. Delivery systems for BMPs: factors contributing to protein retention at an application site. J Bone Joint Surg Am 2001; 83-A(Suppl. 1):S128–35.
[113] Hing KA, Revell PA, Smith N, Buckland T. Effect of silicon level on rate, quality and progression of bone healing within silicate-substituted porous hydroxyapatite scaffolds. Biomaterials 2006;27:5014–26.
[114] Pietak AM, Reid JW, Stott MJ, Sayer M. Silicon substitution in the calcium phosphate bioceramics. Biomaterials 2007;28:4023–32.
[115] Nair MB, Varma H, Shenoy SJ, John A. Treatment of goat femur segmental defects with silica-coated hydroxyapatite–one-year follow-up. Tissue Eng Part A 2010;16:385–91.
[116] Palangadan R, Sukumaran A, Fernandez FB, John A, Varma H. Pulsed laser deposition and in vitro characteristics of triphasic—HASi composition on titanium. J Biomater Appl 2014;28:849–58.
[117] Panzavolta S, Torricelli P, Sturba L, Bracci B, Giardino R, Bigi A. Setting properties and in vitro bioactivity of strontium-enriched gelatin-calcium phosphate bone cements. J Biomed Mater Res Part A 2008;84:965–72.
[118] Peng S, Liu XS, Wang T, Li Z, Zhou G, Luk KD, et al. In vivo anabolic effect of strontium on trabecular bone was associated with increased osteoblastogenesis of bone marrow stromal cells. J Orthop Res Off Publ Orthop Res Soc 2010;28:1208–14.
[119] Capuccini C, Torricelli P, Sima F, Boanini E, Ristoscu C, Bracci B, et al. Strontium-substituted hydroxyapatite coatings synthesized by pulsed-laser deposition: in vitro osteoblast and osteoclast response. Acta Biomater 2008;4:1885–93.
[120] Li ZY, Lam WM, Yang C, Xu B, Ni GX, Abbah SA, et al. Chemical composition, crystal size and lattice structural changes after incorporation of strontium into biomimetic apatite. Biomaterials 2007;28:1452–60.
[121] Xia W, Lindahl C, Lausmaa J, Borchardt P, Ballo A, Thomsen P, et al. Biomineralized strontium-substituted apatite/titanium dioxide coating on titanium surfaces. Acta Biomater 2010;6:1591–600.
[122] Tat SK, Pelletier JP, Mineau F, Caron J, Martel-Pelletier J. Strontium ranelate inhibits key factors affecting bone remodeling in human osteoarthritic subchondral bone osteoblasts. Bone 2011;49:559–67.
[123] Tian M, Chen F, Song W, Song Y, Chen Y, Wan C, et al. In vivo study of porous strontium-doped calcium polyphosphate scaffolds for bone substitute applications. J Mater Sci Mater Med 2009;20:1505–12.
[124] Baier M, Staudt P, Klein R, Sommer U, Wenz R, Grafe I, et al. Strontium enhances osseointegration of calcium phosphate cement: a histomorphometric pilot study in ovariectomized rats. J Orthop Surg Res 2013;8:16.
[125] Simchi A, Tamjid E, Pishbin F, Boccaccini AR. Recent progress in inorganic and composite coatings with bactericidal capability for orthopaedic applications. Nanomed Nanotechnol Biol Med 2011;7:22–39.
[126] Yeo IS, Kim HY, Lim KS, Han JS. Implant surface factors and bacterial adhesion: a review of the literature. Int J Artif Organs 2012;35:762–72.
[127] Ewald A, Hosel D, Patel S, Grover LM, Barralet JE, Gbureck U. Silver-doped calcium phosphate cements with antimicrobial activity. Acta Biomater 2011;7:4064–70.
[128] Li K, Xie Y, Ao H, Huang L, Ji H, Zheng X. The enhanced bactericidal effect of plasma sprayed zinc-modified calcium silicate coating by the addition of silver. Ceram Int 2013; 39:7895–902.
[129] Chen Y, Zheng X, Xie Y, Ding C, Ruan H, Fan C. Anti-bacterial and cytotoxic properties of plasma sprayed silver-containing HA coatings. J Mater Sci Mater Med 2008;19:3603–9.

[130] Surmenev RA. A review of plasma-assisted methods for calcium phosphate-based coatings fabrication. Surf Coatings Technol 2012;206:2035–56.
[131] Drake MT, Clarke BL, Khosla S. Bisphosphonates: mechanism of action and role in clinical practice. Mayo Clin Proc Mayo Clin 2008;83:1032–45.
[132] Guimaraes MB, Bueno RS, Blaya MB, Shinkai RS, Marques LM. Influence of the local application of sodium alendronate gel on osseointegration of titanium implants. Int J Oral Maxillofac Surg 2015;44:1423–9.
[133] Suratwala SJ, Cho SK, van Raalte JJ, Park SH, Seo SW, Chang SS, et al. Enhancement of periprosthetic bone quality with topical hydroxyapatite-bisphosphonate composite. J Bone Joint Surg Am 2008;90:2189–96.
[134] Schindeler A, Little DG. Bisphosphonate action: revelations and deceptions from in vitro studies. J Pharm Sci 2007;96:1872–8.
[135] Wen HB, de Wijn JR, van Blitterswijk CA, de Groot K. Incorporation of bovine serum albumin in calcium phosphate coating on titanium. J Biomed Mater Res 1999;46: 245–52.
[136] Yu X, Qu H, Knecht DA, Wei M. Incorporation of bovine serum albumin into biomimetic coatings on titanium with high loading efficacy and its release behavior. J Mater Sci Mater Med 2009;20:287–94.
[137] Norowski Jr PA, Bumgardner JD. Biomaterial and antibiotic strategies for peri-implantitis: a review. J Biomed Mater Res Part B, Appl Biomater 2009;88:530–43.
[138] Quirynen M, Bollen CM. The influence of surface roughness and surface-free energy on supra- and subgingival plaque formation in man. A review of the literature. J Clin Periodontol 1995;22:1–14.
[139] Madi M, Zakaria O, Noritake K, Fuji M, Kasugai S. Peri-implantitis progression around thin sputtered hydroxyapatite-coated implants: clinical and radiographic evaluation in dogs. Int J Oral Maxillofac Implants 2013;28:701–9.
[140] Piattelli A, Cosci F, Scarano A, Trisi P. Localized chronic suppurative bone infection as a sequel of peri-implantitis in a hydroxyapatite-coated dental implant. Biomaterials 1995; 16:917–20.

Peri-implant biological behavior: clinical and scientific aspects

5

J.E. Maté Sánchez de Val, J.L. Calvo-Guirado, S. Gehrke
Universidad Católica San Antonio (UCAM), Murcia, Spain

5.1 Introduction

The scientific basis of the current implantology was established by Per-Ingvar Brånemark [1,2], who used a titanium chamber to study the blood flow of the rabbit bone, discovering the high biocompatibility of titanium and its capability to be surrounded by the mineralized bone. He used the term "osseointegration," which has remained permanently in the medical language. Osseointegration means living bone tissue attached to the surface of the implant under masticatory loads. This relationship between an artificial device and a living tissue has revolutionized the dental field and is also used today for cranial and maxillofacial reconstruction. Brånemark studies [1,2] formed the basis for the development of an operating protocol for the osseointegration [3].

The bone tissue is subjected to constant evolution, in a continuous process of maturation; this process begins at 6 weeks of embryonic development and continues throughout life. This process of continuous remodeling happens also around implants.

The bonds between implant surfaces and peri-implant bone are physical and chemical. Brånemark [2] found that physical forces, including Van der Waals forces and hydrogen bonds, are involved. On the other hand, covalent and ionic bonds, both chemical in nature, are responsible for the high values of the bond strength. When the titanium surface is exposed to blood, as occurs during surgery, there is a spontaneous formation of calcium and phosphate on the surface. This fact shows a reactivity of the titanium surface with water, mineral ions, and plasma fluids, and in parallel, the low pH of the implant bed accelerates the formation of calcium phosphates on the surface. The oxide surface of the implant is a system of dynamic nature, which plays an important role in the process of bone remodeling [4–6].

The placement of an implant involves the preparation of a bed in the bone, and therefore trauma to the bone. The bone tissue will respond to the trauma by inflammation, repair, and remodeling [7–9]. Osteoblasts will then start producing osteoid matrix that will undergo mineralization [10]. In the first 4 weeks postoperatively, the osteogenic response is massive, reaching a peak in the first 15–20 days. Bone formation continues for another 4–6 weeks, while, simultaneously, initial remodeling processes lead to a gradual adaptation of the newly formed bone. In the eighth postoperative week, the osteogenic activity is drastically reduced, whereas the remodeling activity and morphostructural adaptation of the newly formed bone tissue, reach its highest expression [11]. Simultaneously, there is an increase in the newly formed

Bone Response to Dental Implant Materials. http://dx.doi.org/10.1016/B978-0-08-100287-2.00005-7

bone, which can cover more than 50% of the surface of the implant [12]. It has been experimentally shown that the percentage of bone, directly in contact with the implant surface, reaches an adequate amount only after 3 months; this amount will increase progressively over the next 6–9 months.

5.2 Implant features

5.2.1 Surface

Titanium is considered to be the most appropriate material for the manufacture of dental implants. The response after implant placement is directly influenced by the surface. The rate of bone-to-implant contact (BIC) depends on specific characteristics, such as ionic composition of the metal alloy, topography, roughness, and energy on the implant surface. The chemical composition and topography of titanium implant surfaces play an important role in the rates and extent of osseointegration and in the movement of bone cells toward the modified surface [13].

To improve the BIC values, many new surfaces have been developed over the years. In general, the surface roughness can be divided into three levels: macro-, micro-, and nanoroughness. The macrolevel is believed to be in the range of millimeters to tens of micrometers, and it is directly related to implant geometry (e.g., implants thread design). The microlevel on the other hand, includes surface roughness in the range of 1–10 μm [14]. The nanoroughness is in the nanometer range.

The rough surfaces can be produced by several modification techniques, including either additive or subtractive processes. Additive processes include titanium plasma-sprayed surfaces, hydroxyapatite and other calcium phosphate coatings, ion deposition, and oxidation. On the other hand, electropolishing, mechanical polishing, blasting, etching, and laser microtexturing are considered subtractive processes. Moreover, implant surfaces modification can be obtained by the means of chemical or physical processes.

1. Chemical processes
    a. Ion beam implantation
    b. Silanization
    c. Self-supported monolayer
    d. Microcontact impression
    e. Layers
    f. Etching with different acids or alkalis
2. Physical processes
    a. Sandblasting
    b. Electric beam
    c. Photolitography
    d. Ion beam
    e. Mechanical machining
    f. Electric arc
    g. Laser microetching or microstructuring.

It has been shown that rough implant surfaces have superior properties over the previously used machined surfaces. In addition, both animal studies and human trials have assessed and compared these different surfaces and showed improved and favorable clinical outcomes.

Microrough surfaces also stimulate osteoblast differentiation and were suggested to enhance peri-implant wound healing by the upregulation of genes correlated with regeneration, mesenchymal cell differentiation, and angiogenesis.

Although, currently, the optimum implant surface characteristic cannot be defined, advances in microdesign and surface modifications have improved osseointegration. This, in turn, might maximize the success rates of dental implants and reduce their complications.

5.3 Implant anatomy

5.3.1 Implant neck design

The anatomy and surface treatment of the neck of the implant, together with the type of connection between the implant and the prosthetic components, have been considered as viable alternatives to reduce the crestal bone loss [15] (Fig. 5.1). Regarding the surface treatment of the implant–abutment interface, it remains unclear whether it could influence the peri-implant bone reaction.

Histological investigations show that loading does not affect osteoclast activation in peri-implant–bone [16]. Thus, changes in peri-implant–bone levels during function appear to be unrelated to whether the initial soft and hard tissue healing following implant placement occurred under submerged or nonsubmerged conditions.

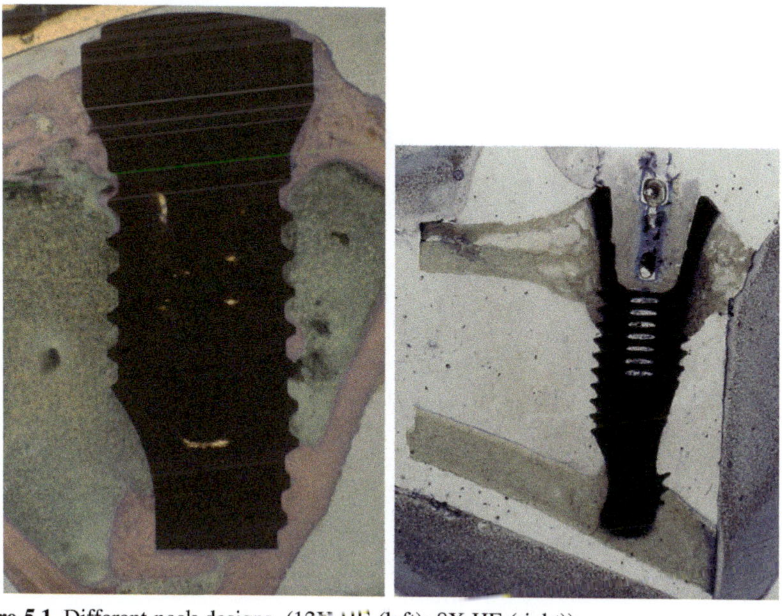

Figure 5.1 Different neck designs. (12X HE (left); 8X HE (right)).

Focusing on implant micro- and macrostructure effects on marginal bone levels, different aspects have been discussed in the literature. Crestal bone changes occur during the early phase of healing after implant placement and loading [17].

Experimental and clinical studies have demonstrated that implants designed with a shorter, smooth coronal collar caused no additional bone loss and might help reduce the risk of an exposed metal implant margin in areas of esthetic concern [18–20]. On the other hand, Shin et al. [21] concluded that a rough surface with microthreads at the implant neck was the most effective design for minimizing marginal bone loss during functional loading.

It has been demonstrated that following implant surgery, remodeling occurs and is characterized by a reduction in bone dimension, both horizontally and vertically [22]. The radiographic marginal bone level showed a mean loss of 0.9 mm at the time of abutment connection and crown placement and a further mean loss of 0.7 mm at 1 year. Similar results were reported in a retrospective study, which showed a range of resorption of 2–3 mm after 1 year depending on arch, jaw region, smoking status, case type, bone quality, surface type, and implant design [23].

It has been suggested that this biological process resulting in the loss of crestal bone height may be altered when the outer edge of the implant–abutment interface is horizontally repositioned inwardly and away from the outer edge of the implant platform. This prosthetic concept has been introduced as "platform switching" and radiographic follow-up has demonstrated a smaller than expected vertical change in the crestal bone height around implants [24].

Furthermore, it is generally accepted that the mechanical status of the bone–implant interface is an important determinant for the establishment and maintenance of the bone–implant interface. As far as implant shape is concerned, design parameters that primarily affect load transfer characteristics include implant diameter and length, as well as thread pitch shape and depth. Bone-retention elements such as microthreads and a rough surface at the implant neck help to stabilize the marginal bone through an interlocking of the implant surface and the crestal bone. Such an implant–bone interlocking inhibits detrimental micromotion and shear forces at the interface and allows an efficient force transfer to the surrounding tissues [25–31].

There is evidence from both experimental and clinical studies that relatively smooth, machined titanium surfaces are associated with additional crestal bone loss [32–34]. Hanggi et al. [20] performed a radiographic evaluation. They observed that there is no additional crestal bone loss when placing implants with their rough/smooth implant border at the bone crest level exhibiting a shorter (1.8 mm) as opposed to a slightly larger (2.8 mm) machined coronal portion over a period of 3 years after implant placement. However, the results of animal studies showed a more pronounced crestal bone resorption in the implants with a polished collar of 1.5 mm in height when compared with the implants with a polished collar of 0.7 mm. These results may be of importance in areas of esthetic concern based upon the principle of the biological width, eventually reducing the risk of an exposed metal implant shoulder.

Nickenig et al. [35] performed a radiographic evaluation of the marginal bone levels adjacent to implants that had either machined-neck or rough-surfaced microthreaded configurations and showed that the microthreaded design was superior in minimizing marginal bone loss during stress-free healing and under functional loading. It was concluded that the use of rough-surfaced microthreaded implants could maintain crestal bone levels.

Finally, related to the microsurface of the implants, in the last few years, there has been a trend to increase the BIC and the stability of the implants through the treatment of the surface with different techniques to create microretentions that can influence the peri-implant bone behavior. Neck microgrooves have demonstrated to be effective to get an increase of the BIC at the contact area, an increase of the bone density, a reduced crestal bone resorption, a better connective tissue attachment, and an increased stability of the implant.

5.3.2 Middle threads configuration

There are different configurations of the middle of the implant, with different anatomy and direction of the threads and different thread pitch and distance from the implant body to the end of the thread (Fig. 5.2).

Similarly, the anatomy of the threads will produce different effects on bone on the compression exerted on it at the time of insertion and the effective contact surface that exists with the peri-implant tissue. It has been shown that different thread configurations will produce different actions. "V" threads and large squares are the most recommended, whereas narrow threads should be avoided.

Similarly, the anatomy of the intermediate threads will have a direct effect on the distribution of forces to the peri-implant bone. When primary stability is a concern, as in cancellous bone, increasing the implant surface area using implants with smaller pitch might be beneficial.

5.3.3 Apex

Finally, apical anatomy influences directly the peri-implant bone response from a point of view that has more to do with biomechanics and compression. Noncutting implants blunt apex will produce higher compression and higher secondary remodeling; whereas tapping implants with sharp apices get less compression.

5.4 BIC percentage

A lot of research in the field of implant dentistry is concerned with the evaluation of the BIC percentage because BIC is the most important factor contributing to implant stability. Numerous authors have specified the factors influencing BIC levels, in particular: original bone density, functional force values exerted on implants, implant materials and shape, surface roughness, implant length and width [36–40] (Fig. 5.3). However, to date no study has responded to the question of what could be the best method for evaluating BIC and no studies have set out to assess the reliability of the various methods of evaluating BIC currently in use. It is a well-known fact that calcium

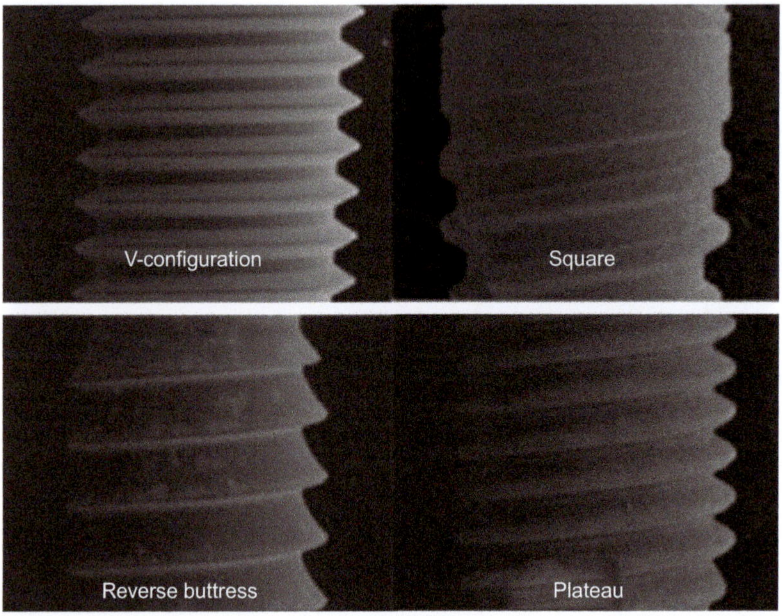

Figure 5.2 Different thread configurations. (SEM 200X).

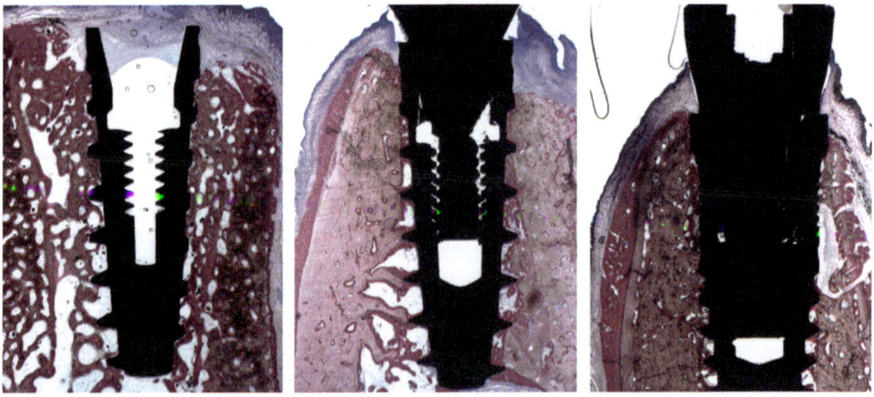

Figure 5.3 BIC evaluated in different bone quality sites. (8X acid fuchsin and toluidine blue (left); 10X acid fuchsin and toluidine blue (centre); 12X acid fuchsin and toluidine blue (right)).

levels are a good indicator of bone quality, so elemental analysis is a good way of assessing the quality of newly formed bone [41,42]. Although there may be good BIC levels, if the newly formed bone is of low quality with a low calcium content, implant retention will be less than expected and long-term stability may be compromised [43]. Studies involving elemental analysis used for this purpose are few; indeed,

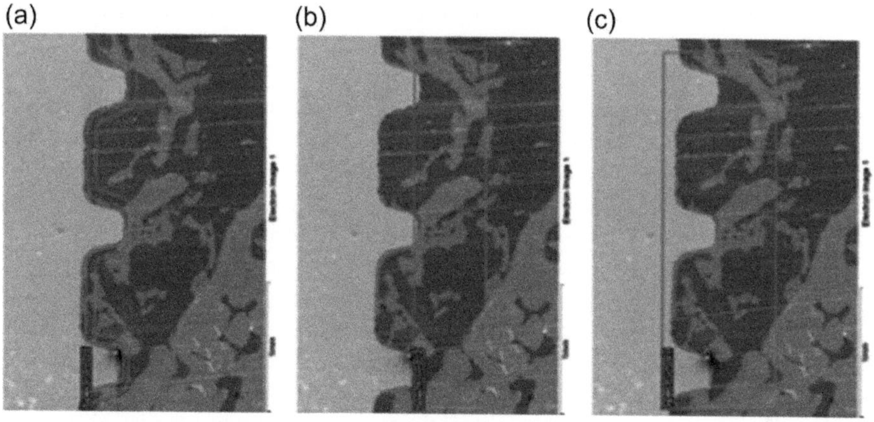

Figure 5.4 Different types of BIC measurements. (SEM 300X).

our review of studies involving BIC evaluation has identified only one that includes elemental analysis.

There are three different ways of measuring BIC. The first consists of measuring the quantity of mineralized bone in direct contact with the implant's titanium surface across the entire threaded area. This we call BIC I (Fig. 5.4a). It measures new bone around the implant threads but does not measure the new bone that joins this to old

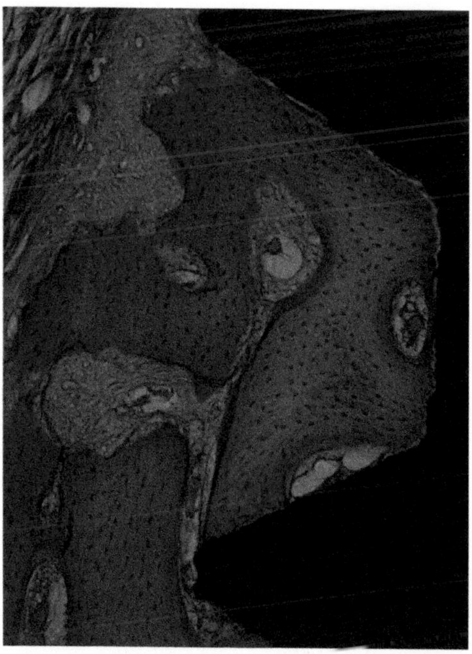

Figure 5.5 Detail of BIC over an implant thread. (100X acid fuchsin and toluidine blue).

bone. BIC II measures BIC along a line that passes from apex to apex of the implant threads (Fig. 5.4b); this measures real BIC but does not take into account BIC between threads. This tends to measure the old bone and some new bone but ignores interthread bone. Last, BIC III measures BIC both in areas around and above the threads and in between threads (Fig. 5.4c).

BIC is a sine qua non condition for the osseointegration of dental implants. It is a fact that BIC will not be the same in the palatine zone as in the buccal zone, as less contact is produced on the buccal side because it is a finer bone wall [44–57].

Most researches use optical microscopes for taking histomorphometric evaluations, but this is not an exact method for obtaining BIC values as measurement is taken from a photo of the microscope image. With the scanning electron microscope, measurement can be carried out directly without the need for intermediary digital imagery.

It must be said that BIC III evaluation is the most certain method for establishing the quantity of formed bone, as the BIC area at which evaluation is carried out includes the area over and above implant threads as well as the areas between threads (Fig. 5.5). All studies should include elemental analysis that helps to assess the quality of BIC and allows to transfer the research outcomes to everyday clinical practice.

References

[1] Brånemark PI, Adell R, Breine U, Lindstrom J, Hallen O, Ohman A. Intra-osseous anchorage of dental prostheses I. Experimental studies. Scand J Plast Reconst Surg 1969;3:81–100.

[2] Brånemark PI, Zarb GA, Albrektsson T, editors. Tissue-integrated prostheses: osseointegration in clinical dentistry. Chicago: Quintessence; 1985.

[3] Brånemark PI, Hansson BO, Adell R, Breine U, Lindstrom J, Hallen O, et al. Osseointegrated implants in the treatment of the edentulous jaw. Experience from a 10-year period. Scand J Plast Reconst Surg Suppl 1977;16:1–132.

[4] Schroder A, Stich H, Straumann F. Uber die anlagerung von Osteozement an einen belasteten implantatkorper. Schweitz Monatssch Zahnheilk 1978;88:1051–8.

[5] Davies JE. Understanding peri-implant endosseous healing. J Dent Educ 2003;67:932–49.

[6] Lang R, Wetzel A, Stich H, Caffesse R. Oral Implant 1994;2(1):191–201. Illinois: Quintessence Publishing Co. Inc.

[7] Osborn JF, Newesely H. Dynamic aspects of the implant-bone interface. In: Heimke G, editor. Dental Implants: materials and systems. Munich: Verlag; 1980. p. 111–23.

[8] Marx RE, Garg AK. Bone structure, metabolism and physiology: its impacts on dental implantology. Implant Dent 1998;7:267–76.

[9] Sennerby L. On the bone tissue response to titanium implants (thesis). Goteborg: University of Goteborg; 1991.

[10] Hobo S, Ichida E, García LT. Osseointegration and occlusal rehabilitation. Chicago: Quintessence; 1991. p. 33–56.

[11] Spector M. Current concepts of bone ingrowth and remodelling. In: Fitzgerald Jr R, editor. Non-cemented total hip arthroplasty. New York: Raven Press; 1988. p. 69–85.

[12] Haider R, Watzek G, Plenk H. Effects of drill cooling and bone structure on IMZ implant fixation. Int J Oral Maxillofac Implants 1993;8:39–91.

[13] Albrektsson T, Brånemark PI, Hansson HA, Lindström J. Osseointegrated titanium implants. Requirements for ensuring a long-lasting, direct bone-to-implant anchorage in man. Acta Orthop Scand 1981;52(2):155–70.
[14] Le Guehennec L, Soueidan A, Layrolle P, et al. Surface treatments of titanium dental implants for rapid osseointegration. Dent Mater 2007;23:844–54.
[15] Hurzeler M, Fickl S, Zuhr O, Wachtel HC. Peri-implant bone level around implants with platform-switched abutments: preliminary data from a prospective study. J Oral Maxillofac Surg 2007;65:33–9.
[16] Assenza B, Scarano A, Petrone G, Iezzi G, Thams U, San Roman F, et al. Osteoclast activity around loaded and unloaded implants: a histological study in the beagle dog. J Oral Implant 2003;29:1–7.
[17] Hermann JS, Buser D, Schenk RK, Higginbottom FL, Cochran DL. Biologic width around titanium implants. A physiologically formed and stable dimension over time. Clin Oral Implants Res 2000;11:1–11.
[18] King GN, Hermann JS, Schoolfield JD, Buser D, Cochran DL. Influence of the size of the microgap on crestal bone levels in non- submerged dental implants: a radiographic study in the canine mandible. J Periodontol 2002;73:1111–7.
[19] Alomrani AN, Hermann JS, Jones AA, Buser D, Schoolfield J, Cochran DL. The effect of a machined collar on coronal hard tissue around titanium implants: a radiographic study in the canine mandible. Int J Oral Maxillofac Implants 2005;20:677–86.
[20] Hanggi MP, Hanggi DC, Schoolfield JD, Meyer J, Cochran DL, Hermann JS. Crestal bone changes around titanium implants. Part I: a retrospective radiographic evaluation in humans comparing two non-submerged implant designs with different machined collar lengths. J Periodontol 2005;76:791–802.
[21] Shin YK, Han CH, Heo SJ, Kim S, Chun HJ. Radiographic evaluation of marginal bone level around implants with different neck designs after 1 year. Int J Oral Maxillofac Implants 2006;21:789–94.
[22] Cardaropoli G, Lekholm U, Wennstrom JL. Tissue alterations at implant-supported single-tooth replacements: a 1-year prospective clinical study. Clin Oral Implants Res 2006;17: 165–71.
[23] Manz MC. Factors associated with radiographic vertical bone loss around implants placed in a clinical study. Ann Periodontol 2000;5:137–51.
[24] Lazzara RJ, Porter SS. Platform switching: a new concept in implant dentistry for controlling postrestorative crestal bone levels. Int J Periodontics Restor Dent 2006;26:9–17.
[25] Lee DW, Choi YS, Park KH, Kim CS, Moon IS. Effect of microthread on the maintenance of marginal bone level, a 3-year prospective study. Clin Oral Implants Res 2007;18:465–70.
[26] Stanford CM. Surface modifications of dental implants. Aust Dent J 2008;53(S1):26–33.
[27] Duyck J, Slaets E, Sasaguri K, Vandamme K, Naert I. Effect of intermittent loading and surface roughness on peri-implant bone formation in a bone chamber model. J Clin Periodontolol 2007;34:998–1006.
[28] Vandamme K, Naert I, Geris L, Vander Sloten J, Puers R, Duyck J. Influence of controlled immediate loading and implant design on peri-implant bone formation. J Clin Periodontol 2007;34:172–81.
[29] Vandamme K, Naert I, Geris L, Vander Sloten J, Puers R, Duyck J. The effect of micromotion on the tissue response around immediately loaded roughened titanium implants in the rabbit. Eur J Oral Sci 2007;115:21–9.
[30] Vandamme K, Naert I, Vander Sloten J, Puers R, Duyck J. Effect of implant surface roughness and loading on peri-implant bone formation. J Periodontol 2008;79:150–7.

[31] Turkyilmaz I, Aksoy U, McGlumphy EA. Two alternative surgical techniques for enhancing primary implant stability in the posterior maxilla: a clinical study including bone density, insertion torque, and resonance frequency analysis data. Clin Implant Dent Relat Res 2008;10:231–7.

[32] Hermann JS, Buser D, Schenk RK, Cochran DL. Crestal bone changes around titanium implants. A histometric evaluation of unloaded non-submerged and submerged implants in the canine mandible. J Periodontol 2000;71:1412–24.

[33] Hermann JS, Schoolfield JD, Nummikoski PV, Buser D, Schenk RK, Cochran DL. Crestal bone changes around titanium implants: a methodologic study comparing linear radiographic with histometric measurements. Int J Oral Maxillofac Implants 2001;16:475–85

[34] Hammerle CH, Bragger U, Burgin W, Lang NP. The effect of subcrestal placement of the polished surface of ITI implants on marginal soft and hard tissues. Clin Oral Implants Res 1996;7:111–9.

[35] Nickenig H-J, Wichmann M, Schlegel KA, Nkenke E, Eitner S. Radiographic evaluation of marginal bone levels adjacent to parallel-screw cylinder machined-neck implants and rough-surfaced microthreaded implants using digitized panoramic radiographs. Clin Oral Implants Res 2009;20:550–4.

[36] Carr AB, Gerard DA, Larsen PE. Histomorphometric analysis of implant anchorage for 3 types of dental implants following 6 months of healing in baboon jaws. Int J Oral Maxillofac Implants 2000;15:785–91.

[37] Cho P, Schneider GB, Krizan K, Keller JC. Examination of the bone-implant interface in experimentally induced osteoporotic bone. Implant Dent 2004;13:79–87.

[38] De Pauw GA, Dermaut LR, Johansson CB, Martens G. A histomorphometric analysis of heavily loaded and non-loaded implants. Int J Oral Maxillofac Implants 2002;17:405–12.

[39] Ivanoff CJ, Sennerby L, Johansson C, Rangert B, Lekholm U. Influence of implant diameters on the integration of screw implants. An experimental study in rabbits. Int J Oral Maxillofac Surg 1997;26:141–8.

[40] Trisi P, Lazzara R, Rebaudi A, Rao W, Testori T, Porter SS. Bone-implant contact on machined and dual acid-etched surfaces after 2 months of healing in the human maxilla. J Periodontol 2003;74:945–56.

[41] Calvo-Guirado JL, Maté-Sánchez JE, Delgado-Ruiz R, Ramírez- Fernández MP. Calculation of bone graft volume using 3D reconstruction system. Med Oral Patol Oral Cir Bucal 2011;16:e260–4.

[42] López-Marí L, Calvo-Guirado JL, Martín-Castellote B, Gomez- Moreno G, López-Marí M. Implant platform switching concept: an updated review. Med Oral Patol Oral Cir Bucal 2009;14:e450–4.

[43] Calvo-Guirado JL, Ramírez-Fernández MP, Gómez-Moreno G, Maté-Sánchez JE, Delgado-Ruiz R, Guardia J, et al. Melatonin stimulates the growth of new bone around implants in the tibia of rabbits. J Pineal Res 2010;49:356–63.

[44] Aloy-Prosper A, Maestre-Ferrin L, Penarrocha-Oltra D, Penarrocha-Diago M. Marginal bone loss in relation to the implant neck surface: an update. Med Oral Patol Oral Cir Bucal 2011;16:e365–8.

[45] Roriz VM, Rosa AL, Peitl O, Zanotto ED, Panzeri H, de Oliveira PT. Efficacy of a bioactive glass-ceramic (Biosilicate) in the maintenance of alveolar ridges and in osseointegration of titanium implants. Clin Oral Implants Res 2010;21:148–55.

[46] Fenner M, Vairaktaris E, Fischer K, Schlegel KA, Neukam FW, Nkenke E. Influence of residual alveolar bone height on osseointegration of implants in the maxilla: a pilot study. Clin Oral Implants Res 2009;20:555–9.

[47] Fugl A, Ulm C, Tangl S, Vasak C, Gruber R, Watzek G. Long-term effects of magnetron-sputtered calcium phosphate coating on osseointegration of dental implants in non-human primates. Clin Oral Implants Res 2009;20:183–8.
[48] Parlar A, Bosshardt DD, Cetiner D, Schafroth D, Unsal B, Haytac C, et al. Effects of decontamination and implant surface characteristics on re-osseointegration following treatment of peri-implantitis. Clin Oral Implants Res 2009;20:391–9.
[49] Song JK, Cho TH, Pan H, Song YM, Kim IS, Lee TH, et al. An electronic device for accelerating bone formation in tissues surrounding a dental implant. Bioelectromagnetics 2009;30:374–84.
[50] Vignoletti F, Johansson C, Albrektsson T, De Sanctis M, San Roman F, Sanz M. Early healing of implants placed into fresh extraction sockets: an experimental study in the beagle dog. De novo bone formation. J Clin Periodontol 2009;36:265–77.
[51] Jeong R, Marin C, Granato R, Suzuki M, Gil JN, Granjeiro JM, et al. Early bone healing around implant surfaces treated with variations in the resorbable blasting media method. A study in rabbits. Med Oral Patol Oral Cir Bucal 2010;15:e119–25.
[52] Lee J, Sieweke JH, Rodriguez NA, Schupbach P, Lindstrom H, Su- sin C, et al. Evaluation of nano-technology-modified zirconia oral implants: a study in rabbits. J Clin Periodontol 2009;36:610–7.
[53] Vidigal Jr GM, Groisman M, Gregorio LH, Soares Gde A. Osseointegration of titanium alloy and HA-coated implants in healthy and ovariectomized animals: a histomorphometric study. Clin Oral Implants Res 2009;20:1272–7.
[54] Calvo-Guirado JL, Gomez-Moreno G, Barone A, Cutando A, Al- caraz-Banos M, Chiva F, et al. Melatonin plus porcine bone on discrete calcium deposit implant surface stimulates osteointegration in dental implants. J Pineal Res 2009;47:164–72.
[55] Calvo-Guirado JL, Gomez-Moreno G, Lopez-Mari L, Guardia J, Marinez-Gonzalez JM, Barone A, et al. Actions of melatonin mixed with collagenized porcine bone versus porcine bone only on osseointegration of dental implants. J Pineal Res 2010;48:194–203.
[56] Calvo-Guirado JL, Ortiz-Ruiz AJ, Negri B, Lopez-Mari L, Rodriguez-Barba C, Schlottig F. Histological and histomorphometric evaluation of immediate implant placement on a dog model with a new implant surface treatment. Clin Oral Implants Res 2010;21:308–15.
[57] Ballo AM, Akca EA, Ozen T, Lassila L, Vallittu PK, Narhi TO. Bone tissue responses to glass fiber-reinforced composite implants. A histomorphometric study. Clin Oral Implants Res 2009;20:608–15.

Implant primary stability and occlusion

6

G. Frisardi[1,2], C. Murray[3], P.P. Valentini[4], E.M. Staderini[5], F. Frisardi[1]
[1]Epochè – Orofacial Pain Centre, Rome, Italy; [2]University of Sassari, Sassari, Italy;
[3]European University College, Dubai, UAE; [4]University Tor Vergata, Rome, Italy;
[5]Western Switzerland Universities of Applied Sciences, Geneva, Switzerland

6.1 Introduction

In tackling topics such as implant-prosthetic rehabilitation, one should first consider characteristics of the biological phenomenon at hand. All biological systems make up the organic system of the human being, from neurophysiological to osteomuscular interactions. As such, these should be considered as "complex systems" comprising a series of elements or components, which interact with each other according to stochastic processes [1–6]. These interactions generate an "emergent behavior" [7] of the complex system, which is unfortunately not predictable from the knowledge of each single isolated component.

Therefore, in discussing primary implant stability, we have to extend our knowledge to a larger network comprising multiple components that interact with one another. These include the biomolecular genesis of bone [8–10], the interface between the implant and bone [11–13], the specific characteristics of the materials, and the shape of the implants [14,15] and occlusal loading of implant fixtures [16,17] among other factors.

A phenomenon termed "fatigue microtrauma" has been proposed as the cause of cervical and progressive bone loss during the modeling process due to excessive occlusal loading of the implant. This microtrauma occurs when the rate of fatigue microdamage exceeds the bone reparative rate, thereby resulting in the irreversible loss of cervical bone [18].

Several physical and mathematical modalities have been used in biomechanical studies to simulate occlusal loading. These include two-dimensional (2D) and three-dimensional (3D) photoelastic models, strain gauge analysis, and 2D and 3D finite element analysis [19,20]. Although these techniques have inherent advantages and weaknesses, they essentially demonstrate the presence of points or areas of relative stress concentration in modeled superstructures, implants, and supporting and surrounding bone structure [21].

Some investigators in bone deformation models have been able to quantify the level of strain and relate this value to the calculated values of fatigue overload. A positive correlation has been verified in both animal and clinical studies as they all demonstrated an increased amount of cervical stress concentration with increased levels of loading when there is off-axis inclination or bending movements [22–24]. Although

Bone Response to Dental Implant Materials. http://dx.doi.org/10.1016/B978-0-08-100287-2.00006-9

these studies are of substantial scientific and experimental importance, due to the inherent stochastic nature of the system under consideration and intrasubject variability of the biomechanical characteristics, many questions remain unanswered.

An implant-prosthetic rehabilitation, therefore, relates to a complex system that is able to adapt to local conditions thereby generating an "adaptive emergent behavior," which simulates a clinically acceptable efficiency of the masticatory system that is physiologically adaptive. To understand this "adaptive emergent behavior," it is necessary to explore at least two essential components underpinning the efficiency of the system.

1. The implant–bone biomechanical primary stability phenomenon through press-fit analysis that we will refer to as "press-fit primary stability"
2. The occlusal primary stability phenomenon named neurognathological functions subsequently referred to as "NGF primary stability"

6.2 Press-fit primary stability

The press-fit phenomenon indicates a mechanical connection of two structures based on the contact pressure. However, a more appropriate definition, "interference-fit" could be used considering that each component mutually interferes to generate the deformation. The press-fit technique, which is adopted to ensure a primary stability condition for endosseous implants, requires the diameter of the hole drilled within the bone to be smaller than the implant major diameter. The bone tissues are affected by a biomechanical phenomenon, which is affected by the mechanical properties of bone, implant materials, the difference between implant and hole diameters and surrounding bone morphology.

Recently, image-based approaches combined with finite element analyses have allowed effective stress–strain investigations within dental implantology. Dental implants can be virtually positioned in realistic models of human jaws reproduced from high definition cone beam computed tomography (CT) image data with respect to the anatomical and physiological structures of the recipient bone. Worldwide, scientists have focused on this topic to improve the success rates of endosseous implants [25–29].

A common goal is to understand the key factors of osseointegration processes following the implant surgery. Some researchers have investigated microdisplacements occurring at the bone–implant interface. Conversely, others have considered load transfer at the interface to be more important in determining the correct mechanical stimulation of osteoblasts, which are assumed to be responsible for bone tissue regeneration and consequent osseointegration of the implant [30,31].

Generally, trabecular microstructures of bone are modeled as homogeneous entities with particular mechanical properties and contiguity assumed at implant–bone interfaces. The contiguity conditions do not allow relative motions between the parts generating a continuum of stress distribution at the interface, where stresses are concentrated.

Limbert et al. [32], as an example, has studied the trabecular microstructure of mandibular bone and the discontinuity at the implant–bone interface by finite element analysis (FEA). Further studies have investigated the preload condition generated by insertion of the abutment screw in the implant for different designs of the screw-abutment system [31].

To date, the selection of drill diameter with respect to the implant geometrical configuration is still performed without any robust scientifically tested criteria. Natali et al. [33] analyzed the press-fit phenomenon occurring in oral implantology using the FEA approach. In this study, the mandibular bone was reconstructed using the CT data and different mechanical properties in the cortical and trabecular regions were observed. However, a more detailed study should also consider the trabecular microstructure of real bone tissue and the contacts associated with the relative movement between the implant and the bone.

In our recent paper [34], an accurate model of human mandibular bone segment was created by processing high-resolution micro-CT data (Fig. 6.1) using image-based tools. The biomechanics of press-fit phenomena was analyzed by FE methods for different drill diameters.

The finite element analysis was conducted for three different drill diameter values.

The drill was modeled assuming a cylindrical shape with different diameter values: $D_A = 2.8$ mm (model A), $D_B = 3.3$ mm (model B), and $D_C = 3.8$ mm (model C) and

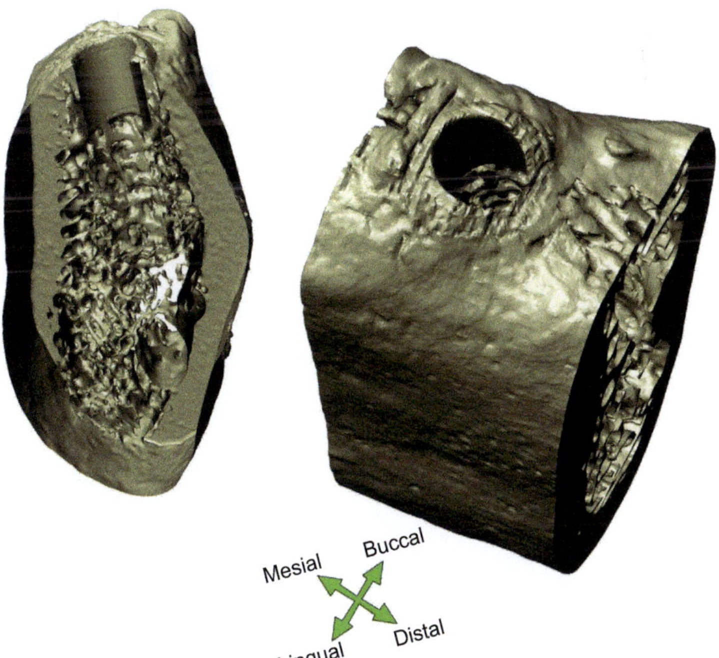

Figure 6.1 Result of the virtual drilling process. ScanIP reimported model: (left) view through cut, (right) full volume.

length $L = 12$ mm. The virtual implant model has been assumed with a cylindrical geometry having height $L = 11$ mm and diameter $D = 4$ mm. The drill models were positioned into the bone model through the use of ScanCAD (Simpleware Ltd., Innovation Centre, Rennes Drive, Exeter, United Kingdom). It allows placement to be driven by the corresponding 3D gray-scale micro-CT images and taking into account the bone structure (Fig. 6.2)

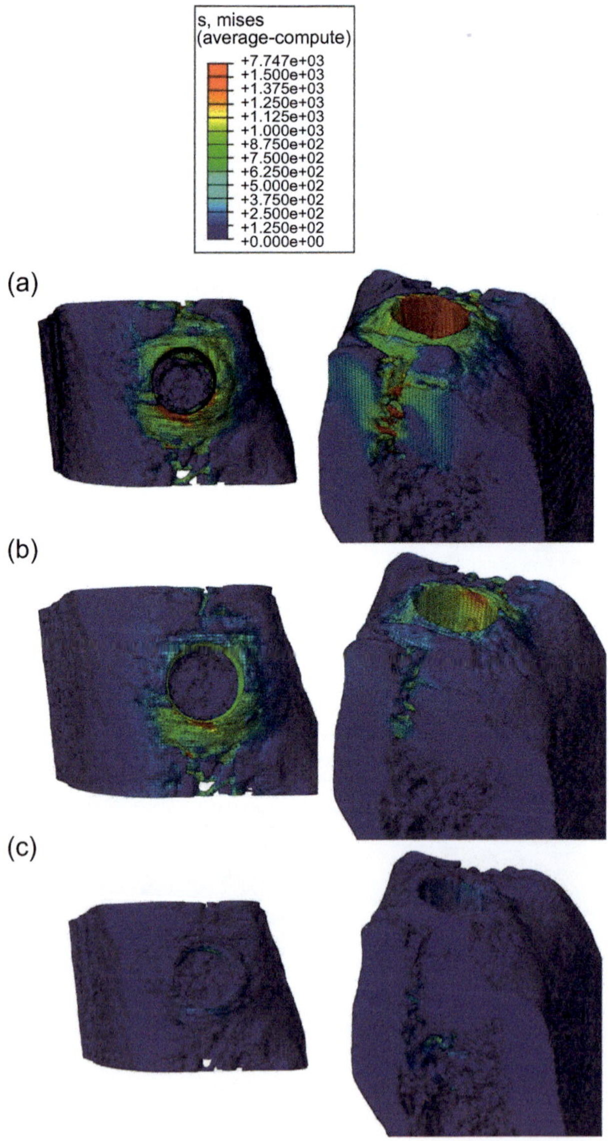

Figure 6.2 Von Mises stress distributions. Top view of the Von Mises stresses induced by bone tissue expansion for models (a), (b), and (c), respectively.

The Von Mises stresses are presented along the buccolingual and mesiodistal planes. In models A and B, the press-fit phenomenon is almost completely supported by the cortical structure, although the implant is in contact with both the cortical and the trabecular bone. The stresses in the trabecular zone are minimal compared to those characterizing the cortical area.

In model C, the stresses are equally distributed across the cortical and trabecular structure reducing the generation of critical and localized loads.

A uniform stress distribution, as reported in model C, is the optimal condition for the osseointegration process allowing a distribution of bone cell stimulation all around the implant. The maximum stresses in models A, B, and C are 12.31, 7.74, and 4.52 GPa, respectively (Figs. 6.2 and 6.3)

High-stress concentrations may induce bone cell necrosis or result in deficient homogeneous osteoblast stimulation, which are both possible causes of implant destabilization [35].

As mentioned before, the press-fit phenomenon indicates a mechanical connection of two structures based on contact pressure.

Generally, the actual viscoelastic behavior of bone tissue implies that the elastic recoil of bone decreases over time (creep phenomenon). The bone deformation and the elastic recoil depend on the density of bone tissue, and cortical bone has less viscoelastic behavior than cancellous bone [36–38].

The results obtained in our studies demonstrate that the cortical bone is stressed and deformed significantly, even with moderate values of interference fit. Figs. 6.2 and 6.3 demonstrate higher Von Mises values in juxtacortical areas than in the cancellous bone structure.

Viscoelastic behavior also depends on the degree of initial elastic deformation of bone when the press-fit is achieved. The "assembly strain" (i.e., the deformation of the bone tissue upon the introduction of the implant) has an effect on both the contact pressure between the bone and implant during the initial press-fit and the rate at which the press-fit is dissipated through deformation and elastic relaxation [39,40].

The data presented in Figs. 6.2 and 6.3 indicate that the only press-fit value at implant preload demonstrating evenly distributed stresses at the bone–implant contact is generated within model C. In contrast, models A and B yield uneven stress distributions at the bone–implant interface. However, the stresses occurring in model C may not yet be high enough to yield the necessary press-fit persisting to ensure the primary stability especially in the situation of immediate implant loading.

Once the initial press-fit is dissipated, the implant is capable of moving in the bone under load. This would suggest the use of an "undersized" approach that only accentuates an elevated cortical bone–implant load using techniques at our disposal.

The intermediate period between the initial press-fit and the healing of osseointegration is typically characterized by a relaxation of press-fit, if this occurs too fast, it could cause implant instability. The bone ingrowth, which leads to osseointegration, is a very susceptible biophysical process especially in the case of immediate loading of full arches [41].

A recent study [42] demonstrated that the undersized drilling technique, also to enhancing primary implant stability, might achieve a translocation of bone particles.

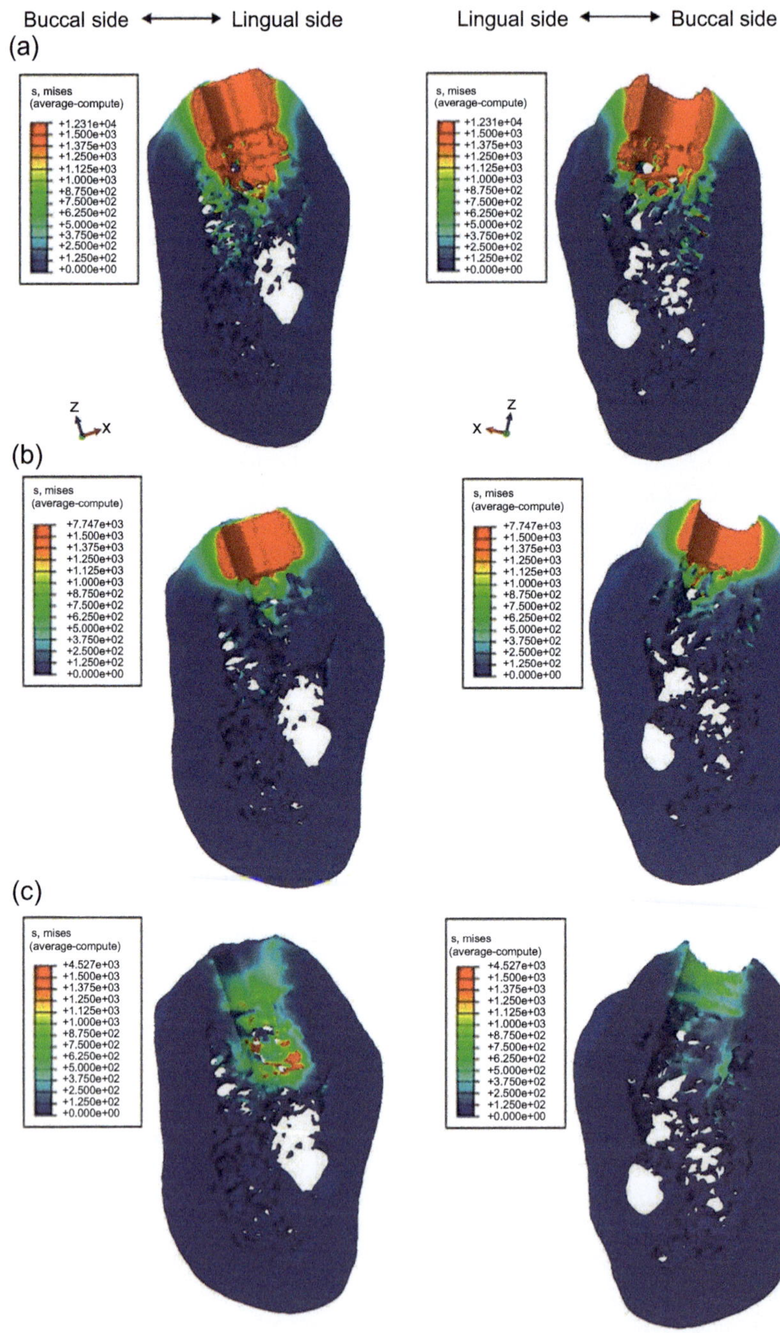

Figure 6.3 Von Mises stresses distribution for the press-fit implant. View of the Von Mises stresses distribution on the opposite sides of the buccolingual virtual cut.

This biological phenomenon, comparable to the autologous bone graft, has a positive influence on the osteogenic response.

In conclusion, our study data identify that the cortical bone plays a significant role in supporting the implant. Therefore, implant stability assessment based solely on the axial displacement may be unreliable as the apparent high implant stability, determined from low axial displacements, may be produced only by the cortical bone in the alveolar region. In this scenario, the success of the implant may be jeopardized by the increased strains in the alveolar region that may lead to peri-implantitis, atrophy, and implant failure.

Naturally, implant stability is also affected by the individual quality of the cancellous bone. Interestingly, the cancellous bone demonstrates the highest strain a few millimeters from the implant and not necessarily in the tissue in direct proximity to the implant. This observation is consistent with experiments previously performed by Gabet et al.(2010) [43].

However, many trabeculae in this region are thin and demonstrate highly variable cross-sectional area along their length. Such trabeculae may, therefore, display certain locations where the loads are excessively concentrated and this may ultimately lead to the destruction of the trabeculae. In the long term, the bone remodeling processes may naturally eliminate these problematic locations. However, this is only the case provided that the implant is embedded in a sufficient quantity of cancellous bone and that the additional bony layer is created around the whole implant during the healing process.

In conclusion, it is our opinion that efforts should be focused on developing a method that is capable of determining relative uniform stresses and strain values across the whole alveolar region and involving the cancellous bone interface in addition to the cortical interface. This surgical method should be geometrically and biomechanically considered as a "differentiated interference-fit" and should be focused on the preparation of the artificial alveolar bone using different surgical steps and diameters of drills.

The following discussion introduces the NGF primary stability concept.

The biomechanic primary stability of the implant–bone interface remains the primum movens in implant surgery approach. Nevertheless, the occlusal load component on the implants remains of critical importance, particularly when rehabilitating a patient using immediate implant loading.

Another important issue is that the evaluation of adjacent bone strength is based upon the calculation of stresses in the bone tissue under masticatory loading. Holmgren et al. [44] suggested using combined (oblique) loads because these are a more realistic representation of bite direction and, for a given force, will reproduce the greatest localized stress in the cortical bone. Following this experimental approach, Demenko et al. [45] determined the "ultimate magnitudes of oblique masticatory force" that were applied at the center of an abutment's upper surface in a 3D asymmetric loading scheme. They concluded that overloading of the cortical bone might occur in the compressed part of the neck zone due to oblique occlusal loading.

This conclusion could be true in a simple biological system. However, as mentioned above, the masticatory forces represent a "complex system" and the resulting occlusal loads are, therefore, more difficult to quantify.

Indeed, the trajectory of these functional motions affects the direction and magnitude of masticatory force with all muscles acting together to generate a resultant force and torque (6 degrees of freedom) with respect to the mandible and maxilla [46].

The moving dynamics of the mandible are expressed in terms of position, velocity, and acceleration. Because the mandible is a 3D body, it possesses both translational and rotational degrees of freedom. Therefore, the location and attitude of the mandible can be defined by three parameters that describe the location of the center of mass and three angles (yaw, pitch, and roll). Because the movement of the mandible is limited, the gimbal lock phenomenon is avoided and the use of Euler's parameters or quaternions is not necessary.

Every moving body, including the mandible, obeys Newton's laws. Movements are caused by forces acting on the mandible and may be active muscle forces or passive (reaction) forces generated by joints, ligaments, and dental elements.

These forces also display six components with linear force (F_x, F_y, F_z) accompanied by torques (M_{yaw}, M_{pitch}, M_{roll}). The resultant forces and torques generate accelerations according to Newton's second law (Fig. 6.4). This accounts for each degree of freedom, emphasizing the fact that the jaw mass also consists of mass and inertia tensor. The inertia tensor depends on the distribution of mass and therefore upon the shape of the mandible and adhering structures [47].

For a mandible of about 0.44 kg of mass, considering a principal reference system and the symmetry of the shape, the principal moments of inertia have been estimated as 8.6, 2.9, and 6.1 kg cm^2 for I_{yaw}(about the z-axis), I_{pitch}(about the y-axis), and I_{roll} (about the x-axis), respectively [48]. Therefore, about three times less muscle torque is required to accelerate the jaw for open–close movements than for laterodeviations.

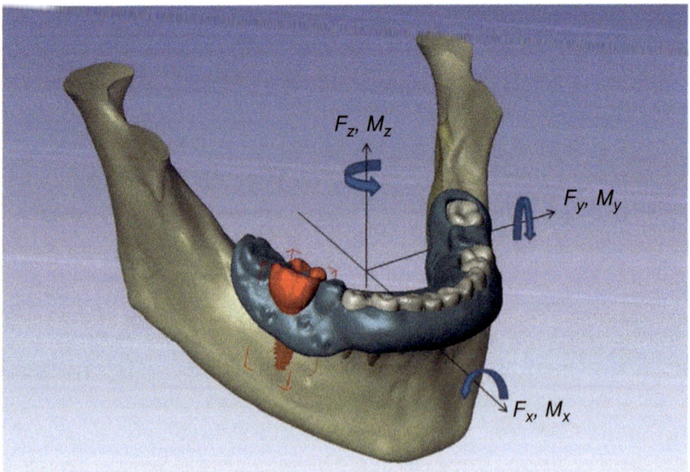

Figure 6.4 Six degrees of freedom for mandibular movement. These forces also display six components with linear force (F_x, F_y, F_z) accompanied by torques (M_{yaw}, M_{pitch}, M_{roll}). All these components generate accelerations according to Newton's second law.

Figs. 6.4 and 6.5 highlight the fundamental characteristics of the masticatory and bone–implant systems and the contextual limits of analysis procedures. Firstly, the implants, as with teeth, are subjected to dynamic forces and torque. The resulting loading force is related to the size of the mass, muscle strength, speed, and instant, impulsive acceleration events of masticatory occlusal contacts.

When applying FEA to dental implants, it is therefore important to consider not only axial loads and horizontal forces (moment-causing loads) but also a combined oblique occlusal loading force because the latter represents more realistic occlusal directions and, for a given force, may result in localized stress in cortical bone [44].

Simultaneously, it needs to be taken into account that maximum recruitment of the motoneural pool is generated during maximum interscuspation [49] and in the first millimeter of lateral excursion (our neurophysiological unpublished data). The occlusal contacts on the implant elements must be multiples to allow the reduction of extra-axial dynamic loads in masticatory cycles [44]. This was confirmed by Eskitascioglu et al. [50] who undertook a study on occlusal loading of the framework's crown and its effect upon the abutment implant bone. These authors performed the study by loading the framework with an average occlusal force of 300 N. Three-point vertical loads were applied at the tip of the buccal cusp (300 N; model A); tip

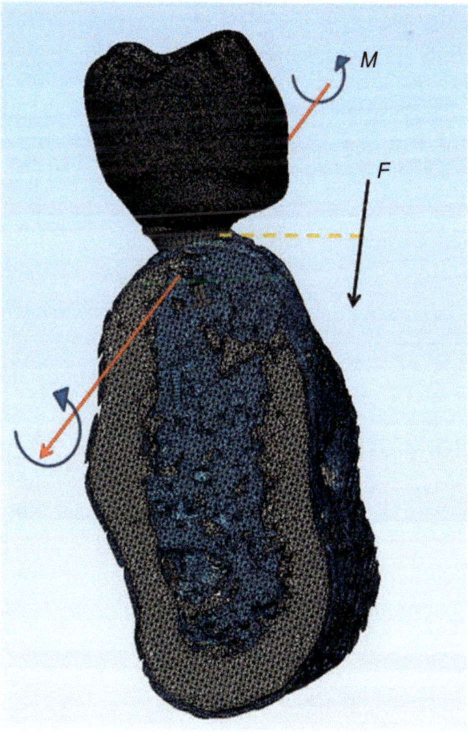

Figure 6.5 Force and torque generated by a muscle (*arrow*) with respect to the center of gravity of the lower jaw.

of buccal cusp (150 N) and the distal fossa (150 N) (model B); the tip of buccal cusp (100 N), distal fossa (100 N), and the mesial fossa (100 N) (model C). They concluded that vertical loading at model B and C produced high stresses on the framework and occlusal surface of the implant-supported fixed partial denture and low stresses distributed to the bone. These types of loads would appear to minimize force transmission to the implant and surrounding bone. Vertical loading at model A produced stresses on the cortical bone and implant, with the low stresses being distributed to the framework and occlusal surface.

To understand the final result of 3D occlusal loading, we have to shift our attention to neuromuscular recruitment and brain functional activity. Using functional magnetic resonance imaging (fMRI), Kimoto et al. [51] compared the change in brain regional activity of four edentulous subjects who wore either mandibular complete dentures (CD) or implant-supported removable overdentures (IOD).

From these fMRI studies, six regions of interest have been identified. These regions are robustly activated by gum-chewing in dentate subjects regardless of their age and include the primary sensorimotor cortex, supplementary motor area, insula, thalamus, cerebellum, and prefrontal cortex [52,53].

The ROIs analysis identified that chewing with IOD resulted in a decrease in the maximum beta value in comparison to chewing with CD in the prefrontal cortex, primary sensorimotor cortex, and cerebellum. There are several possible explanations for the observed phenomenon. As for the latter two regions concerning motor execution, the reduction of brain activity might reflect more smooth manipulation of the masticatory organ while chewing with IOD than with CD. However, the interesting consequence of this hypothesis is that chewing is a maintained rhythmic pattern under the control of the "central pattern generator" located in the pons and medulla [54].

This last suggestion introduces a basic contribution of the mesencephalic structures in managing the bite strength, so that the trigeminal electrophysiological approach could be considered as a basic element in the field of implant-prosthetic rehabilitation to immediate loading.

For this reason, we proposed a new paradigm in implantoprosthetic rehabilitation called "neurognathological functions," which we describe as NGF primary stability.

6.3 NGF primary stability

For a correct evaluation of masticatory function, a precise knowledge of the forces involved in this action and the resulting movements is required. Although these can be easily and accurately measured with various instruments, the real underlying problem is in the assessment of masticatory muscle control from a neurophysiopathological point of view.

The cortical projections to trigeminal motoneurons are believed to be bilateral and symmetric. Interestingly, using electrical or magnetic brain stimulation through the intact scalp [55,56], it is possible to evoke motor responses in masticatory muscles.

The root-motor evoked potentials (R-MEPs), therefore, could be considered an organic response as they are not modulated by central or peripheral mono and polysynaptic drives and demonstrate an absolute stability giving important information about the anatomical symmetry and integrity of the trigeminal motor system.

The NGF involves the study of muscular-evoked potentials on the muscles after direct bilateral electrical stimulation of the motor roots of the trigeminal motor system. This electrophysiological event has been called bilateral R-MEPs ($_b$R-MEPs) by transcranial electrical stimulation. The maximum absolute neural energy evoked, the symmetry, and the synchrony properties of the resulting $_b$R-MEPs have been studied using measures such as latency, amplitude, and integrated area of the signal. This technique could allow us, from a neurophysiopathological perspective, a better assessment of masticatory function and to verify the possibility to consider the $_b$R-MEPs as a "normalization factor."

6.3.1 Electrophysiological procedure

The tests have been performed using an electromyographic device (Nemus-NGF, EBNeuro, Firenze, Italy) [57,58]. Considering the safety limitations, we computed the energy delivered for each single pulse in our application through this formula:

$$E = P \cdot \Delta t = R \cdot I^2 \cdot \Delta t = 2.5 \text{ mJ} \tag{6.1}$$

Where E is the energy; P is the power; Δt is the duration of the pulse.

As two electrostimulators were used, the limits were 10 times lower than those stated in international electrotechnical commission regulations.

The electrodes were arranged as described below. A common anode to the two electrostimulators was placed at the vertex, whereas a cathode electrode was placed on each side at 11 cm along the line joining the vertex to the acoustic meatus in the parietal region. The electrical stimulus consisted of a square wave lasting 250 μs at a voltage of ≅ 300 V and maximum current of 100 mA.

Fig. 6.6 demonstrates the distribution of the electric field inside the intracranial brain tissue of an analysis performed through a generic finite element (FE) process (SimNibs method), only as a descriptive model (data not reported) [59].

Briefly, FE models consisted of around 1.7 million tetrahedral solid element. Mesh resolution was selectively enhanced in gray matter (GM), white matter (WM), skull, and the cerebrospinal fluid (CSF) regions with an average tetrahedron volume of 1 mm^3. Electrical conductivities (σ) were assigned to different tissue types where (skin) $\sigma = 0.465$ S/m, (skull) $\sigma = 0.010$ S/m, (CSF) $\sigma = 1.654$ S/m, (GM) $\sigma = 0.276$ S/m, and (WM) $\sigma = 0.126$ S/m [60].

The electrode arrangement is shown in Fig. 6.6(a). The maximum current spreads below the cathodes (red color) in the parietal cortex (Fig. 6.6(b)). Conversely, in the region of the skull base close to the trigeminal motor root, only a small amount of current is present (Fig. 6.6(c), black arrows). Fig. 6.6(d) shows the current density that spreads below the skull.

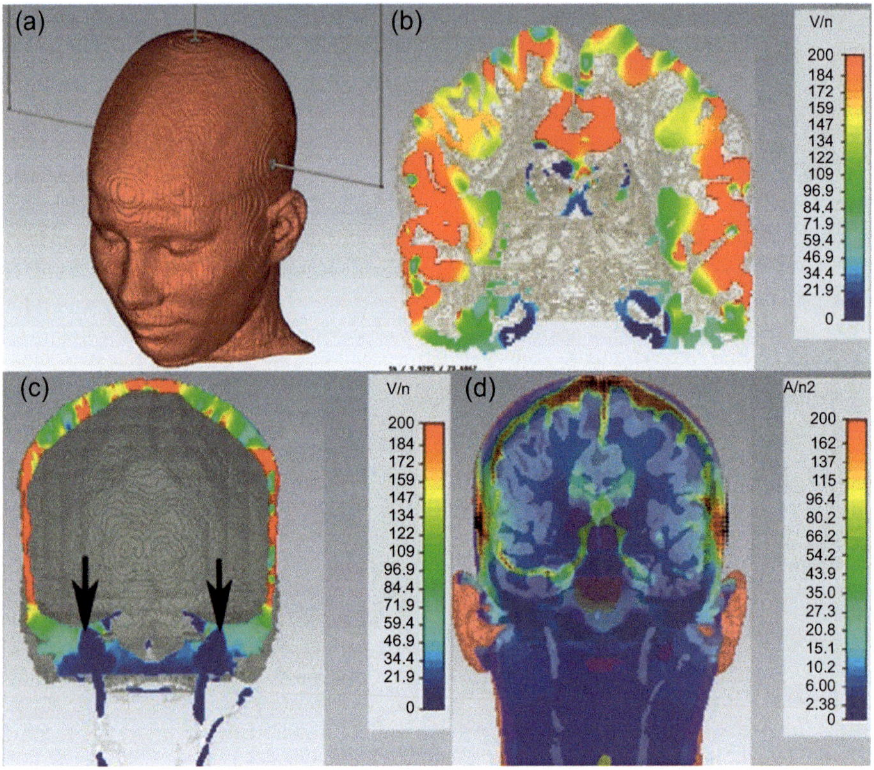

Figure 6.6 The figure shows the arrangement of the electrodes on the skull (a), the distribution of electric fields inside the intracranial brain tissue (b), the low current intensity around the trigeminal roots (c), and current density below the skull (d).

We underline how a minimal amount of electric current inside the brain tissue is required to saturate the motor trigeminal root compared to the amount of current needed to evoke a response by the trigeminal motor cortex below the cathode. This is one of the reasons that led us to choose this type of peripheral-evoked response rather than cortical, which has a higher threshold and less stability in terms of neuromuscular response. We recorded simultaneously the motor-evoked potentials of both the right and left trigeminal roots from the right and left masseter muscles through two paired surface electrodes. The EMG device was set with 20-ms time window width, with 2 mV per division and a filter bandwidth of 2 Hz−2 kHz.

The onset latency, the peak-to-peak amplitude, and the integral area of 10 trials of motor-evoked potentials for each side of each subject were analyzed (data not reported). Fig. 6.7 shows the neuromuscular responses of a subject with the measurements of latency, peak-to-peak amplitude, and integral area. The high symmetry of the $_{b}$R-MEPs can be observed from the perfect symmetry of amplitude that builds, through a complex algorithm, an organic symmetry Gaussian curve reproduced in the bottom right corner. This organic symmetry Gaussian curve will be considered as "normalization factor."

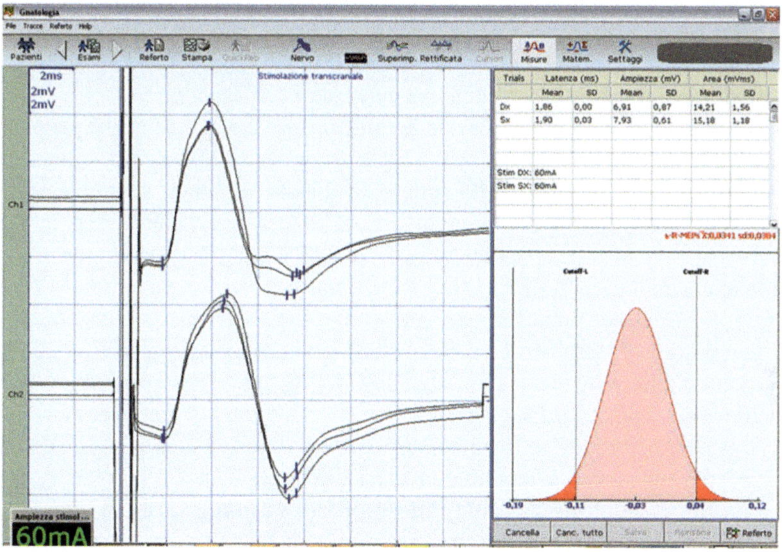

Figure 6.7 Display of the amplitude symmetry and organic symmetry Gaussian curve derived from $_{b}$R-MEPs.

6.3.2 Organic symmetry

To share the concept of organic symmetry of the trigeminal motor system, it is additionally necessary to address some fundamental points about the masticatory system's functionality according to experimental animal studies. A reflex opening of the mandible resulting from the simultaneous relaxation of jaw closers and contraction of jaw openers, not only helps to avoid injuries to the oral tissues but also contributes toward coordinating rhythmic masticatory movements [61].

Previous studies [62] have identified that peripheral stimulation evokes inhibitory postsynaptic potentials in bilateral jaw-closure motor neurons. This bilateral inhibition is mediated, at least in part, by supra- and juxta-trigeminal neurons with bifurcating axons projecting to both the right and the left masseter motor neurons. The goal of a recent study [63] was to morphologically analyze how the functional symmetry of the masticatory system might be reflected in the organization of premotor neurons and how it could potentially mediate excitation of jaw-opener motor neurons.

It has been demonstrated that in the masticatory system, where symmetrical motor output is the rule, using neurons with bifurcating axons as a premotor element might be a common strategy for mediation of both peripheral and central signals.

The concept of organic symmetry is not restricted solely to the masticatory system but can be found in complex neuronal processes in which the output is the result of the sensorimotor drive of the central and peripheral nervous systems.

6.3.3 Functional symmetry

Regarding jaw reflexes, we have also studied the jaw jerk (JJ) and masseteric silent period (MSP) to determine a "functional symmetry Gaussian curve."

The JJ was elicited by placing the index finger over the middle of the patient's chin and the index finger then tapped with a reflex hammer equipped with a piezoelectric sensor recording the level of EMG activity. Subjects held their mandibles in a very slightly clenched intercuspal position ($_{ip}$JJ). Subjects were then asked to perform five maximal clenches, each lasting up to 3 s, with the mandible held in the intercuspal position to obtain the mean EMG value at maximal voluntary contraction (MVC). During these $_{ip}$JJ tests, the subjects were guided by visual feedback to ensure that their EMG levels were maintained at 20% of the MVC. Electromyographic signals were recorded simultaneously (50-ms time-window width, 100 μV per division, filter bandwidth 20–2 kHz) using surface electrodes on the right and left masseter muscles, with an electromyographic device (Nemus-NGF, EBNeuro). The JJ was averaged over 20 trials, and the peak-to-peak amplitude measured.

The resulting data from this study show a perfect symmetry of the JJ in a healthy subject in the latency, amplitude, and integral area [64]. This symmetry is capable of building a functional symmetry Gaussian curve (Fig. 6.8).

In the same way, we performed analyses of the MSP and through a more complex algorithm (data not reported) we built a "functional symmetry Gaussian curve" (Fig. 6.9).

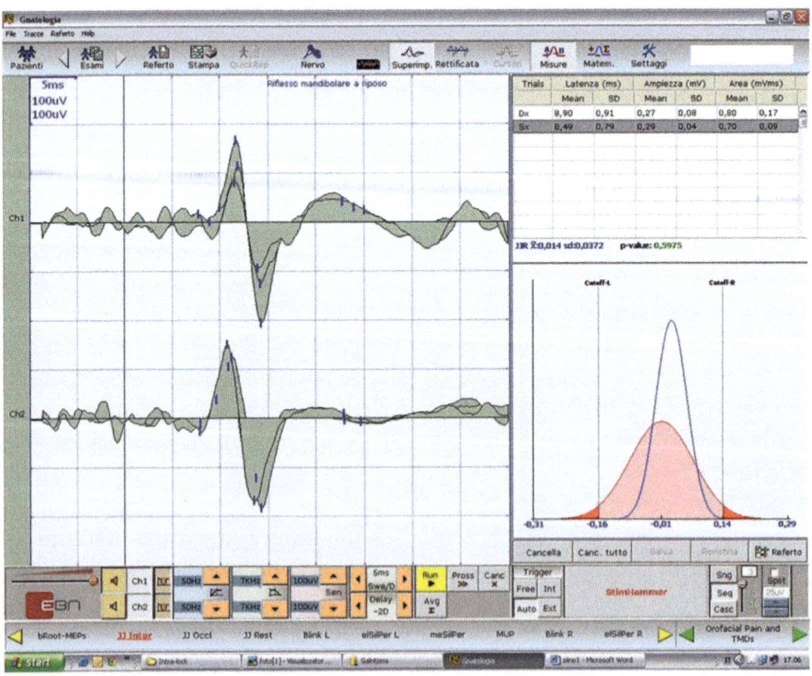

Figure 6.8 The amplitude symmetry and functional symmetry Gaussian curve derived from $_{ip}$JJ of a healthy patient.

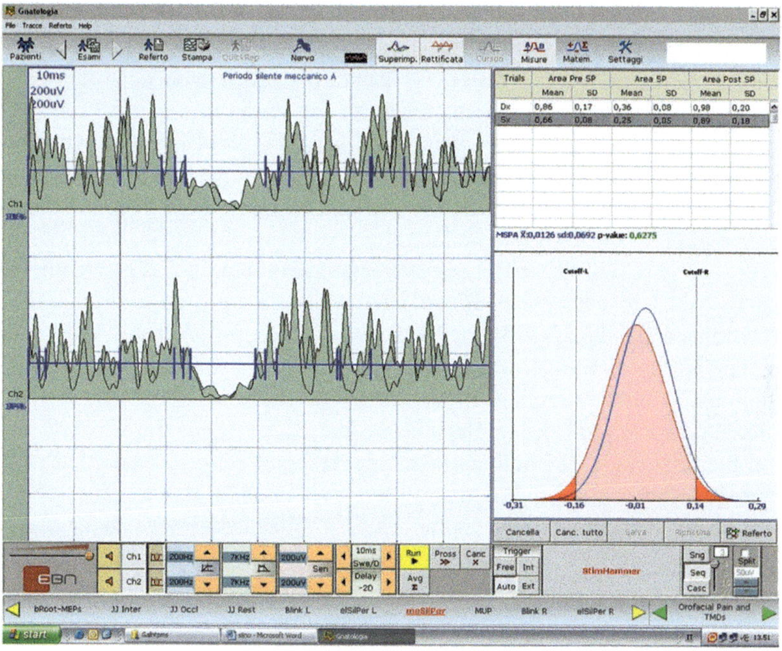

Figure 6.9 The amplitude symmetry and functional symmetry Gaussian curve derived from the MSP.

In conclusion, this paradigm has been developed to quantify the trigeminal anatomic symmetry and refer to it, the jaw reflex responses coming from various positions and level of the bite of the mandible.

Obviously, when both the organic and functional Gaussian curves of symmetry overlap, then the occlusal loads are distributed in a symmetrical, stable, and simultaneous manner, which demonstrates maximum efficiency of the masticatory system.

Nevertheless, some questions arise:

1. Is it desirable to obtain similar results for patients undergoing implant-prosthetic rehabilitation?
2. Is there any way to determine a symmetric, stable, and simultaneous centric occlusion in the implant-prosthetic rehabilitation patient with immediate loading?

The answer to the first question is "Yes." Despite the absence of periodontal receptors in implant rehabilitation, the trigeminal reflexes remain intact and symmetrical. This means that the peripheral input should be carefully considered in managing the occlusal scheme during implantoprosthetic rehabilitation especially in immediate implant loading rehabilitation.

It is desirable that the electrophysiological responses, as discussed previously for healthy subjects, are symmetrical because this event would indicate a symmetry, synchronicity, and stability of the occlusal position or centric occlusion. The symmetric, synchronous, and stable occlusal position in centric occlusion would avoid excessive and asymmetric height of some cusps and consequently avoid any overloading of individual implants.

A series of articles has described the influence of experimental occlusal overload on peri-implantitis in monkeys (*Macaca fascicularis*). In the first article of this series, it was reported that bone resorption was not observed around implants when occlusal trauma was produced by a superstructure that was in supraocclusal contact with an excess occlusal height of approximately 100 μm provided there was no inflammation in the peri-implant tissue [65].

In the second part of the study, experimental inflammation was created in the peri-implant tissue, and occlusal overload was produced by a superstructure with an excess occlusal height of 100 μm. Notable bone resorption was observed around the implant with the passage of time. These results suggested that, also to the control of inflammation in peri-implant tissue, traumatic occlusion may play a role in the bone breakdown around the implant in the presence of peri-implant inflammation [66]. In the final study, the authors investigated the effect of exerting various levels of traumatic force with inflammation-free peri-implant tissue upon bone level changes around implants. The supraoccluding prostheses were defined as being excessively high by 100, 180, and 250 μm. The results elucidated that bone resorption around implants tended to increase when the excessive height of the superstructure was 180 μm or more. This suggests that the threshold of the excessive height of the superstructures at which peri-implant tissue breakdown may start is approximately 180 μm [67]. Therefore, there is a real possibility of bone resorption occurring around the implants from excessive occlusal trauma, even when no inflammation is present within the peri-implant tissue.

At this point, centric occlusion and the occlusal contacts come into play in a predominant way and the biomechanical features of occlusal contacts are important in understanding the contributory role of occlusion in masticatory function. Cusp-fossa contact is the typical pattern of occlusion between upper and lower teeth. This includes static relations, such as during clenching and dynamic relations when mandibular tooth contact in function along the maxillary occlusal pathways, as during mastication.

During clenching in the maximum intercuspal (ICP) position, cuspal inclines may take the role of distributing the occlusal forces in multidirections. This helps prevent excessive point pressures on each tooth. During chewing movement on the functional side, the mandible moves slightly from buccal through the maximum ICP to the contralateral side. The part of the chewing cycle where occlusal contacts occur and the pathways taken by the mandible with teeth in occlusal contact are determined by the morphology and position of the teeth. The degree of contact is associated with the activity of the jaw muscles. In conclusion, in addition to the standard occlusal concepts of centric relation/centric occlusion and group function/cuspid protection relation, biomechanics in static and dynamic cusp-fossa relationships should be assessed to develop an understanding of occlusal harmony. Such harmony should include no interfering or deflective contacts during functional occlusal contact [68–70].

Therefore, the question arises: Is there any means of determining a symmetric, synchronous, and stable centric occlusion in the implant-prosthetic rehabilitation for immediate loading of implants?

We can answer that currently, through trigeminal electrophysiological innovative paradigm, this goal can now be achieved through an unconventional centric relation recording called neuro-evoked centric relation used in the masticatory rehabilitation using the $_b$R-MEPs.

6.4 Neuro-evoked centric relation

The NGF paradigm relating to the neuro-evoked centric relation entirely changes the concept of interpretation of centric occlusal registrations being based on a vector trigeminal neuromotor phenomenon. In doing so, it bypasses the conventional methods of kinematic centers (KC) and/or techniques such as transcutaneous electric neural stimulation (TENS) or myomonitor. Indeed, both methods include specific limitations and errors that can trigger an irritative spine in the implant-prosthetic rehabilitative processes, particularly in immediate loading implant cases. The KC, for example, has been proposed as a standardized reference point to represent condylar movements of the TMJ [71,72]. The KC has been presented as being situated in the center of a spherical condyle [73], and researchers thought it to be the only condylar point performing solely translatory movements "parallel" to the articular eminence during mandibular movements [72], with trajectories allegedly showing the smallest variability [74].

The KC trajectories were also believed to reflect variations in intra-articular distances [75] because during symmetric unloaded opening/closing movements, the opening trajectories were closer to the articular eminence than were the closing ones.

Such studies, as well as those using other condylar reference points, have the major drawback of being performed without relating the trajectories to the shape of the fossa. Therefore, the anatomical and functional significance of the kinematic center remains obscure, and it seems premature to infer variations in intra-articular distances solely from the trajectories of the KC as proposed [75].

Dynamic stereometry permits the 3D reconstruction of the anatomy of the TMJ and its animation with real kinematics acquired with 6 degrees of freedom [76]. The system, therefore, allows the movement of the whole condyle within the fossa to be visualized and variations in the true distances between the condyle and fossa surfaces to be measured as movement progresses [77–79]. Thus, the system permits the elucidation of the significance of the KC because it relates its trajectories during any mandibular movement to the joint anatomy.

Gallo et al. [80] tested whether the KC lies in a peculiar anatomical point and whether its trajectory reflects intra-articular distance. In 11 asymptomatic individuals (seven females, four males, aged 24–37 years), four opening/closures and four protrusion/retrusions were tracked with dynamic stereometry. In a 3D lattice (0.5 mm grid) constructed solidly around each condyle, the KC was the point with maximal cross-correlation between opening–closing and protrusion–retrusion paths. KC trajectories were more cranial on closing than on opening, consistent with intra-articular distances being smaller on closing than on opening. However, KCs were never located on condylar main axes (distance, 4.5 ± 2.9 mm), and they did tnot coincide with points best-approximating fossa shapes (distance, 12.5 ± 6.4 mm). The KC's anatomical and functional significance, therefore, appears to be highly questionable.

Regarding myomonitor in dental practice, the use of TENS appears to be limited to the alleviation of fatigue and pain from the jaw muscles and the establishment of contact as well as noncontact postural positions of the mandible [81−83]. Concerning the mandibular contact position created by TENS, it was the aim of these researchers to determine the mechanism by which the myomonitor instrument causes muscle contraction. Because the shortest latency of the masseteric H-reflex is 4.60 ms, the authors concluded that masseteric motor nerves are directly stimulated as a so-called M-response. Consequently, the results and conclusions of these studies are essentially the same as those of Dao et al. [81], in that TENS caused direct activation of alpha-motor nerves without eliciting reflex responses. These authors confirmed that the mandibular contact positions elicited by TENS are approximately 2 mm anterior to the most retruded contact position of the mandible, also referred to as forced centric relation occlusion.

This anterior position of 2 mm is precisely the result of the direct stimulation, or so-called M-response, only of the masseter muscle so that it has a protrusive component. To reach the infratemporal fossa and/or oval foramen to depolarize muscles innervated by trigeminal nerve would evoke a root response. To obtain this target, we require a high voltage electric stimulus with a short square wave of roughly 100 ns.

Hence, the first procedure is to check for saturation of the motor trigeminal fiber response or root-MEPs. At 20, 30, and 40 mA we can see a recorded onset latency of 2.4, 2.4, and 2.3 ms, respectively, and even increasing the amperage we observe a decrease in latency of 2.1 ms to 50 mA, 2 ms to 70 mA, and 1.9 ms to 80, 90 and 100 mA (Fig. 6.10).

These differences in latency up to the maximal current density depend on the capacitive components of the tissues encountered by the intracranial current flow [59,60,84]. The EMG amplitude saturation of the trigeminal motor root is the first step to being

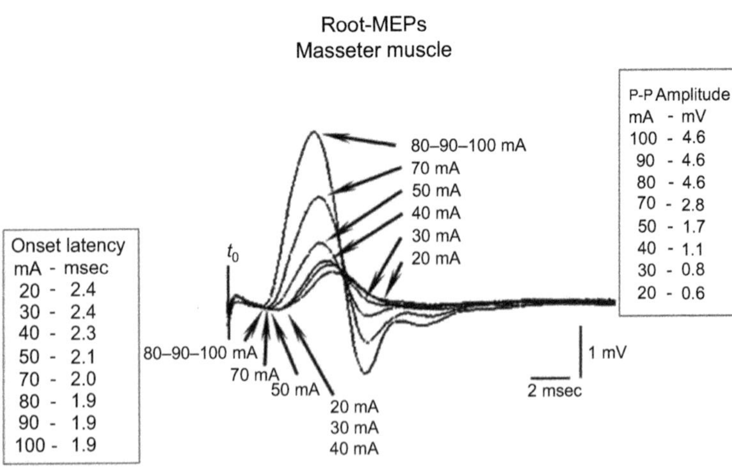

Figure 6.10 Signal saturation of the root with respect to latency and amplitude.

performed, even before clinically interpreting a delay in latency and to perform a symmetric elevation in centric occlusion of the mandible.

In fact, at delivered amperage of 80, 90, and 100 mA, the P–P amplitude remains at 4.6 mV. The amplitude value of 4.6 mV and the onset latency of 1.9 ms correspond to the maximum absolute values of neural energy elicited by the motor of the trigeminal nervous system and the spatial result corresponds to a coactivation of closer muscles innervated by the trigeminal system [57]. Of course, the amplitude can be chosen to be equivalent to the integral area, depending on the purpose of the study.

After this electrophysiological scheme, to determine a symmetric, stable, and synchronous centric occlusion by avoiding the discrepancies and external disturbances transferred from manual maneuvers by the operator or incongruous maneuvers such as myomonitor, we developed an electrophysiological method capable of determining a physiological centric relation called "neuro-evoked centric relation."

To explain this neuro-evoked centric relation, we present a case report in which the added value of this innovative and unconventional implant-prosthetic rehabilitation tool is demonstrated.

6.5 Case reports

6.5.1 Case report in the delayed loading procedures

As you can see in Fig. 6.11 it shows an implant-prosthetic rehabilitation using eight NobelReplace implants of 3.5 and 4.3 mm diameter placed in the maxilla through a NobelGuide surgical procedure (NobelBiocare, Gothenburg, Sweden), in which the correlation between neurophysiological trigeminal responses, according to the paradigm NGF, and occlusal adjustments can be appreciated. Fig. 6.11(a–c) reveals the surgical procedures and finalization of the rehabilitation framework in zirconia ceramics. In Fig. 6.11(d), the centric occlusal contacts are marked through blue articulation paper and for disclusion contacts, in red. The corresponding trigeminal reflex responses are also presented and a significant asymmetry of jaw jerk is evident.

Fig. 6.11(g–i) shows the coupling between the occlusal parameters and the neurophysiological symmetries responding to the requirements dictated by the NGF paradigm. An occlusal adjustment resulting from sandblasting the occlusal surfaces is clearly visible in the new occlusal contacts marked in blue, which were previously absent. The new contacts maintain a disclusive path and we lay out how the system responds with the marked trigeminal symmetry of the JJ amplitude and the silent period. A further confirmation is deduced from the overlapping of the organic and functional Gaussian curves symmetry.

This trigeminal neurophysiological symmetry (NGF paradigm) confirms, with irrefutable numerical data, that the occlusal loads are redistributed in a symmetrical, synchronous, and stable manner over the whole occlusal arch. The maximum efficiency of an implant-prosthetic rehabilitation performed through a detailed surgical primary stability (press-fit procedure) and an occlusal primary stability (NGF paradigm) would ensure the success of the implant-prosthetic rehabilitation, responding to the dictates of a "biological complex system."

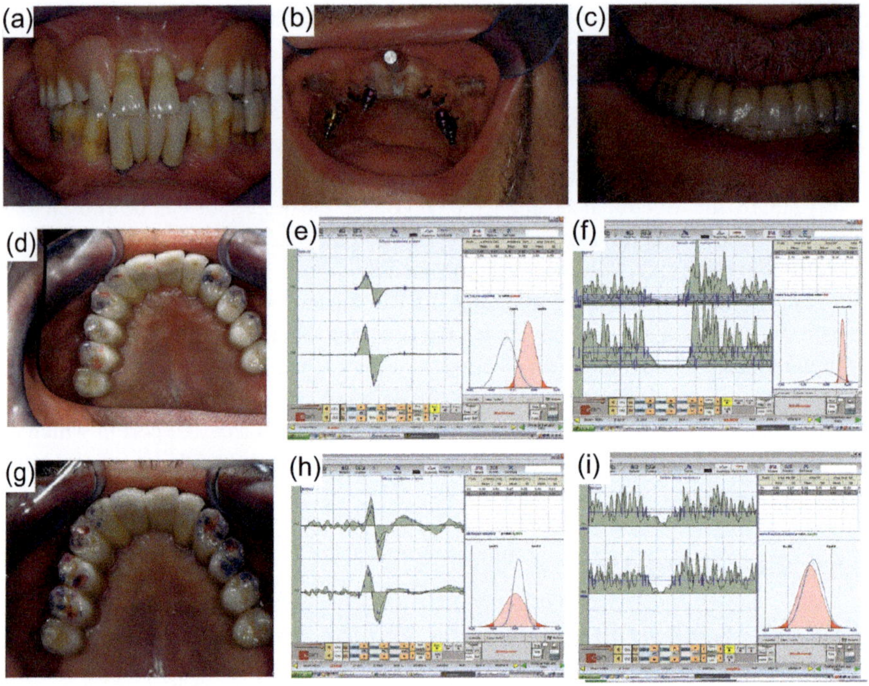

Figure 6.11 The figures show the correlation between the occlusal adjustments and neurophysiological trigeminal responses, according to the NGF paradigm, during an implantprosthetic rehabilitation. (a–c) Rehabilitative procedures; (d–f) trigeminal electrophysiology before occlusal adjustments; (g–i) trigeminal electrophysiology after occlusal adjustments.

In the next case report, an implantoprosthetic rehabilitative procedure with immediate loading was performed with the determination of neuro-evoked centric relation and the neurophysiological control already mentioned.

6.5.2 Case report in the immediate loading procedures

The patient had undergone a NobelGuide-guided surgical procedure for the placement of six implants, NobelReplace narrow (NobelBiocare, Gothenburg, Sweden), and extraction of teeth 11 and 21. A prosthesis was planned with immediate loading in 24 h following surgery. Fig. 6.12(a) shows that the first implant-prosthetic rehabilitative step was to reach the goal of primary stability by distributing the strain and stress equally on the trabeculae and cortical bone. To avoid cortical interference, it is better to prepare previously the cortical bone volume through cortical drills and to check the maximum insertion torque by dimensional screw tap.

After this first step of preparing the cortical volume, we proceeded to dimensioning of the trabecular bone volume with appropriate undersize procedures to achieve the right balance of " differentiated interference fit."

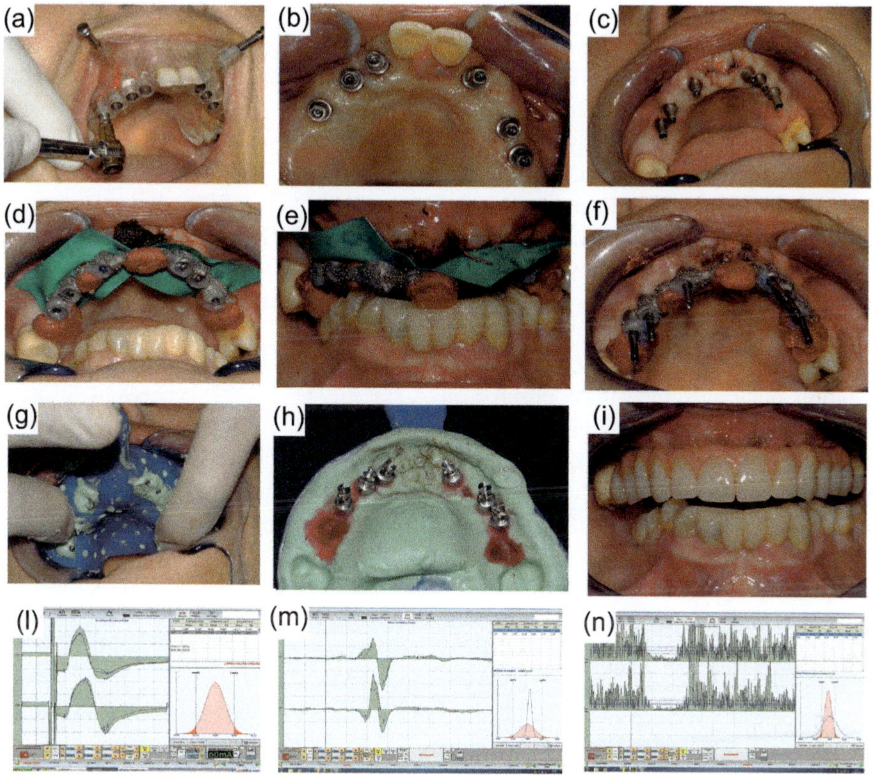

Figure 6.12 Implantoprosthetic rehabilitative procedures in an immediate loading it is not clear (a–i) and neurophysiological trigeminal correlation (l–n).

Fig. 6.12(b) shows the six provisional abutments positioned on the multiunits, previously modified in the laboratory based on the master cast that was produced from the surgical mask. The surgical intervention was then completed with the tooth extractions (Fig. 6.12(c)).

However, the primary stability of bone–implant interface is static, therefore, not subjected to dynamic, extra-axial, and extra-symmetrical occlusal loads, as previously mentioned. In the case of implant-prosthetic rehabilitation through the immediate load, it is necessary to distribute the occlusal loads, originated by neuromotor recruitment activity of masticatory muscles, in a symmetrical, synchronous, and stable manner. A spatial and temporal asynchronous contact phase in maximum intercuspation cannot be permitted. Therefore, the neurognathological functions of the primary stability phase determining the neuro-evoked centric relation is introduced. To reach this target, it is necessary to complete the surgical phase so far performed by inserting the chrome-cobalt structure previously fabricated in the laboratory on the master cast model from the NobelGuide surgical mask (Fig. 6.12(d)). Thereafter, centric registration was recorded by positioning self-curing resin at predefined areas where the antagonist teeth would contact during mandibular closure caused by bilateral motor evoked potentials of the trigeminal roots called neuro-evoked centric relation (Fig. 6.12(e)). This centric registration technique produces a symmetric, synchronous, and stable jaw elevation. The neuro-evoked centric relation through this method simulates the natural neuromuscular coactivation of chewing functions.

Because structural stability is guaranteed by the abutments cemented to the chrome-cobalt structure, once the neuromotor primary stability is performed, the next step was to transfer the whole structure to the laboratory. To obtain a defined master cast, the abutment screws were replaced by guide pins (Fig. 6.12(f)).

A detailed impression was then taken and transferred to the laboratory for the final technical stages and delivery of the prosthesis 24 h after the surgical intervention (Fig. 6.12(g) and (h)).

Fig. 6.12(i) shows the implant-prosthetic rehabilitation 24 h after the surgical intervention, but it must meet the occlusal primary stability requirements checked through a careful control of the trigeminal reflexes.

During the first days of healing, the nociceptive system physiologically tends to inhibit or otherwise reduce the entity of neuromotor recruitment. However, an occlusal discrepancy greater than 180 nm in the height of cusps or asynchronous contacts, as previously mentioned [54], could result in overload, bone damage, and implant instability. Therefore, it is necessary that the trigeminal reflexes respond symmetrically.

Fig. 6.12(l) shows the individual symmetry of $_{b}$R-MEPs that corresponds to an organic Gaussian curve considered as "normalization factor," whereas Fig. 6.12(m) and (n) shows the functional symmetry of JJ and MSP.

The perfect overlapping of the Organic and Functional Gaussian Curve implies that a balanced occlusion has been created that can distribute the occlusal load symmetrically, synchronously and stably across all the implants. Also, this takes into account that the maximum plateau of the motoneural recruitment is obtained in maximum intercuspation, whereas the occlusal loads decrease significantly even at 1 mm of laterality.

The EMG traces of the mechanical silent period (Fig. 6.12 (n)) are divided in two sections called preanalysis and postanalysis. The first is not contaminated by sensorimotor input, while the second one includes the facilitatory and inhibitory processes from the central and peripheral drive. Also for the mechanical silent period the organic and functional Gaussian curves appear overlapped. This neurophysiological overlapping indicates an optimized symmetry of the occlusal load.

6.6 Conclusions

In this chapter, we have focused on primary implant stability, not only from a biomechanical bone–implant perspective, but also taking into account neuromotor function that could generate occlusal dynamic, asymmetric, and extra-axial loads.

If the "differentiated press-fit" achieves a distribution of the torque and thereby of stress and strain within all the alveolar bone in contact with the implant, through neuro-evoked centric relation and comparison of electrophysiological trigeminal functional symmetries (functional) with organic ones (anatomic), we can at least quantify the degree of the distribution of occlusal loads on the whole implant-prosthesis rehabilitation.

References

[1] Kanamaru T, Aihara K. Stochastic synchrony of chaos in a pulse-coupled neural network with both chemical and electrical synapses among inhibitory neurons. Neural Comput 2008;20:1951−72.
[2] Lagang M, Srinivasan L. Stochastic optimal control as a theory of brain-machine interface operation. Neural Comput 2013;25:374−417.
[3] Nelken I. Analysis of the activity of single neurons in stochastic settings. Biol Cybern 1988;59:201−15.
[4] Savtchenko LP, Gogan P, Korogod SM, Tyc-Dumont S. Imaging stochastic spatial variability of active channel clusters during excitation of single neurons. Neurosci Res 2001; 39:431−46.
[5] Usami H, Tsukada M, Sato R. The probabilistic and stochastic analysis of the mutual inhibitory network with the mathematical models of single neurons (author's transl). Iyodenshi To Seitai Kogaku 1978;16:169−76.
[6] Yamamoto T, Smith CE, Suzuki Y, Kiyono K, Tanahashi T, Sakoda S, et al. Universal and individual characteristics of postural sway during quiet standing in healthy young adults. Physiol Rep 2015;3.
[7] Tommasini SM, Wearne SL, Hof PR, Jepsen KJ. Percolation theory relates corticocancellous architecture to mechanical function in vertebrae of inbred mouse strains. Bone 2008;42:743−50.
[8] Jepsen KJ. Systems analysis of bone. Wiley Interdiscip Rev Syst Biol Med 2009;1:73−88.
[9] Kulterer B, Friedl G, Jandrositz A, Sanchez-Cabo F, Prokesch A, Paar C, et al. Gene expression profiling of human mesenchymal stem cells derived from bone marrow during expansion and osteoblast differentiation. BMC Genomics 2007;8:70.
[10] Rachmiel A, Leiser Y. The molecular and cellular events that take place during craniofacial distraction osteogenesis. Plast Reconstr Surg Glob Open 2014;2:e98.
[11] Leucht P, Monica SD, Temiyasathit S, Lenton K, Manu A, Longaker MT, et al. Primary cilia act as mechanosensors during bone healing around an implant. Med Eng Phys 2013; 35:392−402.
[12] Liu B, Chen S, Cheng D, Jing W, Helms JA. Primary cilia integrate hedgehog and Wnt signaling during tooth development. J Dent Res 2014;93:475−82.
[13] Wazen RM, Currey JA, Guo H, Brunski JB, Helms JA, Nanci A. Micromotion-induced strain fields influence early stages of repair at bone-implant interfaces. Acta Biomater 2013;9:6663−74.
[14] Bandyopadhyay A, Espana F, Balla VK, Bose S, Ohgami Y, Davies NM. Influence of porosity on mechanical properties and in vivo response of Ti6Al4V implants. Acta Biomater 2010;6:1640−8.
[15] Tomisa AP, Launey ME, Lee JS, Mankani MH, Wegst UG, Saiz E. Nanotechnology approaches to improve dental implants. Int J Oral Maxillofac Implants 2011;26(Suppl.): 25−44. discussion 45−9.
[16] Chang M, Chronopoulos V, Mattheos N. Impact of excessive occlusal load on successfully-osseointegrated dental implants: a literature review. J Invest Clin Dent 2013; 4:142−50.
[17] Isidor F. Loss of osseointegration caused by occlusal load of oral implants. A clinical and radiographic study in monkeys. Clin Oral Implants Res 1996;7:143−52.
[18] Gross MD. Occlusion in implant dentistry. A review of the literature of prosthetic determinants and current concepts. Aust Dent J 2008;53(Suppl. 1):S60−8.

[19] Kasai K, Takayama Y, Yokoyama A. Distribution of occlusal forces during occlusal adjustment of dental implant prostheses: a nonlinear finite element analysis considering the capacity for displacement of opposing teeth and implants. Int J Oral Maxillofac Implants 2012;27:329–35.
[20] Simeone P, Trerotola M, Urbanella A, Lattanzio R, Ciavardelli D, Di Giuseppe F, et al. A unique four-hub protein cluster associates to glioblastoma progression. PLoS One 2014; 9:e103030.
[21] Janovic A, Saveljic I, Vukicevic A, Nikolic D, Rakocevic Z, Jovicic G, et al. Occlusal load distribution through the cortical and trabecular bone of the human mid-facial skeleton in natural dentition: a three-dimensional finite element study. Ann Anat 2015; 197:16–23.
[22] Ishigaki S, Nakano T, Yamada S, Nakamura T, Takashima F. Biomechanical stress in bone surrounding an implant under simulated chewing. Clin Oral Implants Res 2003;14: 97–102.
[23] Lai HC, Zhang ZY, Zhang BW, Zhang JZ, Zhang FQ, Xue M. Characteristics of stress distribution on bone adjacent to implants under three different loading directions. Shanghai Kou Qiang Yi Xue 2002;11:253–5.
[24] Pellizzer EP, Falcon-Antenucci RM, De Carvalho PS, Sanchez DM, Rinaldi GA, De Aguirre CC, et al. Influence of implant angulation with different crowns on stress distribution. J Craniofac Surg 2011;22:434–7.
[25] Al-Sukhun J, Kelleway J, Helenius M. Development of a three-dimensional finite element model of a human mandible containing endosseous dental implants. I. Mathematical validation and experimental verification. J Biomed Mater Res A 2007;80:234–46.
[26] Al-Sukhun J, Lindqvist C, Helenius M. Development of a three-dimensional finite element model of a human mandible containing endosseous dental implants. II. Variables affecting the predictive behavior of a finite element model of a human mandible. J Biomed Mater Res A 2007;80:247–56.
[27] Field C, Li Q, Li W, Swain M. Biomechanical response in mandibular bone due to mastication loading on 3-Unit fixed partial dentures. J Dent Biomech 2010;2010: 902537.
[28] Muhlberger G, Svejda M, Lottersberger C, Emshoff R, Putz R, Kuhn V. Mineralization density and apparent density in mandibular condyle bone. Oral Surg Oral Med Oral Pathol Oral Radiol Endod 2009;107:573–9.
[29] Schwartz-Dabney CL, Dechow PC. Edentulation alters material properties of cortical bone in the human mandible. J Dent Res 2002;81:613–7.
[30] Bonnet AS, Postaire M, Lipinski P. Biomechanical study of mandible bone supporting a four-implant retained bridge: finite element analysis of the influence of bone anisotropy and foodstuff position. Med Eng Phys 2009;31:806–15.
[31] Park JK, Choi JU, Jeon YC, Choi KS, Jeong CM. Effects of abutment screw coating on implant preload. J Prosthodont 2010;19:458–64.
[32] Limbert G, Van Lierde C, Muraru OL, Walboomers XF, Frank M, Hansson S, et al. Trabecular bone strains around a dental implant and associated micromotions—a micro-CT-based three-dimensional finite element study. J Biomech 2010;43:1251–61.
[33] Natali AN, Carniel EL, Pavan PG. Dental implants press fit phenomena: biomechanical analysis considering bone inelastic response. Dent Mater 2009;25:573–81.
[34] Frisardi G, Barone S, Razionale AV, Paoli A, Frisardi F, Tullio A, et al. Biomechanics of the press-fit phenomenon in dental implantology: an image-based finite element analysis. Head Face Med 2012;8:18.

[35] Bishop NE, Hohn JC, Rothstock S, Damm NB, Morlock MM. The influence of bone damage on press-fit mechanics. J Biomech 2014;47:1472–8.
[36] Lakes RS, Katz JL. Viscoelastic properties of wet cortical bone—II. Relaxation mechanisms. J Biomech 1979;12:679–87.
[37] Lakes RS, Katz JL. Viscoelastic properties of wet cortical bone—III. A non-linear constitutive equation. J Biomech 1979;12:689–98.
[38] Lakes RS, Katz JL, Sternstein SS. Viscoelastic properties of wet cortical bone—I. Torsional and biaxial studies. J Biomech 1979;12:657–78.
[39] Brown CU, Norman TL, Kish 3rd VL, Gruen TA, Blaha JD. Time-dependent circumferential deformation of cortical bone upon internal radial loading. J Biomech Eng 2002; 124:456–61.
[40] Shultz TR, Blaha JD, Gruen TA, Norman TL. Cortical bone viscoelasticity and fixation strength of press-fit femoral stems: finite element model. J Biomech Eng 2006; 128:7–12.
[41] Degidi M, Daprile G, Piattelli A. RFA values of implants placed in sinus grafted and nongrafted sites after 6 and 12 months. Clin Implant Dent Relat Res 2009;11:178–82.
[42] Tabassum A, Walboomers XF, Wolke JG, Meijer GJ, Jansen JA. Bone particles and the undersized surgical technique. J Dent Res 2010;89:581–6.
[43] Gabet Y, Kohavi D, Voide R, Mueller TL, Muller R, Bab I. Endosseous implant anchorage is critically dependent on mechanostructural determinants of peri-implant bone trabeculae. J Bone Min Res 2010;25:575–83.
[44] Holmgren EP, Seckinger RJ, Kilgren LM, Mante F. Evaluating parameters of osseointegrated dental implants using finite element analysis—a two-dimensional comparative study examining the effects of implant diameter, implant shape, and load direction. J Oral Implantol 1998;24:80–8.
[45] Demenko V, Linetskiy I, Nesvit K, Shevchenko A. Ultimate masticatory force as a criterion in implant selection. J Dent Res 2011;90:1211–5.
[46] Koolstra JH, Van Eijden TM. Three-dimensional dynamical capabilities of the human masticatory muscles. J Biomech 1999;32:145–52.
[47] Wakeling JM, Nigg BM. Modification of soft tissue vibrations in the leg by muscular activity. J Appl Physiol (1985) 2001;90:412–20.
[48] Koolstra JH, Van Eijden TM. Biomechanical analysis of jaw-closing movements. J Dent Res 1995;74:1564–70.
[49] Gibbs CH, Mahan PE, Lundeen HC, Brehnan K, Walsh EK, Sinkewiz SL, et al. Occlusal forces during chewing—influences of biting strength and food consistency. J Prosthet Dent 1981;46:561–7.
[50] Eskitascioglu G, Usumez A, Sevimay M, Soykan E, Unsal E. The influence of occlusal loading location on stresses transferred to implant-supported prostheses and supporting bone: a three-dimensional finite element study. J Prosthet Dent 2004;91:144–50.
[51] Kimoto K, Ono Y, Tachibana A, Hirano Y, Otsuka T, Ohno A, et al. Chewing-induced regional brain activity in edentulous patients who received mandibular implant-supported overdentures: a preliminary report. J Prosthodont Res 2011;55:89–97.
[52] Onozuka M, Fujita M, Watanabe K, Hirano Y, Niwa M, Nishiyama K, et al. Mapping brain region activity during chewing: a functional magnetic resonance imaging study. J Dent Res 2002;81:743–6.
[53] Onozuka M, Fujita M, Watanabe K, Hirano Y, Niwa M, Nishiyama K, et al. Age-related changes in brain regional activity during chewing: a functional magnetic resonance imaging study. J Dent Res 2003;82:657–60.

[54] Barker AT, Jalinous R, Freeston IL. Non-invasive magnetic stimulation of human motor cortex. Lancet 1985;1:1106–7.
[55] Lund JP, Kolta A. Generation of the central masticatory pattern and its modification by sensory feedback. Dysphagia 2006;21:167–74.
[56] Merton PA, Morton HB. Stimulation of the cerebral cortex in the intact human subject. Nature 1980;285:227.
[57] Frisardi G. The use of transcranial stimulation in the fabrication of an occlusal splint. J Prosthet Dent 1992;68:355–60.
[58] Frisardi G, Ravazzani P, Tognola G, Grandori F. Electric versus magnetic transcranial stimulation of the trigeminal system in healthy subjects. Clinical applications in gnathology. J Oral Rehabil 1997;24:920–8.
[59] Windhoff M, Opitz A, Thielscher A. Electric field calculations in brain stimulation based on finite elements: an optimized processing pipeline for the generation and usage of accurate individual head models. Hum Brain Mapp 2013;34:923–35.
[60] Opitz A, Windhoff M, Heidemann RM, Turner R, Thielscher A. How the brain tissue shapes the electric field induced by transcranial magnetic stimulation. Neuroimage 2011; 58:849–59.
[61] Shigenaga Y, Yoshida A, Mitsuhiro Y, Tsuru K, Doe K. Morphological and functional properties of trigeminal nucleus oralis neurons projecting to the trigeminal motor nucleus of the cat. Brain Res 1988;461:143–9.
[63] Yoshida A, Yamamoto M, Moritani M, Fukami H, Bae YC, Chang Z, et al. Bilateral projection of functionally characterized trigeminal oralis neurons to trigeminal motoneurons in cats. Brain Res 2005;1036:208–12.
[62] Nakamura Y, Nagashima H, Mori S. Bilateral effects of the afferent impulses from the masseteric muscle on the trigeminal motoneuron of the cat. Brain Res 1973;57:15–27.
[64] Frisardi G, Chessa G, Sau G, Frisardi F. Trigeminal electrophysiology: a 2 x 2 matrix model for differential diagnosis between temporomandibular disorders and orofacial pain. BMC Musculoskelet Disord 2010;11:141.
[65] Miyata T, Kobayashi Y, Araki H, Motomura Y, Shin K. The influence of controlled occlusal overload on peri-implant tissue: a histologic study in monkeys. Int J Oral Maxillofac Implants 1998;13:677–83.
[66] Miyata T, Kobayashi Y, Araki H, Ohto T, Shin K. The influence of controlled occlusal overload on peri-implant tissue. Part 3: a histologic study in monkeys. Int J Oral Maxillofac Implants 2000;15:425–31.
[67] Miyata T, Kobayashi Y, Araki H, Ohto T, Shin K. The influence of controlled occlusal overload on peri-implant tissue. Part 4: a histologic study in monkeys. Int J Oral Maxillofac Implants 2002;17:384–90.
[68] Hidaka O, Iwasaki M, Saito M, Morimoto T. Influence of clenching intensity on bite force balance, occlusal contact area, and average bite pressure. J Dent Res 1999;78:1336–44.
[69] Kim Y, Oh TJ, Misch CE, Wang HL. Occlusal considerations in implant therapy: clinical guidelines with biomechanical rationale. Clin Oral Implants Res 2005;16:26–35.
[70] Wang M, Mehta N. A possible biomechanical role of occlusal cusp-fossa contact relationships. J Oral Rehabil 2013;40:69–79.
[71] Naeije M. Measurement of condylar motion: a plea for the use of the condylar kinematic centre. J Oral Rehabil 2003;30:225–30.
[72] Yatabe M, Zwijnenburg A, Megens CC, Naeije M. The kinematic center: a reference for condylar movements. J Dent Res 1995;74:1644–8.
[73] Huddleston Slater JJ, Visscher CM, Lobbezoo F, Naeije M. The intra-articular distance within the TMJ during free and loaded closing movements. J Dent Res 1999;78:1815–20.

[74] Yatabe M, Zwijnenburg A, Megens CC, Naeije M. Movements of the mandibular condyle kinematic center during jaw opening and closing. J Dent Res 1997;76:714–9.
[75] Huddleston Slater JJ, Lobbezoo F, Naeije M. Mandibular movement characteristics of an anterior disc displacement with reduction. J Orofac Pain 2002;16:135–42.
[76] Krebs M, Gallo LM, Airoldi RL, Palla S. A new method for three-dimensional reconstruction and animation of the temporomandibular joint. Ann Acad Med Singap 1995;24: 11–6.
[77] Fushima K, Gallo LM, Krebs M, Palla S. Analysis of the TMJ intraarticular space variation: a non-invasive insight during mastication. Med Eng Phys 2003;25:181–90.
[78] Gallo LM, Nickel JC, Iwasaki LR, Palla S. Stress-field translation in the healthy human temporomandibular joint. J Dent Res 2000;79:1740–6.
[79] Gossi DB, Gallo LM, Bahr E, Palla S. Dynamic intra-articular space variation in clicking TMJs. J Dent Res 2004;83:480–4.
[80] Gallo LM, Gossi DB, Colombo V, Palla S. Relationship between kinematic center and TMJ anatomy and function. J Dent Res 2008;87:726–30.
[81] Dao TT, Feine JS, Lund JP. Can electrical stimulation be used to establish a physiologic occlusal position? J Prosthet Dent 1988;60:509–14.
[82] Kawazoe Y, Kotani H, Maetani T, Yatani H, Hamada T. Integrated electromyographic activity and biting force during rapid isometric contraction of fatigued masseter muscle in man. Arch Oral Biol 1981;26:795–801.
[83] Konchak PA, Thomas NR, Lanigan DT, Devon RM. Freeway space measurement using mandibular kinesiograph and EMG before and after TENS. Angle Orthod 1988;58: 343–50.
[84] Thielscher A, Opitz A, Windhoff M. Impact of the gyral geometry on the electric field induced by transcranial magnetic stimulation. Neuroimage 2011;54:234–43.

Clinical bone response to dental implant materials

7

O.T. Jensen
University of Utah School of Dentistry, Salt Lake City, UT, United States

Clinical bone response to surgically placed dental implants at the time of or soon after insertion (preosseointegration) relates to biomechanical factors. This would include surgical insertion technique, such as drilling and nondrilling approaches, bone quality factors, including bone density, and use of adjacent graft material and device capabilities related to implant force generation upon placement as part of early- and late-stage healing biocompatibility. Each of these three aspects is strategically applied to obtain initial primary stability, which must persist through the demineralization phase of bone injury, permitting implants depending on the surface topography to remain passive long enough for bone modeling to progress to a unifying callus and then onto load responsive (maintenance) osseointegration [1,2].

Following early bone modeling, at about 5 or 6 weeks, basic multicellular unit remodeling commences replacing woven bone with a more dense lamelized bone. The process of osseointegration continues to increase the bone mineral density proximate to the implant body for up to 2 years and it is proportionate to load as the *mechanostat* seeks to minimize stress and strain caused by the lack of stress dampening of the titanium root analog. A "steady state" of osseointegration is achieved where there is nearly equal gain and loss of mineral, without substantial change in volumetric bone mass. Unlike the relatively narrow lamina dura adjacent to a periodontal ligament (PDL) of a tooth, there is nearly direct bone contact—dense bone that may extend for several millimeters away from a titanium element—but no PDL-like space. Ankylotic bone response is a desired property of dental implant design and responsive biology. Interestingly, very long-term implants can sometimes have a hypodense area several millimeters away from the implants, suggestive of a relative stress-dampening capacity [3,4].

7.1 Bone response to dental implants

Early events for bone healing around a newly inserted implants are affected by the nanotechnology and perhaps bioactive chemical modifications of the titanium surfaces now "roughened" to increase the surface area and bioactivity for osteogenesis. Such treatments can significantly increase the osteogenic activity by inducing the focal adhesion development [5]. However, the basic early finding of bone modeling in the first few weeks of healing is described as contact osteogenesis and distance osteogenesis, both affected by implant surface tension and wettability [6]. In any case, a recent review noted

Bone Response to Dental Implant Materials. http://dx.doi.org/10.1016/B978-0-08-100287-2.00007-0

that the surgical injury of alveolar bone induces a cascade of healing events starting with the clot formation. When the inflammation is not present osseointegration is manifest by an increase in gene expression from osteogenesis, angiogenesis, and neurogenesis [7]. The rate of bone healing progression in animals demonstrates near complete healing by 4–6 weeks. In one dog model, the 1-week gap bone fill was about 5%, after 2 weeks about 30%, and after 3 weeks close to 50% [8]. Human healing rate is perhaps 1.5× slower. By 2 months, the dead bone is removed by osteoclasis or creeping substitution, so that in humans, nonvital or damaged bone in the site preparation is likely removed during woven bone formation at about 6 weeks [8]. One study, however, showed that the degradation of residual bone particles acts as a nidus for the new bone formation with osteoblasts sometimes lining particles as osteoid is formed and therefore nonvital bone is removed as a later event during remodeling [9].

Bone strain that is nonphysiologic or mildly overloading (about 2000–3000 microstrain) leads to the bone gain, which is manifested as hypermineralization or increased bone mineral content around an implant. Compared with a ligament attached tooth, the titanium bone screw is in a prolonged state of mild overload—the body is constantly increasing the bone mineral content until the system reaches a state of less strain near the physiological load (about 2000 microstrain). There is a narrow window, between 2000 and 3000 microstrain, where damaged bone is repairable, but above which it leads to the pathological overload and the bone repair mechanisms are overcome (Fig. 7.1). This concept is difficult to comprehend with fixed implant devices as

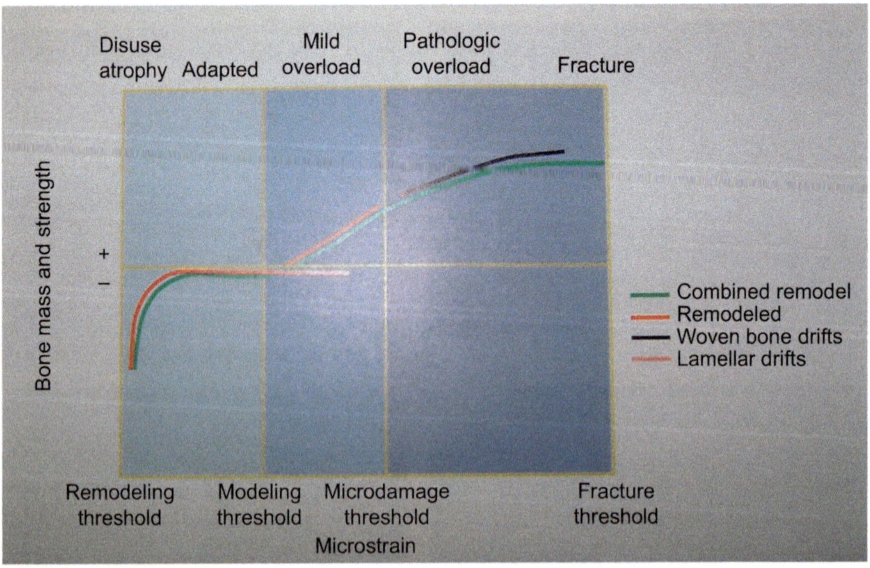

Figure 7.1 Bone response plotted by measuring bone gain or loss, which is a function of bone strength, against bone microstrain over time. The graphic is useful to visualize bone strength and mass changes that occur in dynamic living bone. (Disuse atrophy is about 50–150 microstrain; mild overload is about 2000–3000 microstrain and bone fracture is around 25,000 microstrain.)

dentists think in terms of teeth and avoidance of deflective contacts, particularly lateral loads as being detrimental to the bone–PDL–tooth interface. Although with oral implants, this is not the case. In fact, an example of this is lateral orthodontic force actually increasing the bone mineral density around an implant anchor. Bone strain should not exceed a threshold of force that might lead to microfractures that cannot be repaired physiologically, within the strain rate history. If it exceeds this threshold, it eventually leads to fatigue fracture–induced osteoclasis and the loss of bone mineral density. This rarely happens in dental implant constructions, but when it does marginal bone contact and osseointegration fail. Most often device mechanical failure precedes this event leading instead to component failure, or rarely, implant fixture fracture. A peri-implant lesion appears clinically as a peri-implantitis infection, bacteria being an opportunistic cofactor of the final throes of mechanical implant–bone contact failure [10,11].

Interestingly, the need for a certain number of millimeters of osseointegration has been shown to be counterintuitively small. That is, the implant root-form titanium screw need not be as long or as wide as a tooth root and by a long ways. In fact, the very first implants placed by Branemark were short implants 7–10 mm in length with perhaps only 5 mm of vertical osseointegration even after the long-term function in excess of 30 years. Short implants have been found to last as long as long implants [1]. The common use of short implants now suggest, once again, that tooth-oriented thinking does not apply to the titanium bone screw, which can replace teeth with perhaps as little as 4 mm of vertical height of osseointegration and still maintain the stability over time. So now, instead of implants being placed as tooth root analogs they are placed as fixed anchors of much reduced length such as 5–7 mm in length as the biomechanical capability of bone repair under load is sufficient for this length of implant. Furthermore, the implant is placed for each tooth unit lost and is not required biomechanically from the standpoint of the bone; now three or four implants (splinted) are commonly used to restore edentulous arches. As few as two implants, as small as 15–20 mm of total circumferential osseointegration, can restore a complete arch [12–14].

It is thought that as less as 16 mm of total cortical bone contact is sufficient in four implants for the immediate function restoration of the complete arch as evident by high levels of maxillary atrophy (Class C, Class D) using transsinus or zygomatic implants for immediate function. At some threshold minimum in both the mandible and the maxilla there is simply not enough cortex for immediate mechanical fixation function, and, therefore, the potential to progress toward osseointegration. This threshold is thought to be 4 mm of circumferential cortical bone per implant [15–19].

Once peri-implantitis infection progresses, unlike in periodontal disease, there is direct contact of the bacterial lesion to the underlying bone. Periodontal probing will extend all the way down to the bone unlike probing periodontal lesions around teeth, yet progressive bone loss is relatively slow due to lack of a PDL space. On the other hand, poor bone-to-implant contact (poor osseointegration) or implant dehiscence can lead to the rapid progression of the disease. Also, some rough surface peri-implant lesions progress more quickly than others in the presence of peri-implantitis [20].

In addition to the mechanical, the hematological response, including neurohumeral, immunological, and the blood clotting cascade, helps to determine whether or not the implant will progress toward intimate woven bone healing. For example, implant surfaces, which form intimate blood clot between the bone preparation and the newly inserted implant, form a greater percent of osseointegration than implant–bone interfaces that do not. Although, these are biological, nontechnical events, they are impacted by the clinical placement. Burning or overheating the bone will cause fibrinolysis of the clot and prevent the formation of osseointegration. So technical efforts can set in motion the healing events that prevent osseointegration.

Site preparation can be done by sequential drilling, blunt osteotome, or piezosurgery. The endpoint clinical bone response is similar, although the mechanism of healing is different. It is important to understand the difference in bone quality as dense bone, Type I bone, has no need for condensation or an underdrilling technique. Although less dense trabecular bone such as Type III bone is more conducive to bone condensation, underdrilling, or even addition of free graft material into the site preparation in order to get implant stability. It is uncertain if peizosurgery, which leaves a clean cavity for implant placement compared to the blunt osteotome method or a drilling method, is superior in any given setting of bone quality. Drilling results in free osseous debris and microfractured walls, which requires additional biological energy to repair but still leads to undiscernible differences in osseointegration from a clinical standpoint when compared to piezosurgery. Osteotome condensation of bone laterally and apically adds bone mineral stock simultaneous to implant placement to provide mechanical fixation for implants placed into trabecular bone. The loose particles of osseous debris in the implant osteotomy site although do not substantially contribute to bone formation directly, particles are almost always resorbed delaying bone modeling contact to the implant. Therefore, delayed implant placement is often recommended especially in complex osteotomy settings such as for alveolar split cases combined with osteotome intrusion of the sinus floor as illustrated in Fig. 7.2. So, the bone is quite facile in the development of osseointegration despite differing methods of achieving an osteotomy [21–23].

Late-term bone response is related to implant material characteristics including surface topography and the functional response to oral environmental stress typified by durability of the osseogingival attachment and peri-implant maintenance of health.

In a small percentage of cases bone does not form primary union leading to early loss of the implant—perhaps about 3% of the time. Although causation is multifactorial, it remains unknown exactly why bone modeling arrests and osseointegration does not develop. Tightness of fit is one factor to consider. Bone, an anisotropic structure, carries within it potential energy such that bone presses against the newly inserted titanium screw as much as the screw pushes against it. Implants placed into a split alveolus do not have a tight fit as the potential energy of the bone is expended kinetically by the splitting of the alveolus, so that the physical energy of the bone to compress against implants is lost. The same thing happens when an implant causes an alveolar plate fracture during insertion. So, an important factor in the stability is controlling the potential energy of bone. Similarly, cancellous bone has less compressive ability than cortical bone and therefore less insertion torque. So the failure of osseointegration due to inadequate primary stability is less in the cancellous bone.

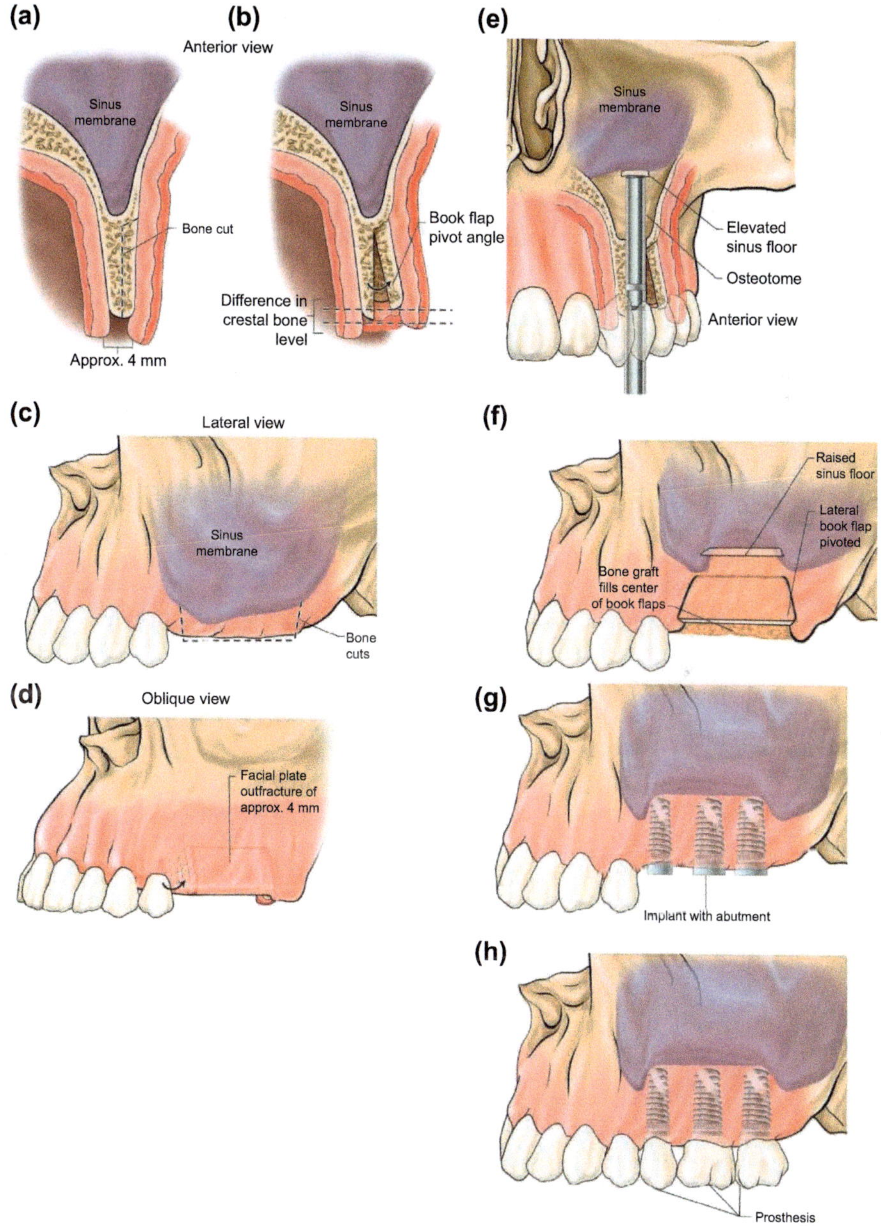

Figure 7.2 Demonstrated graphically is the alveolar split combined with sinus floor intrusion by osteotome from an anterior and lateral view. (a), (b), and (e) show the crestal exposure, the alveolar split, and the sinus floor intrusion from a cross-sectional view. (c), (d), (f), and (g) show a lateral view showing the sinus floor intrusion and subsequent implant placement. Delayed implants placement is advocated in this setting due to the complex osteotomy created making simultaneous implant placement inadvisable.

There probably is an optimal implant insertion torque for which osseointegration may develop. At the extremes of insertion force it is possible that too much force could damage the bone in too tight of fit. This likely occurs at very high torque values, well above 200 Ncm, but could be as low as 50 Ncm in sensitive individuals. On the other hand, the bone is so porous that it does not require drilling, that is, implants can be placed without instrumentation, but this leads to poor fixation potential. Osseointegration occurs even in low insertion torque settings as long as primary stability is maintained such that low insertion torque implants essentially catch up with high insertion torque implants with regard to osseointegration content [24–26].

One of the basic principles in placement is to provide at least 1 mm of circumferential bone around the implant. This is easy to accomplish accurately with open-flap procedures. However, with closed-flap *trans*-gingival placement the implant may be placed too buccal or lingual causing dehiscence. There is a greater risk of this in non-direct vision techniques such as computer-generated-guided surgery. Off-axis angle deviation from computer planned placement has been reported to be 6 degrees or more such that implants can inadvertently be placed with a dehiscence [20,22].

D factor measure of stress dampening by the molecular monolayer of proteins adsorbed to the surface of an implant in the days following placement indicates the degree of wettability. Wettability is a description of the surface activity, the likelihood of protein adsorption, a very important first step toward osseointegration [23].

Surface roughness has been shown to be important, as described by the Sa value in microns, which is the average height of surface roughness, with turned implants having less than 0.5 μm and the so-called rough surface implants 1–2 μm in height. The clinical significance of roughness is related to exposure or nonexposure of the roughened surface to the bone. In the bone, the surface that is rough has more surface area, and, therefore, more binding power—a potentially stronger integration. However, when exposed to the oral cavity a rough surface attracts plaque and leads to peri-implantitis. So the decision to place implants level to the crest or perhaps 1 mm deep of the crest will ensure rough surface bone contact. However, in animal experiments, the biological width has been shown to re-establish to a baseline level of about 3 mm indicating bone remodeling despite subcrestal placement of implants. But this is better than the high profile placement in which 1 mm or more of implant body is supracrestal adding long-term risk for peri-implantitis. One of the important reasons for preparation of the all-on-four bone shelf is positioning implant platforms flush to the newly formed bone level to ensure stable long-term osseous coverage of implant threads.

The most common error in placement of exposed implant surface is dehiscence. This may be particularly problematic on the lingual of the lower arch and on the buccal of the upper arch as bone response typically is not induced to cover the exposed implant threads. Exposed threads should be treated by guided bone regeneration if the implant cannot be repositioned. And, if there is a deficiency of fixed gingival tissue a connective tissue graft is ideally indicated [27,28].

Selection of the implant is important as greater length and diameter aid in gaining better torque and often times reduce bone stress overall. However, the diameter and length should not be excessive, particularly the diameter, which may encroach upon adjacent tooth periodontium, leading to spacing deficiency between implants for crestal bone support. Thread pitch should generally be shallow for the ease of placement following screw-tapping into Type I bone, whereas deeper threads are better suited for cancellous bone. Parallel walled versus tapered implants are another selection criteria important for developing primary implant stability, the tapered implant being preferred in soft bone or tapered bone locations that have concavities or potential tooth root encroachment apically. There are so many variables when technically approaching an osseous dimension that standardization of procedure is almost impossible such that surgical/operative judgment becomes the final arbiter [29,30].

Other factors that may arrest bone healing concern the surface properties of the implant, including wettability, texture of the surface, addition of carbonates or protein polymers, and properties of adsorption of the initial protein biolayer.

One clinical decision to be considered is the placement of abutments in a platform switch relation, which has been shown to decrease slightly crestal bone resorption by preventing epithelial migration beyond the connection interface. Pocket depth should be less and osseous support for papillary form enhanced. This may be particularly important in adjacent implant placement [31].

The prosthetic use of cement that is inadvertently expressed subgingivally can lead to the bone loss and failure of the prosthesis, suggesting a preferred use for screw retention or abutments that do not require cement for fastening such as the nitinol (memory metal) abutment (Fig. 7.3) [32,33].

Medical history is important particularly for unarrested severe periodontal disease, uncontrolled diabetes, high-dose radiation therapy, high-dose bisphosphonate

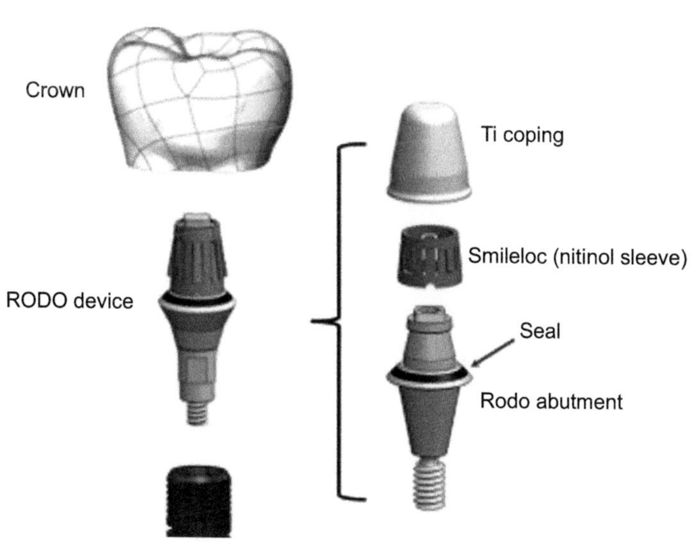

Figure 7.3 The nitinol abutment avoids the need for screw retention or cementation as shown above. (Nitinol, an intermetallic compound made of nickel and titanium, is heat phase sensitive and therefore can secure a crown over an implant with greater retention than cement and yet be retrievable by heating, a function shape memory recovery force.)

accumulation, and damage from cigarette smoking. The net effect is compromise of bone vitality mostly due to decreased blood supply suggesting poor bone healing capacity leading to inadequate osseointegration. So once again, the clinician must use good judgment on patient selection [34].

In summary, the clinical bone response to implant placement is multifactorial not the least of which are methods of bone manipulation done by the surgeon in preparation for insertion of the implant. Thereafter, a cascade of healing events proceeds not only related to clinical surgical/prosthetic management but also to host healing capacity. Long-term consequence of devices in the bone is related to the initial insertion method, subsequent clinical management, as well as patient factors including compliance, all manifested over time in the hard tissue response to the foreign body.

References

[1] Hao J, Zhang Y, Jing D, Shen Y, Tang G, Huang S, et al. Mechanobiology of mesenchymal stem cells: a perspective into mechanical induction of MSC fate. Act Biomater July 2015; 20:1−9.

[2] Ferguson SJ, Langoff JD, Voelter K, con Rechenberg B, Schamweber D, Bierbaum S, et al. Biomechanical comparison of different surface modification of dental implants. Int J Oral Maxillofac Implants 2008 November−December;23(6):1037−46.

[3] Frost HM. The Utah paradigm of skeletal physiology: a overview of its insights for bone, cartilage and cartilaginous tissue organs. J Bone Miner Metab 2000;31:77−88.

[4] Albrektsson T. What is osseointegration? Branemark osseointegration award. Academy of Osseointegration; Titanium Society Speech; March 14, 2014.

[5] Kim HS, Kim YJ, Jang JH, Park JW. Surface engineering of nanostructured titanium implants with bioactive ions. J Dent Res March 9, 2016 [Epub ahead of print].

[6] Larsson WC, Thomson P, Arnosson BO, Tengvall P, Rodahl M, Lausmaa J, et al. Bone response to surface modified titanium implants: studies on the early tissue response to implants with different surface characteristics. J Biomater 2013:412−42.

[7] Salvi GE, Bosshardt DD, Lang NP, Abrahamsson I, Berglundh T, Linde J, et al. Temporal sequence of hard and soft tissue healing around titanium dental implants. Periodontol 2000 June 2015;68(1):135−52.

[8] Favero R, Lang NP, Salata LA, Martins Neto EC, Caroprese M, Botticelli D. Sequential healing events of osseointegration at UnicCa and SLActive implant surfaces: an experimental study in the dog. Clin Oral Implants Res February 2016;(2):203−10.

[9] Simion M, Benigni M, Al-Hezaimi K, Kim DM. Early bone formation adjacent to oxidized and machined implant surfaces: a histological study. J Periodontics Restor Dent January−February 2015;35(1):9−17.

[10] Carter DR. Mechanical loading histories and cortical bone remodeling. Calcif Tissue Int 1984;(Suppl. 1):1547−51.

[11] Frost HM. Strain and other mechanical influences on bone strength and maintenance. Curr Opin Orthop 1997;8:60−70.

[12] Sho JY, Gu YX, Qiao SC, Zhuang LF, Zhang XM, Lai HC. Clinical evaluation of short 6 mm implants alone, short 8 mm implants combined with osteotome sinus floor elevation and standard 10 mm implants combined with osteotome sinus floor elevation in posterior maxilla: a study protocol for a randomized controlled trial. Trials July 30, 2015;16:324.

[13] Nisand D, Picard N, Rocchietta L. Short implants compared to implants in vertically augmented bone: a systematic review. Clin Oral Implants Res June 30, 2015;26(Suppl. 11):170−9. Epub.

[14] Vidya Bhat S, Premkumar P, Kamalakanth Sheony K. Stress distribution around single short dental implants: a finite element study. J Indian Prosthodont Soc December 2014; 14(Suppl. 1):161−7.

[15] Carnizzaro G, Felice P, Soardi E, Ferri V, Leone M, Lazzarini M, et al. Immediate loading of 2 (all-on-2) versus 4 (all-on-4) implants placed with a flapless technique supporting mandibular cross-arch fixed prostheses: 1 year results from a pilot randomized controlled trial. Eur J Oral Implantol 2013;6(2):121−31. Summer.

[16] Graves S, Mahler BA, Javid B, Armellini D, Jensen OT. Maxillary all-on-4 therapy using angled implants: a 16 month clinical study of 110 implants in 276 jaws. Dent Clin North Am October 2011;55(4):779−94.

[17] Jensen OT, Adams MW. Anterior sinus grafts for angled implants placement for severe maxillary atrophy as an alternative to zygomatic implants for full arch fixed restoration: technique and report of 5 cases. J Oral Maxillofac Surg July 2014;72(7): 1268−80.

[18] Jensen OT. Complete arch site classification for all-on-4 immediate function. J Prosthet Dent October 2014;112(4):741−51.

[19] Jensen OT, Adams MW. Secondary stabilization of maxillary M-4 treatment with unstable implants for immediate function: biomechanical consideration and report of 10 cases after 1 year in function. Int J Oral Maxillofac Implants March−April 2014;29(2): e232−240.

[20] Renvert S, Giovannoli JL. Periimplantitis. Paris, France: Quintessence Pub; 2015. 260pp.

[21] Pereira CC, Geath WC, Meorin-Nogueira L, Garcia-Junior IR, Okamoto R. Piezosurgery applied to implant dentistry: clinical and biological aspects. J Oral Implatol July 2014. Spec No. 401−8. Review.

[22] Pinchasov G, Juodzbalys G. Graft-free sinus augmentation procedure: a literature review. J Oral Maxillofac Res April 1, 2014;5(1) [e].

[23] Rashad A, Sadr-Eshkevari P, Weuster M, Schmitz I, Prochonow N, Maurer P. Material attrition and bone micromorphometry after conventional and ultrasonic implant site preparation. Clin Oral Implants Res August 24, 2013;(Suppl. A1000):110−4.

[24] Duyck J, Roesems R, Cardoso MV, Oqawa T, De Villa Camargos G, Candamme K. Effect of insertion torque on titanium implant osseointegration: an animal experimental study. Clin Oral Implants Res February 2015;26(2):191−6.

[25] Barone A, Alfonsi F, Derchi G, Tonelli P, Toti P, Marchionni S, et al. The effect of insertion torque on the clinical outcome of single implants: a randomized clinical trial. Clin Implants Relat Res June 2015;18(3):588−600 [Epub ahead of print].

[26] Lee SY, Kim SJ, An HW, Kim HS, Ha DG, Ryo KH, et al. The effect of the thread depth on the mechanical properties of the dental implant. J Adv Prosthodont April 2015;7(2): 115−21.

[27] Rungcharassaeng K, Caruso JMF, Dan JY, Schutyser F, Boumans T. Accuracy of computer-guided surgery: a comparison of operator experience. J Prosthet Dent June 2015; 114(3):407−13 [Epub ahead of print].

[28] Kasemo B, Gold J. Implant surfaces and interface processes. Adv Dent Res June 1999;13: 8−20. Review. Implant Dent. 2015 Aug;24(4):422−6.

[29] Timmerman A, Keestra JA, Couke W, Teughels W, Quirynen M. The outcome of oral implant placed in bone with limited bucco-oral dimensions: a three-year follow-up study. J Clin Periodontl March 2015;42(3):311−8.

[30] Romanos G, Grizas E, Nentwig GH. Association of keratinized mucosa and periimplant soft tissue stability around implants with platform switching. Implant Dent August 2015; 24(4):422–6.

[31] Cooper LF, Reside G, Standford C, Barawacz C, Feine J, Abi Nader S, et al. Multicenter randomized comparative trial of implants with different abutment interfaces to replace anterior maxillary teeth. Int J Oral Maxillofac Implants May–June 2015;30(3):622–32.

[32] Shapoff CA, Lahey BJ. Crestal bone loss and the consequences of retained excess cement around dental implants. Compend Contin Educ Dent February 2012;33(2):94–101.

[33] Pautke C, Kolk A, Brokate M, Wehrstedt JC, Kneissl F, Miethke T, et al. Development of novel implant abutments using the shape memory alloy nitinol: preliminary results. J Oral Maxillofac Implants May–June 2009;24(3):477–83.

[34] Kotsakis GA, Ionnou AL, Hinrichs JE, Romanos GE. A systematic review of observational studies evaluating implant placement in the maxillary jaws of medically compromised patients. Clin Implant Dent Relat Res June 2015;17(3):598–609.

The effect of loading on peri-implant bone: a critical review of the literature

8

J. Duyck [1,2], *K. Vandamme* [1,2]
[1]KU Leuven, Leuven, Belgium; [2]U.Z. St. Raphaël, Leuven, Belgium

8.1 Introduction

In the nineties, the so-called mechanical "overloading" was considered to be one of the main reasons for peri-implant bone loss and implant failure [1]. Excessive surgical trauma together with an impaired healing ability, premature loading, and infection were pointed out to be the most common causes of early implant losses (= prior to functional loading). Progressive chronic marginal infection (peri-implantitis) and overload in conjunction with the host characteristics on the other hand were thought to be the major etiological factors causing late failures [2]. The fact that mechanical overloading was recognized as a risk factor for oral implant success generated a lot of research to gain insight into the role of mechanical loading on the establishment and the maintenance of oral implant osseointegration.

Since Wolff's law [3], there is a consensus that mechanical loading affects bone size and architecture. Mechanical loading evokes stress and strain in the bone, which can be bone stimulating (anabolic) or negative for the net bone tissue (catabolic). The latter has been supported by correlations between exerted forces and bone response [4–6]. Frost's mechanostat [6] relates four levels of mechanical strain magnitude to the bone response: (1) disuse atrophy (50–100 $\mu\varepsilon$), (2) steady state (100–1500 $\mu\varepsilon$), (3) mild overload (1500–3000 $\mu\varepsilon$), and (4) fatigue failure (>3000 $\mu\varepsilon$). If fatigue failure occurs, the load can theoretically be classified to what is called overload. Fractures occur in the bone at a strain level of about 25,000 $\mu\varepsilon$, depending upon the type of stress–strain testing (compressive, tensile, shear) as well as the exact type of bone that is being tested (anisotropic, cortical, cancellous…). Frost's mechanostat, however, overlooks the importance of other load parameters besides load magnitude. Other parameters such as frequency [5], duration [7], rest periods between load bouts, [8] etc., also play a significant role in the bone response to loading.

It seems only logical that the above-mentioned evidence on the bone response to loading also applies to the bone surrounding oral implants. Nevertheless, load-bearing oral implants perforate into the oral cavity, and it is a rather complex interplay of mechanical, microbial, patient, surgery, and implant-related factors which determines the resulting peri-implant bone response. In addition, the clinical trend to functionally load implants before osseointegration, puts the mechanical loading effect on peri-implant bone in a different context. In case of early or immediate loading,

Bone Response to Dental Implant Materials. http://dx.doi.org/10.1016/B978-0-08-100287-2.00008-2

mechanical loading is superimposed onto the healing processes during implant osseointegration. As it is anticipated that the mechanisms and kinetics of the mechanobiological events of the peri-implant tissues are largely dependent on the timing of loading relative to the osseointegration state, these will be discussed separately in this paper.

This chapter is not a systematic review, but rather joins and interprets the scientific literature on the impact of mechanical loading on oral implant prognosis and differentiates between the impact of loading prior to and after the establishment osseointegration. Clinical as well as animal experimental studies reporting on the outcome of dental/oral implants subjected to immediate load and so-called overload were therefore considered.

8.2 Implant loading prior to osseointegration

Immediately after oral implant installation, the process of osseointegration is initiated, through the classical wound healing cascade, followed by combined bone remodeling and bone regeneration [9—11]. As the size of the osteotomy site is generally smaller than the implant outer diameter, some parts of the implant are in direct contact with the host bone. In those areas of direct bone contact, bone remodeling occurs. In the areas without direct bone contact, tissue—and most preferably bone—regeneration occurs. Bone regeneration in the initially bone-free areas can be accomplished by bone apposition from the host bone or by de novo bone formation.

New bone formation requires bone cell differentiation. Genetic, biochemical, as well as mechanical factors affect the way multipotent mesenchymal stromal cells (MSCs) differentiate into multiple lineages such as osteoblasts, adipocytes, and chondrocytes [12]. MSCs are originally derived from the bone marrow [13], although they have now been isolated from many adult stromal tissues [14]. Carter et al. [15] reviewed some of the mechanobiological principles that are thought to guide the differentiation of mesenchymal tissue into bone, cartilage, or fibrous tissue during the initial phase of regeneration. Cyclic motion and the associated shear stresses cause cell proliferation and the production of a large callus in the early phases of fracture healing. For intermittently imposed loading in the regenerating tissue, (1) direct intramembranous bone formation is permitted in areas of low stress and strain, (2) low to moderate magnitudes of tensile strain and hydrostatic tensile stress may stimulate intramembranous ossification, (3) poor vascularity can promote chondrogenesis in an otherwise osteogenic environment, (4) hydrostatic compressive stress is a stimulus for chondrogenesis, (5) high tensile strain is a stimulus for the net production of fibrous tissue, and (6) tensile strain with a superimposed hydrostatic compressive stress will stimulate the development of fibrocartilage. Finite element models confirmed that the patterns of tissue differentiation observed in fracture healing and distraction osteogenesis followed these fundamental mechanobiological concepts [15], although the precise role of mechanical forces in stem cell function and differentiation is still unraveled [16].

The mechanobiology of fracture healing illustrates the potential effect of mechanical loading on cell differentiation and tissue formation. Although the osteotomy required for implant installation can be considered as a fracture-like bone trauma, there is no evidence to accept that the same mechanobiology applies to healing peri-implant tissues.

8.2.1 Clinical research

The available literature on the impact of immediate loading on prosthesis failure, implant failure, and marginal bone loss, compared with conventional loading, was evaluated in a systematic review by Esposito et al. [17]. Furthermore, the review reported on the potential differences between immediate occlusal and nonocclusal loading and between direct and progressive loading with regard to the peri-implant bone response. Twenty-six of the 45 identified studies were included, reporting on 1217 patients with 2120 implants in total. Eighteen randomized controlled clinical trials (RCTs) comparing immediate versus delayed loading were included. In the studies, mainly implants supporting overdentures (seven studies) or solitary crowns (10 studies) were evaluated. There was only one study reporting on implants supporting a fixed full prosthesis. Three of the included studies had a too low level of evidence. In the remaining 15 RCTs no difference in either prosthesis or implant failure was observed between the two loading conditions. Furthermore, the six RCTs considering immediate versus early loading did not reveal differences either. Finally, insufficient evidence was found for different peri-implant tissue responses between immediate occlusal and nonocclusal loading and between direct and progressive loading. The systematic review article concluded that in general the quality of the clinical evidence concerning the impact of different timings of loading on the implant outcome is low. However, the authors recognized that the majority of the studies included mainly "ideal" participants (e.g., absence of parafunctional habits, high primary stability, good bone quality), thereby suggesting that the implant treatment outcome is not necessarily applicable to the general patient population.

In line with the findings of Esposito et al. [17], more recent systematic reviews and meta-analyses confirm that no significant impact of time of loading on implant or prosthetic outcomes [18] for single tooth replacements [19,20], partial [21], and full-arch prostheses [22] is observed. A systematic review on the impact of the loading protocol in mandibular overdenture treatment by Schimmel et al. [23] based on 58 included articles, however, indicates that early and conventional loading protocols are better documented and seem to result in fewer implant failures during the first year of function compared with immediate loading protocols.

Primary implant stability is an important factor in achieving predictable treatment outcomes in early/immediate loading protocols [24,25]. The implant–bone interlocking created by primary implant stability inhibits detrimental micromotion and related shear forces at the interface on the one hand and allows an efficient transfer of potentially stimulating forces to the surrounding tissues on the other hand [26–28]. Since primary implant stability directly depends on the mechanical connection between the implant and the surrounding bone, it can be strongly influenced by the implant design [29], the bone quality and quantity [30], and the surgical technique (drill diameter; depth of the preparation; tapping of the implant site) [31,25]. In this context, undersized implant site preparation may increase primary implant stability [32]. The insertion of the implant after undersized osteotomy surgery requires a considerable force, which is referred to as the insertion torque. Considering that primary implant stability is influenced by the mechanical interlocking between the implant and the receiving host bone bed, it has been suggested that the implant success can be accelerated and/or enhanced by a surgical protocol applying high insertion torques [33]. Indeed, in a clinical split-mouth study by Ottoni et al. [34], significantly more implant failures were noted for immediately loaded implants installed with a low (20 N cm) compared with a high (>32 N cm) insertion torque. For the conventionally loaded implants, however, the insertion torque displayed no effect on the implant outcome. The impact of the primary implant stability on the outcome of immediately loaded implants has been confirmed in a more recent study [35], where again a significant decrease in implant failure was observed for implants inserted with a high (>80 N cm) compared with a medium (25–35 N cm) insertion torque. On the other hand, other studies have suggested that high insertion torque values produce strong compressive forces onto the peri-implant bone, an altered mechanical strain environment, and the potential induction of deleterious effects on the local microcirculation and bone cellular responses, which may lead to bone necrosis and ultimately to a retarded or compromised implant osseointegration [36,37]. Thus, although a high primary implant stability under immediate loading is a prerequisite, low levels of compressive stresses and strains immediately after implant placement are preferred concomitantly [29].

To evaluate the effect of the implant insertion torque on the peri-implant bone healing process, an animal study was undertaken by the authors' research group evaluating peri-implant bone remodeling and regeneration around unloaded implants installed with a high (>50 N cm) compared with a very low (<10 N cm) insertion torque [38]. The different insertion torques were achieved by varying the bone cavity dimension relative to the implant dimension. It was observed that the low insertion torque implant group healed with considerable de novo bone formation, thereby catching up, already in the early osseointegration stage, the initial inferior amount of contact of the implant with the bone compared with high insertion torque implants. High insertion torque implant installation not only provided an initial higher bone-to-implant contact, but was moreover anabolic for the bone surrounding the implant. A negative impact of the strain environment created because of the high insertion torque for implant installation on the biological process of osseointegration could not be observed, at least not at the tissue level. The study, however, cannot give a clear answer of which condition is preferred for clinical application and factors such as the bone quality, quantity, and loading scheme, among others, should be taken into account.

8.2.2 Animal experimental research

Different animal models have been developed by the BIOMAT Research Group (KU Leuven, Belgium) to investigate the impact of immediate and early implant loading on the peri-implant tissue response. For the animal studies described below, immediate versus early implant loading was defined as well-controlled loading of the implant by a custom-designed external loading device starting at the day itself or 1 day after implant installation versus 1 week postsurgery.

A first model for investigation of the sensitivity of peri-implant tissue differentiation to well-controlled immediate implant loading is the bone chamber methodology for the rabbit [39]. The bone chamber primarily consists of dual-structure perforated hollow cylinders with a centrally positioned implant to be installed in the rabbit proximal tibia. Through the perforations, the bone can grow into the bone chamber. The implant, located in the center of the bone chamber, is displaced in a well-controlled manner by means of a loading device. Several bone chamber studies (each of them consisting of several experiments) were performed exploring the effect of immediate loading of the implant design and surface properties in immediate loading conditions and of the magnitude of micromotion on the peri-implant tissue response [26,27,40–43]. The main findings of these studies are described: (1) controlled immediate implant loading can accelerate the tissue mineralization in the vicinity and at the surface of the implant; (2) the screw-threaded implant design promoted osseointegration by providing a favorable local mechanical environment for bone formation at the implant surface compared with the unthreaded implant design; (3) an adequate force transfer from the loaded implant to the surrounding tissues was enhanced for roughened implant surfaces favoring a good tissue interlocking and resulting in a stimulation of bone formation (Fig. 8.1).

Another animal model for investigation of the peri-implant tissue response to immediate loading is based on the guinea pig model with bicortically anchored, tibial implants as described by Jansen and de Groot [44] and modified by Slaets et al. [11] for the rabbit. In contrast to the bone chamber model, where neoformation of trabecular bone occurs within the chamber, this model can be classified as a cortical bone model investigating the impact of the loading on the bone remodeling in the host cortical bone and on peri-implant bone formation in the marrow zone. The other major difference with the bone chamber model is the nonaxial implant loading direction (compared

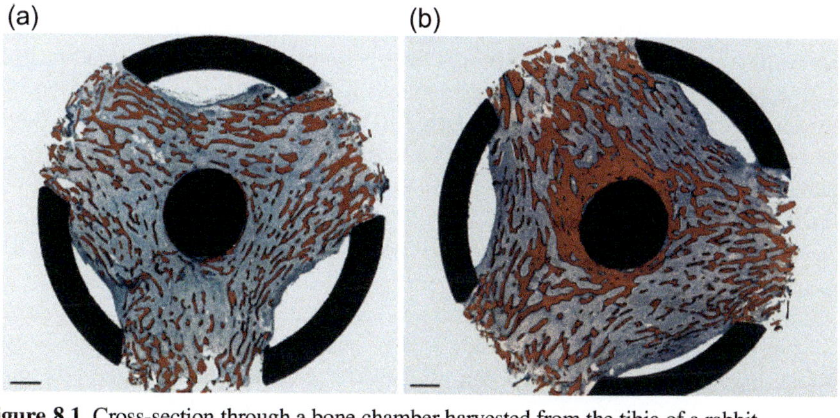

Figure 8.1 Cross-section through a bone chamber harvested from the tibia of a rabbit, illustrating bone tissue architecture around an unloaded (a) and a loaded (30 μm vertical displacement) (b) implant. Stevenel's blue and Von Gieson's picrofuchsin stain; bar, 500 μm [42].

with the axial load application in the bone chamber), resulting in bending moments, with one implant side under compressive loading, and causing stress gradients along the implant surface. It was observed that a well-controlled immediate implant loading did not cause large differences in the sequence of biological events leading to osseointegration in cortical bone, as there was the formation of a hematoma and an altered nuclear morphology of osteocytes surrounding the implantation site, followed by an intensive bone remodeling and the formation of new bone leading to the osseointegration of the implant. At early time points, an endosteal and periosteal bone neoformation was found, whereas the cortex itself hosted damaged osteocytes. At later time points, bone neoformation was also found at the cortical level itself. Differences between loaded and unloaded implants were observed with larger reactions for the endosteal and periosteal bone for the immediately loaded implants at intermediate time points. But at the endpoint of the experiment, bone formation at the cortical level was reduced around the immediately loaded implants compared with the unloaded ones.

The original guinea pig model was used by De Smet et al. [45] for application of early implant loading. Implants were installed bicortically with primary stability on the medial surface of the tibia near the ankle joint. The implants made direct contact with the host bone of the upper and lower cortices, whereas the midpart of the implant faced the bone marrow cavity. The percutaneous part of the implant fitted the mechanical stimulation lever, and mechanical stimulation was started 1 week after implant installation. The influence of specific mechanical parameters, that is, the duration, amplitude, rate, and frequency of loading, of the early implant loading regime on peri-implant bone remodeling in the cortical host bone and on the bone formation in the marrow zone was investigated. The exact strain at the upper cortical implant interface in response to loading was experimentally calculated from cadaver strain gauge measurements. Findings can be summarized as follows: (1) the guinea pig model as a model for cortical bone remodeling and medullar tissue differentiation to early implant loading was validated. Application of moderate loads during implant osseointegration promoted bone formation in the adjacent bone marrow cavity, at the implant side under compression loading, but did not affect the cortical bone; (2) the positive effect of early mechanical stimulation increased with increasing force amplitude and decreasing frequency. The most pronounced stimulation of bone formation in the marrow surrounding the implant was observed for low-frequency stimulation (3 Hz) with low level peri-implant strains (350−540 $\mu\varepsilon$); (iii) the strain levels exerting an anabolic effect on the peri-implant bone lie far beneath the level of minimum effective strain resulting in bone formation, as proposed by Frost [46]. This finding confirms that extrapolation of the gathered knowledge on the parameters of mechanically mediated bone modeling to the bone biology around osseointegrating implants should be performed with caution.

In another animal model, the potential of high-frequency loading on peri-implant tissue regeneration and osseointegration was evaluated in Wistar rats. The tested loading regimes differed in loading magnitude, frequency, duration, and mode (whole-body vibration, direct implant loading, and indirect implant loading).

First, three consecutive experiments were performed to assess the effect of indirect high-frequency loading via whole-body vibration on peri-implant bone remodeling

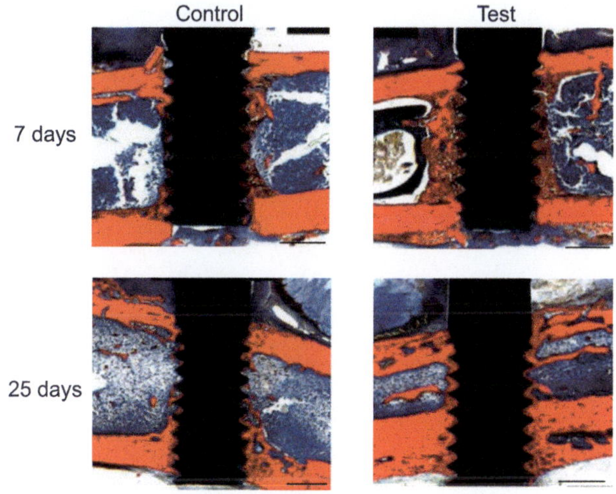

Figure 8.2 Histological sections of implant from the rats that underwent whole-body vibration (test) compared with the unloaded rats (control) after 7 and 25 days of healing. Stevenel's blue and Von Gieson's picrofuchsin stain; scale bars, 1 mm [47].

[47–49]. Both bone-to-implant contact and peri-implant bone fraction increased significantly in the case of loading with a stepwise frequency band from 12 to 150 Hz at 0.3 g for 10 min/day [47] (Fig. 8.2).

When the loading session was shortened to 1 min 15 s, 2 min 30 s, 5 min, and twice 1 min 15 s (with a 4-h load-free time interval), the stimulating effect of high-frequency loading on bone-to-implant contact and peri-implant bone fraction was confirmed [48]. Among the tested loading conditions, the session with a load-free interval presented the most significant effect.

To investigate the combined effect of whole-body vibration frequency and acceleration, different loading protocols were tested. For all combinations (i.e., 12–30 Hz at 0.3 g, 70–90 Hz at 0.3 g, 70–90 Hz at 0.075 g, 130–150 Hz at 0.3 g, and 130–150 Hz at 0.043 g), the loading combination with the highest frequency and acceleration (e.g., 130–150 Hz at 0.3 g) displayed the most favorable effect on bone-to-implant contact and peri-implant bone fraction, compared with the other test groups [49].

Besides whole-body vibration, another indirect loading protocol was performed whereby an implant-containing long bone was compressed through its axis with forces ranging between 0.5 N and 20 N [50] (Fig. 8.3). The controlled compression was applied at both high (40 Hz) and low (2 Hz) frequency. Higher loading magnitudes (and accompanying elevated tissue strains) were required under low-frequency loading to provoke an anabolic peri-implant bone response compared with high-frequency loading. A sustained period of loading at high-frequency was needed to induce enhanced osseointegration.

Also the effect of direct implant loading was evaluated by means of a displacement controlled implant loading through the implant axis [51] (Fig. 8.4). Four loading regimes were applied in this study: (1) (high frequency low magnitude) HF-LM,

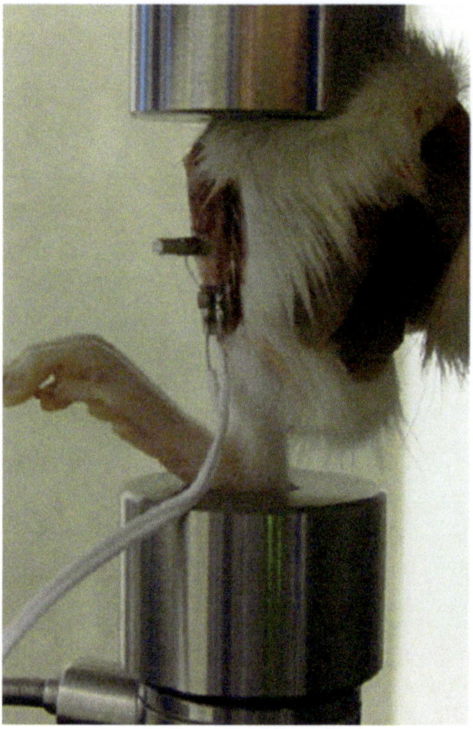

Figure 8.3 Indirect implant loading by means of compression of the implant-containing bone (tibia) through its long axis [50].

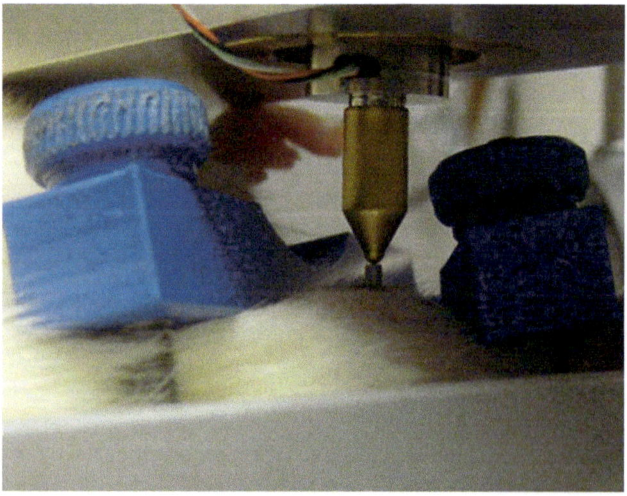

Figure 8.4 Direct implant loading [51].

40 Hz−8 μm; (2) HF-HM, 40 Hz−16 μm; (3) LF-LM, 8 Hz−41 μm; (4) LF-HM, 8 Hz−82 μm. The stimulatory effect of immediate implant loading on bone-to-implant contact was only observed in case of high-frequency (40 Hz), low-magnitude (8 μm) loading. The applied load regimes failed to influence the peri-implant bone fraction.

This series of studies confirmed the role of mechanical loading in peri-implant bone regeneration and remodeling. Although an influencing role was observed for all loading modes, the anabolic effect of whole-body vibration was superior.

Detailed information about the quantification of the mechanical parameters from the results of clinical studies on immediate and early loading is lacking because none of these studies have actually targeted these factors in a quantitative manner. Therefore, the results of the series of controlled and quantified implant loading animal studies contribute to the advanced understanding of the mechanobiology of implants subjected to immediate or early loading. Evidence was provided for the sensitivity of bone formation and resorption to the mechanical conditions at the peri-implant site. Implant loading can be performed immediately or early after the insertion without disturbing the biological osseointegration process and can be beneficial for peri-implant bone formation. An optimal bone response to immediately or early loaded implants may thus be determined not only by the primary stability of the implant and by the host bone characteristics, but also by the individual loading parameters and by an optimized load transfer through appropriate implant design and surface features. These findings should reinforce continued well-designed and fundamental research on immediate and early implant loading, as this loading protocol benefits many patients to a great extent.

8.3 Implant loading after osseointegration

Once implants are integrated and placed by attaching a prosthetic superstructure, they are subjected to various influences such as patient habits (e.g., smoking, nutrition, parafunction, microbial load, mechanical load). It is not feasible to measure the sole effect of implant loading and literature does not provide insight into the effect of mechanical loading alone on peri-implant tissue response or implant outcome. Nevertheless, review studies report high survival rates and limited peri-implant bone loss after medium-term [96] and long-term [97] function of oral implants, thereby indicating that physiological loading does not per se compromises osseointegration. Nevertheless, mechanical loading has long been looked at as a potential threat to osseointegration [1].

A systematic review on the effect of occlusal overload on bone/implant loss was published by our group in 2012 [52]. This article evaluated studies on the effect of (over) load of already osseointegrated implants on peri-implant bone loss and/or implant failure.

8.3.1 *Clinical research*

Clinical observations have fed the idea that occlusal forces on osseointegrated oral implants can result in marginal bone loss or even implant failure [53,2]. Several studies, therefore, evaluated the effect of the so-called overload on peri-implant bone behavior and implant prognosis. The term "implant overload" as often used in literature, however, can be misleading for several reasons. First, although occlusal implant loading can be measured at the level of the prosthesis/abutment, it is uncertain what the resultant stresses and strains are at the level of the bone–implant interface. Numerical models that simulate occlusal load transfer to the bone–implant interface indicate that a certain occlusal load can result in varying stresses and strains at the interface depending on the chosen boundary conditions (e.g., bone mechanical properties, fixation of the simulated bone to the implant). So as long as stresses and strains cannot be measured at the interface itself, the impact of a certain occlusal load on the interface remains uncertain. Second, even if the overload magnitude (>3000 με) as coined by Frost [6] is considered, it overlooks the influence of the other load parameters (such as loading frequency, duration, etc.) that are known to affect peri-implant bone behavior and implant prognosis. The above-mentioned aspects should be kept in mind when reading literature on implant overload.

In the review on occlusal overload and bone/implant loss [52], the review of Klineberg et al. [54], although possessing a high level of evidence owing to its design, was excluded, because it only indirectly dealt with the issue of overloading since they specifically searched for the choice of a particular occlusal design in tooth and implant supported prostheses and full dentures.

Three clinical trials characterized by high evidence-ranked study designs were found; one randomized controlled trial [55], one controlled clinical trial [56], and one crossover study [57]. Jofré et al. [55] and van Kampen et al. [57] both dealt with the effect of maximum bite forces on the marginal bone loss in two-implant mandibular overdentures. A real effort to quantify forces was performed in these studies, but this was done at prosthesis level thereby leaving the magnitude of overload at the implant level undefined. Vigolo and Zaccaria [56] compared splinted (single tooth replacement) with unsplinted (fixed partial prostheses) implants in the posterior maxilla. In none of the above-mentioned review/studies was bone loss related either to the magnitude of the bite forces or to the splinting of the implants. An additional nine cohort studies (four pro- and five retrospective studies) and four case series were discussed in the systematic review, although they were excluded due to high risk of bias. Eventually all these clinical studies could neither evidence nor refute a cause-and-effect relationship between bone loss and the so-called overload as they were considered to be prone to high risk of bias. Either they lacked any definition for measuring occlusal overload or wear was used as a surrogate for occlusal overload although wear is not the result of grinding only (quid; erosion, abrasion, material selection, etc.). Alternatively, the anticipation of the overload status was based on the absence of bilateral contact in the posterior area in the maximal intercuspal position and the lack of balanced occlusion during excursions or on the patients' reporting of bruxism.

Fifteen review articles on the topic have been published so far. These were excluded from the systematic review because they did not meet the inclusion criteria. However, their conclusions are briefly summarized here. The review articles did report both on clinical and on animal studies. Two review articles did not deal with overload but with adaptive bone modeling and remodeling of functionally loaded implants [58,59]. For the remaining 13 articles, two opposite trends could be distinguished. One group of authors reported that although the results were conflicting and bias was at high risk, animal experimental studies have shown that occlusal loads might result in marginal bone loss around oral implants or complete loss of osseointegration. In clinical studies an association between the loading conditions and marginal bone loss around oral implants or complete loss of osseointegration has been mentioned, but a causative relationship has not been shown [60]. Cehreli and Akça [61] concluded that overloading and stress shielding have often been cited as the primary biomechanical factors leading to marginal bone loss around implants, although there is no consensus on these factors. Eventually, Lobbezoo et al. [62,63], Johansson et al. [64], and Manfredini et al. [65] all concluded that there is a lack of support to refute a causal relationship between bruxism and implant failure. The other group of authors [1,66–71] all suggested overload to be an etiological factor in peri-implant bone loss. Therefore, although this occlusal overload concept does not negate other factors related to marginal bone loss, it was anticipated that the restorative dentist is able to impact this condition more extensively than most or any other factors. Methods to decrease occlusal stress to the implant prosthesis are therefore warranted.

In general, the level of clinical evidence on the impact of mechanical load on peri-implant bone behavior and implant failure is low and inconclusive. One may wonder if overload as such can ever be applied in clinical studies, because the opportunity to test such a hypothesis in humans remains inappropriate and unethical. Most of the knowledge in this field, therefore, is derived from animal experimental studies.

8.3.2 Animal experimental research

The studies of Hoshaw [72] and Isidor [73,74] were the first to indicate a possible role of implant overload in peri-implant bone loss and implant failure. In, for example, Isidor's studies [73,74], five implants were placed in each of four monkeys. Two implants per animal were "overloaded" by means of supraocclusion, whereas the other three were infected using ligatures. A total of 75% of the overloaded implants became mobile, whereas marginal bone loss but lack of mobility was observed around the infected implants. Also we found marginal bone resorption when loading dynamically beyond 4000 microstrain (Fig. 8.5) in the rabbit tibiae [75]. Such high strains were exerted through application of 1.5 kg on a distance of 50 mm from the implant top in the proximodistal direction by means of a beam mounted on the implant (Fig. 8.6). Finite element analyses (Figs 8.7 and 8.8) indicate highest strains in the direction of the loading, which results in bone resorption as confirmed by histological (Fig. 8.5) and microcomputed tomography analyses (Fig. 8.9).

Chambrone et al. [76] published a systematic review in 2010 on animal studies evaluating the effect of occlusal load on the peri-implant tissue health of osseointegrated implants. The authors reported that, despite the application of stringent inclusion and exclusion criteria, the selected studies still were at high risk of bias. The following conclusions were drawn: (1) it is not well established if an excessive occlusal load catabolically affects osseointegration when adequate plaque control is performed. Inversely, overload seems to increase bone density around dental implants; (2) overload might play a key role in the development of peri-implant tissue breakdown

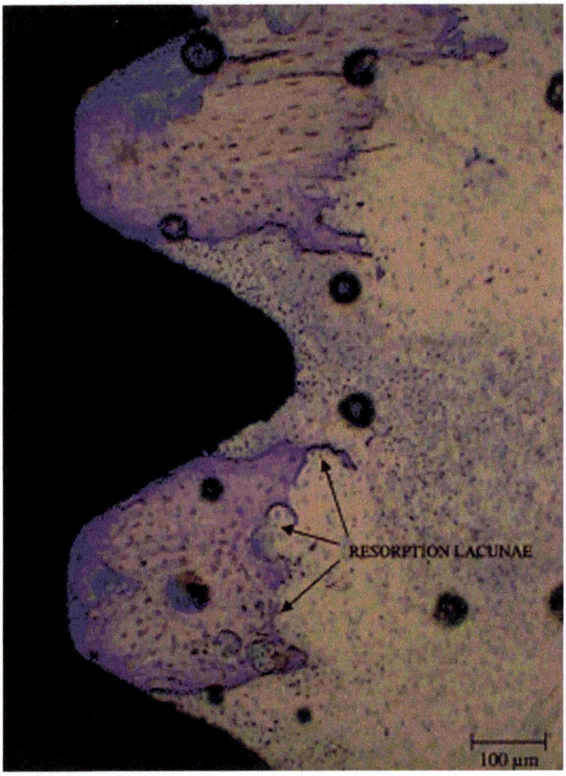

Figure 8.5 Picture of remaining bone around the marginal part of a dynamically loaded implant showing resorption lacunae starting lateral to the implant surface due to high strains ($\geq$4000 microstrain) in the peri-implant bone. Toluidine blue staining; scale bar, 100 μm [75].

when plaque accumulation is present; (3) although studies with a well-designed methodology were selected, few were available for meta-analysis and no RCTs were conducted. The main reason for exclusion of all but two animal studies in the referred review was the fact that splinted instead of single implants were used. One may wonder if this is a valid exclusion criterion since overload cannot be the exclusivity of single restorations only.

For the review by Naert et al. [52], two unburdened exclusion criteria were used: (1) the absence of a strict control hygiene program (minimum 3×/week) and (2) the absence of a genuine control condition in the experimental design. The rationale for claiming meticulous plaque control is self-evident: the causal relationship between oral plaque and peri-implant bone loss has repeatedly been demonstrated (see for review [77,78]) and bacterial load as a confounding covariant warrants exclusion when addressing the question of mechanical overload as a trigger for peri-implant bone loss. The second requirement, a genuine control condition, forced the authors to exclude many studies. A control condition was considered genuine or sham when the experimental test (e.g., loading) condition was fully replicated, except for the

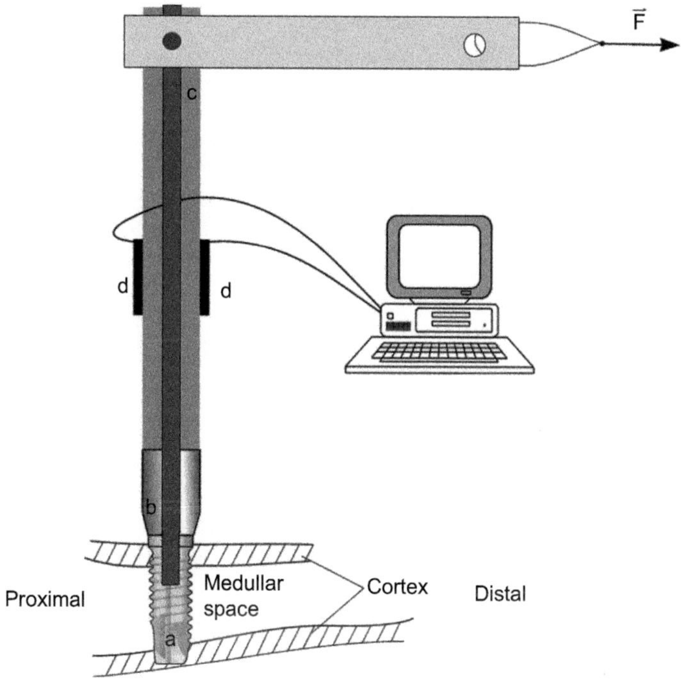

Figure 8.6 Schematical drawing of the dynamic loading device: (a) test implant, (b) 7-mm standard abutment, (c) metal beam that is mounted on the abutment, (d) strain gauges which record the deformation of the beam (connection with a personal computer allows recording and visualization of the data) [75].

parameter under investigation (overload). This implies that the control implants must have undergone abutment surgery (submerged implants were excluded), should have been exposed to the same microflora, should have received the same plaque-control regime, must have been restored with an identical prosthetic suprastructure, and must have been subjected to physiological loading, either through occlusal or food bolus contact. Three split-mouth studies were included in the review [79–83]. All studies were performed in the dog at the same anatomical site. Implants were placed 12 weeks after extraction of the teeth in the mandibular premolar region and a strict hygiene protocol was respected. Similar implant types with slightly varying dimensions were used: Hi-Tec screw-type machined (10.0 × 3.75 mm [83]), Brånemark (7.0 × 3.75 mm [79]), and ITI hollow-screw nonsubmerged implants (8.0 × 3.3 mm, [80]). All implants received delayed loading (12–16 weeks of healing). Dynamic "overload" in the study of Kozlovsky et al. [83] was performed via a supraocclusal contact pattern resulting in an increased anterior vertical dimension of at least 3 mm. To do so, the same abutments, but with varying lengths, were used as prosthesis for both physiologically and supra-occlusal loaded implants, thereby offering an acceptable sham-control group. A total of 16 loaded implants for two experimental "overload" conditions resulted in eight implants/condition. Follow-up

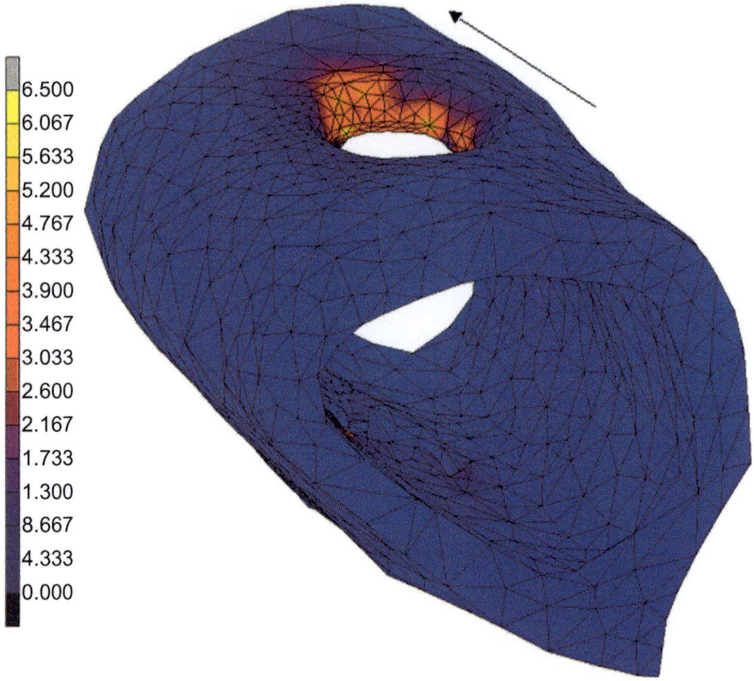

Figure 8.7 Equivalent strain (microstrain) distribution in bone, surrounding a dynamically loaded implant. Highest strains occur at the distal (compressive) side. The *arrow* indicates the load direction [75].

was repeated at 3, 6, 9, and 12 months. In the study of Hürzeler et al. [79], dynamic overload was created through a splint cemented on the antagonistic front teeth and attached to an orthodontic wire construction fixed on the remaining mandibular teeth, resulting in supraocclusal contacts. The occlusion of the implants not subjected to trauma was maintained normal, thereby offering an adequate sham-control group. A total of 20 implants for two experimental load conditions resulted in 10 implants/condition. The experiment lasted 16 months. Moreover, for both referred studies, the experimental set-up was such that the influence of overload could also be tested in ligature-induced peri-implantitis conditions. An equal number of implants as mentioned above, i.e., 16 and 20 implants for Kozlovsky et al. [83] and for Hürzeler et al. [79], respectively, installed at the contralateral mandibular side, received plaque retentive ligatures, which remained in place throughout the whole experiment. Static "overload" was performed in the study of Gotfredsen et al. [80] and more recently by Ikumi et al. [84]. No detrimental effects of these static loads on the osseointegration were observed. Gotfredsen et al. [80] even noted an anabolic loading effect.

Although different exclusion/inclusion criteria were set in the systematic review by Naert et al. [52], the findings corroborate well with those of Chambrone et al. [76]. Indeed, there is a lack of association between overload and peri-implant tissue loss in healthy conditions. However, the term "overload" is often used inappropriately,

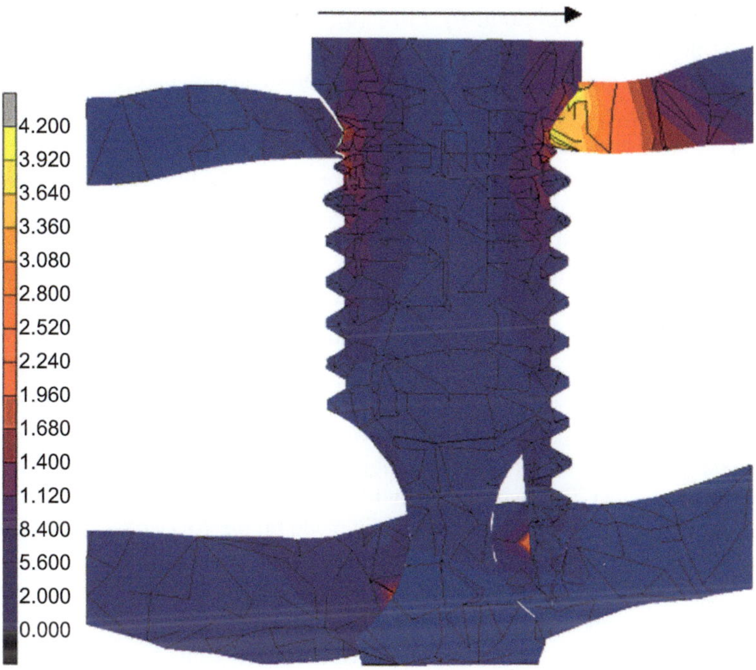

Figure 8.8 Equivalent strain (microstrain) distribution in a cross-section taken in a plane parallel to the load direction through the implant center. The *arrow* indicates the load direction [75].

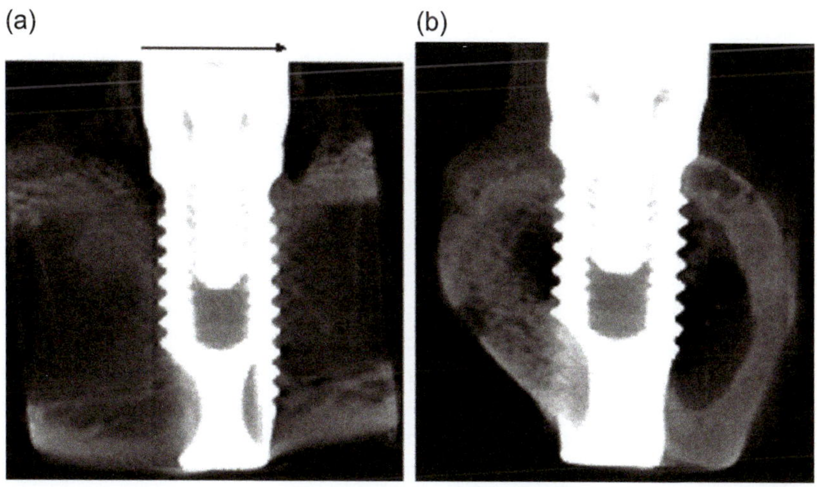

Figure 8.9 Two-dimensional microcomputed tomography image of a dynamically loaded implant, parallel (a) and perpendicular (b) to the long axis of the tibia. The *arrow* indicates the load direction [75].

since according to the definition by Frost [6], overload should lead to a catabolic reaction of the bone. As shown by Kozlovsky et al. [83] and Gotfredsen et al. [80] an anabolic rather than a catabolic effect of "overload" in bacterial unchallenged peri-implant bone tissues was found. Thus it is anticipated that the strains in the peri-implant bone evoked by the so-called "overload," either by dynamic or by static loading, were lying within the strain window of mild overload, resulting in bone gain. Once again, this emphasizes that the use of correct semantics is of crucial importance when communicating and interpreting results.

When the tissues surrounding the bone were exposed to inflammation, the same strain magnitude was shown to be catabolic, as observed by Kozlovsky et al. [83] where "overloading" aggravated the plaque-induced bone resorption. Hürzeler et al. [79] did not observe bone gain or bone loss in uninflamed versus inflamed peri-implant tissues in response to "overloading." The reasons may be related to the rather limited orthodontic spring forces used onto these implants. Although initially named as "mechanical trauma forces" in their study objectives, the authors appreciated the forces as physiological when discussing their findings.

Once again, an important remark has to be made on the "overload" definition used in the reported clinical and animal studies. Even when one raises the occlusion with 3–4 mm, increases the crown/implant ratio's or isolates bruxers from nonbruxers, as long as the stresses and strains are not measured at the bone–implant interface one may only speculate about the real effect of the latter. Clinical indices concerning the magnitude, the direction, the frequency, etc., are not available as they are for plaque accumulation and peri-implant mucositis [85]. This renders it very difficult to correlate occlusal loading and peri-implant tissue reaction. Animal experimental research, however, has this potential and several methodologies with external loading devices enabling well-controlled and well-defined load application to explore the peri-implant tissue response to mechanical stimuli have been proposed [39,72,75, 86–88]. In particular, loading devices used in extra-oral set-up offer excellent control of the mechanical loading history. However, the latter studies were considered as nonrelevant for the systematic reviews as the extra-oral implant site does not harbor the oral microflora. On the other hand, the majority of the searched animal studies with an intraoral implant location were defectively designed owing to the lack of randomization and the lack of genuine control conditions. This opens perspectives and motivates incentives for establishing guidelines and quality assessment tools for animal experimental research (such as the ARRIVE guidelines [89]). It needs to be kept in mind, however, that no matter how well-designed and performed an animal experimental study is, the results cannot simply be extrapolated to the clinical situation due to the many differences between animals and humans.

It is further worth mentioning that even when an animal study investigating the effect of overload on peri-implant bone tissue would meet all criteria to be classified as low-risk bias, it is still impossible to measure the exact strains the peri-implant tissues are exposed to. Strain gauges experiments have tried to do so [90–92], although these are *in se* invalid as the measured strains are strains at the bone surface level and not at the bone–implant interface itself. Hence, for a better understanding of the biomechanical conditions validated numerical modeling data can be of value.

Finally, besides the peri-implantitis and the overloading hypothesis, Chvartsaid et al. [93] proposed the healing/adaptation theory for explaining implant failure and/or bone loss. They claim that marginal bone loss and implant failure depend on similar mechanisms, with only the magnitude of the trauma deciding whether an implant may fail or/and will result in marginal bone loss. The healing/adaptation theory sees adverse loading or peri-implantitis to be, at best, part of the problem behind marginal bone loss. Other factors are also involved such as; (1) poor surgical techniques, (2) poor host beds owing to genetical disorders, drug abuse, disease or previous irradiation, (3) too much strain from implant misfit, bone cell adjustment or prosthodontic errors, or (4) smoking, allergies, or similar conditions that disturb bone cells or their vascular supply. According to Wennerberg and Albrektsson [94], ongoing marginal bone loss may in case of implant micromovements evolve into something that may be termed as secondary peri-implantitis. This secondary problem may, of course, need clinical treatment. They hasten to say that this theory is more generally applicable to the true clinical situation than are hypotheses of isolated peri-implantitis or overloading, the alleged reasons for marginal bone loss in many experimental articles. The current review offers ammunition for this phrasing.

8.4 Concluding remarks

In this review, studies with various levels of evidence were discussed as—especially on the topic of peri-implant bone overload—very few or no studies with a high level of evidence such as systematic reviews or randomized clinical trials are available. Therefore, also animal experimental research was considered to evaluate this clinically relevant topic.

The available literature indicates that immediate loading as such does not compromise the establishment of osseointegration, although primary stability appears to be an important determining factor. Animal experimental studies [26,27,40–43] indicate that interfacial micromotion compromises the establishment of implant osseointegration. These findings from animal studies corroborate with these from clinical studies [24,25,34,35] by underlining the importance of sufficient primary stability for the implant prognosis as this secures the healing tissue against excessive interfacial micromotion.

Whereas several animal studies [72–75] report a detrimental effect of excessive load on peri-implant bone after osseointegration, this could not be observed in clinical studies. This indicates that it is unlikely that implant overload is the reason for peri-implant bone loss as it presents in many clinical cases. It does not necessarily mean, however, that implant loading cannot affect peri-implant bone. It is unlikely that excessive loads as applied in the described animal experiments would not lead to peri-implant bone breakdown in clinical situations. Scientific obstacles (e.g., in vivo quantification and qualification of the induced peri-implant strains) and ethical objections, however, impede performing clinical research that allows us to answer the question whether implant "overload" can lead to peri-implant bone loss and implant failure. We are, therefore, unable to scientifically prove a possible detrimental effect of excessive implant loads in the same way as we are unable to prove that Frost's mechanostat [6] would not apply to the peri-implant bone.

Acknowledgment

Wiley (© 2014 John Wiley & Sons Ltd) is gratefully acknowledged for granting permission to use the article authored by J. Duyck and K. Vandamme, published in the *Journal of Oral Rehabilitation* [95].

References

[1] Esposito M, Hirsch JM, Lekholm U, Thomsen P. Biological factors contributing to failures of osseointegrated oral implants. (I). Success criteria and epidemiology. Eur J Oral Sci 1998;106:527−51.

[2] Esposito M, Hirsch JM, Lekholm U, Thomsen P. Biological factors contributing to failures of osseointegrated oral implants. (II). Etiopathogenesis. Eur J Oral Sci 1998;106:721−64.

[3] Wolff JD. Das Gesetz der Transformation der Knochen. Berlin: A. Hirschwald; 1892.

[4] Duncan RL, Turner CH. Mechanotransduction and the functional response of bone to mechanical strain. Calcif Tissue Int 1995;57:344−58.

[5] Hsieh YF, Turner CH. Effects of loading frequency on mechanically induced bone formation. J Bone Miner Res 2001;16:918−24.

[6] Frost HM. A 2003 update of bone physiology and Wolff's Law for clinicians. Angle Orthod 2004;74:3−15.

[7] Farr JN, Blew RM, Lee VR, Lohman TG, Going SB. Associations of physical activity duration, frequency, and load with volumetric BMD, geometry, and bone strength in young girls. Osteoporos Int 2011;22:1419−30.

[8] Robling AG, Hinant FM, Burr DB, Turner CH. Improved bone structure and strength after long-term mechanical loading is greatest if loading is separated into short bouts. J Bone Miner Res 2002;17:1545−54.

[9] Berglundh T, Abrahamsson I, Lang NP, Lindhe J. De novo alveolar bone formation adjacent to endosseous implants. Clin Oral Implants Res 2003;14:251−62.

[10] Slaets E, Carmeliet G, Naert I, Duyck J. Early cellular responses in cortical bone healing around unloaded titanium implants: an animal study. J Periodontol 2006;77:1015−24.

[11] Slaets E, Carmeliet G, Naert I, Duyck J. Early trabecular bone healing around titanium implants: a histologic study in rabbits. J Periodontol 2007;78:510−7.

[12] Cook D, Genever P. Regulation of mesenchymal stem cell differentiation. Adv Exp Med Biol 2013;786:213−29.

[13] Pittenger MF, Mackay AM, Beck SC, Jaiswal RK, Douglas R, Mosca JD, et al. Multilineage potential of adult human mesenchymal stem cells. Science 1999;284:143−7.

[14] da Silva Meirelles L, Chagastelles PC, Nardi NB. Mesenchymal stem cells reside in virtually all post-natal organs and tissues. J Cell Sci 2006;119:2204−13.

[15] Carter DR, Beaupré GS, Giori NJ, Helms JA. Mechanobiology of skeletal regeneration. Clin Orthop Relat Res 1998;355S:S41−55.

[16] Castillo AB, Jacobs CR. Mesenchymal stem cell mechanobiology. Curr Osteoporos Rep 2010;8:98−104.

[17] Esposito M, Grusovin MG, Maghaireh H, Worthington HV. Interventions for replacing missing teeth: different times for loading dental implants. Cochrane Database Syst Rev March 28, 2013;3:CD003878.

[18] Xu L, Wang X, Zhang Q, Yang W, Zhu W, Zhao K. Immediate versus early loading of flapless placed dental implants: a systematic review. J Prosthet Dent October 2014;112(4):760–9. http://dx.doi.org/10.1016/j.prosdent.2014.01.026. Epub 2014 May 13.

[19] Benic GI, Mir-Mari J, Hämmerle CH. Loading protocols for single-implant crowns: a systematic review and meta-analysis. Int J Oral Maxillofac Implants 2014;29(Suppl.): 222–38. http://dx.doi.org/10.11607/jomi.2014suppl.g4.1 [Review].

[20] Moraschini V, Porto Barboza E. Immediate versus conventional loaded single implants in the posterior mandible: a meta-analysis of randomized controlled trials. pii:S0901-5027(15)00273-8 Int J Oral Maxillofac Surg August 8, 2015. http://dx.doi.org/10.1016/j.ijom.2015.07.014 [Epub ahead of print].

[21] Schrott A, Riggi-Heiniger M, Maruo K, Gallucci GO. Implant loading protocols for partially edentulous patients with extended edentulous sites—a systematic review and meta-analysis. Int J Oral Maxillofac Implants 2014;29(Suppl.):239–55. http://dx.doi.org/10.11607/jomi.2014suppl.g4.2 [Review].

[22] Papaspyridakos P, Chen CJ, Chuang SK, Weber HP. Implant loading protocols for edentulous patients with fixed prostheses: a systematic review and meta-analysis. Int J Oral Maxillofac Implants 2014;29(Suppl.):256–70. http://dx.doi.org/10.11607/jomi.2014suppl.g4.3.

[23] Schimmel M, Srinivasan M, Herrmann FR, Müller F. Loading protocols for implant-supported overdentures in the edentulous jaw: a systematic review and meta-analysis. Int J Oral Maxillofac Implants 2014;29(Suppl.):271–86. http://dx.doi.org/10.11607/jomi.2014suppl.g4.4.

[24] Szmukler-Moncler S, Salama H, Reingewirtz Y, Dubruille JH. Timing of loading and effect of micromotion on bone-dental implant interface: review of experimental literature. J Biomed Mater Res 1998;43:192–203.

[25] Tabassum A, Meijer GJ, Walboomers XF, Jansen JA. Evaluation of primary and secondary stability of titanium implants using different surgical techniques. Clin Oral Implants Res 2013. http://dx.doi.org/10.1111/clr.12180 [Epub ahead of print].

[26] Vandamme K, Naert I, Geris L, Vander Sloten J, Puers R, Duyck J. Histodynamics of bone tissue formation around immediately loaded cylindrical implants in the rabbit. Clin Oral Implants Res 2007;18:471–80.

[27] Vandamme K, Naert I, Geris L, Vander Sloten J, Puers R, Duyck J. Influence of controlled immediate loading and implant design on peri-implant bone formation. J Clin Periodontol 2007;34:172–81.

[28] Turkyilmaz I, McGlumphy EA. Influence of bone density on implant stability parameters and implant success: a retrospective clinical study. BMC Oral Health 2008;24:8–32.

[29] Freitas-Júnior AC, Rocha EP, Bonfante EA, Almeida EO, Anchieta RB, Martini AP, et al. Biomechanical evaluation of internal and external hexagon platform switched implant-abutment connections: an in vitro laboratory and three-dimensional finite element analysis. Dent Mater 2012;28:e218–228.

[30] Beer A, Gahleitner A, Holm A, Tschabitscher M, Homolka P. Correlation of insertion torques with bone mineral density from dental quantitative CT in the mandible. Clin Oral Implants Res 2003;14:616–20.

[31] Javed F, Romanos GE. The role of primary stability for successful immediate loading of dental implants. A literature review. J Dent 2010;38:612–20.

[32] Campos FE, Gomes JB, Marin C, Teixeira HS, Suzuki M, Witek L, et al. Effect of drilling dimension on implant placement torque and early osseointegration stages: an experimental study in dogs. J Oral Maxillofac Surg 2012;70:e43–50.

[33] Trisi P, Perfetti G, Baldoni E, Berardi D, Colagiovanni M, Scogna G. Implant micromotion is related to peak insertion torque and bone density. Clin Oral Implants Res 2009;20: 467–71.

[34] Ottoni JM, Oliveira ZF, Mansini R, Cabral AM. Correlation between placement torque and survival of single-tooth implants. Int J Oral Maxillofac Implants 2005;20:769–76.

[35] Cannizzaro G, Leone M, Ferri V, Viola P, Federico G, Esposito M. Immediate loading of single implants inserted flapless with medium or high insertion torque: a 6-month follow-up of a split-mouth randomised controlled trial. Eur J Oral Implantol 2012;5:333–42.

[36] Duyck J, Corpas L, Vermeiren S, Ogawa T, Quirynen M, Vandamme K, et al. Histological, histomorphometrical, and radiological evaluation of an experimental implant design with a high insertion torque. Clin Oral Implants Res 2010;21:877–84.

[37] Coelho PG, Granato R, Marin C, Bonfante EA, Freire JN, Janal MN, et al. Biomechanical evaluation of endosseous implants at early implantation times: a study in dogs. J Oral Maxillofac Surg 2010;68:1667–75.

[38] Duyck J, Roesems R, Vivan Cardoso M, Ogawa T, De Villa Camargos G, Vandamme K. Effect of insertion torque on titanium implant osseointegration: an animal experimental study. Clin Oral Implants Res 2013. http://dx.doi.org/10.1111/clr.12316 [Epub ahead of print].

[39] Duyck J, De Cooman M, Puers R, Van Oosterwyck H, Vander Sloten J, Naert I. A repeated sampling bone chamber methodology for the evaluation of tissue differentiation and bone adaptation around titanium implants under controlled mechanical conditions. J Biomech 2004;37:1819–22.

[40] Duyck J, Vandamme K, Geris L, Van Oosterwyck H, De Cooman M, Vandersloten J, et al. The influence of micro-motion on the tissue differentiation around immediately loaded cylindrical turned titanium implants. Arch Oral Biol 2006;51:1–9.

[41] Duyck J, Slaets E, Sasaguri K, Vandamme K, Naert I. Effect of intermittent loading and surface roughness on peri-implant bone formation in a bone chamber model. J Clin Periodontol 2007;34:998–1006.

[42] Vandamme K, Naert I, Geris L, Vander Sloten J, Puers R, Duyck J. The effect of micro-motion on the tissue response around immediately loaded roughened titanium implants in the rabbit. Eur J Oral Sci 2007;115(1):21–9. Erratum in: Eur J Oral Sci 2007;115:167.

[43] Vandamme K, Naert I, Vander Sloten J, Puers R, Duyck J. Effect of implant surface roughness and loading on peri-implant bone formation. J Periodontol 2008;79:150–7.

[44] Jansen JA, de Groot K. Guinea pig and rabbit model for the histological evaluation of permanent percutaneous implants. Biomaterials 1988;9:268–72.

[45] De Smet E, Jaecques SV, Jansen JJ, Walboomers F, Vander Sloten J, Naert IE. Effect of constant strain rate, composed of varying amplitude and frequency, of early loading on peri-implant bone (re)modelling. J Clin Periodontol 2007;34:618–24.

[46] Frost HM. Bone "mass" and the "mechanostat": a proposal. Anat Rec 1987;219:1–9.

[47] Ogawa T, Zhang X, Naert I, Vermaelen P, Deroose CM, Sasaki K, et al. The effect of whole body vibration on peri-implant bone healing in rats. Clin Oral Implants Res 2011 Mar;22(3):302–7.

[48] Ogawa T, Possemiers T, Zhang X, Naert I, Chaudhari A, Sasaki K, et al. Influence of loading time on the impact of whole body vibration on peri-implant bone healing: a histomorphometrical study on rat. J Clin Periodontol 2011 Feb;38(2):180–5.

[49] Ogawa T, Vandamme K, Zhang X, Naert I, Possemiers T, Chaudhari A, et al. Stimulation of titanium implant osseointegration through high frequency vibration loading is enhanced when applied at high acceleration. Calcif Tissue Int November 2014;95(5):467–75.

[50] Zhang X, Vandamme K, Torcasio A, Ogawa T, van Lenthe GH, Naert I, et al. In vivo assessment of the effect of controlled high- and low-frequency mechanical loading on peri-implant bone healing. J R Soc Interface 2012 Jul 7;9(72):1697−704.

[51] Zhang X, Torcasio A, Vandamme K, Ogawa T, van Lenthe GH, Naert I, et al. Enhancement of implant osseointegration by high-frequency low-magnitude loading. PLoS One 2012;7(7):e40488.

[52] Naert I, Duyck J, Vandamme K. Occlusal overload and bone/implant loss. Clin Oral Implants Res 2012;(Suppl. 6):95−107.

[53] Adell R, Lekholm U, Rockler B, Brånemark PI. A 15-year study of osseointegrated implants in the treatment of the edentulous jaw. Int J Oral Surg 1981;10:387−416.

[54] Klineberg I, Kingston D, Murray G. The bases for using a particular occlusal design in tooth and implant-borne reconstructions and complete dentures. Clin Oral Implants Res 2007;18S3:151−67.

[55] Jofré J, Hamada T, Nishimura M, Klattenhoff C. The effect of maximum bite force on marginal bone loss of mini-implants supporting a mandibular overdenture: a randomized controlled trial. Clin Oral Implants Res 2010;21:243−9.

[56] Vigolo P, Zaccaria M. Clinical evaluation of marginal bone level change of multiple adjacent implants restored with splinted and nonsplinted restorations: a 5-year prospective study. Int J Oral Maxillofac Implants 2010;25:1189−94.

[57] van Kampen F, Cune M, van der Bilt A, Bosman F. The effect of maximum bite force on marginal bone loss in mandibular overdenture treatment: an in vivo study. Clin Oral Implants Res 2005;16:587−93.

[58] Stanford CM. Biomechanical and functional behavior of implants. Adv Dent Res 1999;13: 88−92.

[59] Stanford CM, Brand RA. Toward an understanding of implant occlusion and strain adaptive bone modeling and remodeling. J Prosthet Dent 1999;81(5):553−61.

[60] Isidor F. Influence of forces on peri-implant bone. Clin Oral Implants Res 2006;17(S2): 8−18.

[61] Cehreli MC, Akca K. Mechanobiology of bone and mechanocoupling of endosseous titanium oral implants. J Long Term Eff Med Implants 2005;15:139−52.

[62] Lobbezoo F, Brouwers JE, Cune MS, Naeije M. Dental implants in patients with bruxing habits. J Oral Rehabil 2006;33:152−9.

[63] Lobbezoo F, Van Der Zaag J, Naeije M. Bruxism: its multiple causes and its effects on dental implants - an updated review. J Oral Rehabil 2006;33:293−300.

[64] Johansson A, Omar R, Carlsson GE. Bruxism and prosthetic treatment: a critical review. J Prosthodont Res 2011;55:127−36.

[65] Manfredini D, Bucci MB, Sabattini VB, Lobbezoo F. Bruxism: overview of current knowledge and suggestions for dental implants planning. Cranio 2011;29:304−12.

[66] Duyck J, Naert IE, Van Oosterwyck H, Van der Sloten J, De Cooman M, Lievens S, et al. Biomechanics of oral implants: a review of the literature. Technol Health Care 1997;5:253−73.

[67] Duyck J, Naert I. Failure of oral implants: aetiology, symptoms and influencing factors. Clin Oral Investig 1998;2:102−14.

[68] van Steenberghe D, Naert I, Jacobs R, Quirynen M. Influence of inflammatory reactions vs. occlusal loading on peri-implant marginal bone level. Adv Dent Res 1999;13:130−5.

[69] Oh TJ, Yoon J, Misch CE, Wang HL. The causes of early implant bone loss: myth or science? J Periodontol 2002;73:322−33.

[70] Misch CE, Suzuki JB, Misch-Dietsh FM, Bidez MW. A positive correlation between occlusal trauma and peri-implant bone loss: literature support. Implant Dent 2005;14: 108−16.

[71] Sakka S, Coulthard P. Implant failure: etiology and complications. Med Oral Patol Oral Cir Bucal 2011;16(1):e42–44.
[72] Hoshaw SJ, Brunski JB, Cochran GVB. Mechanical loading of Brånemark implants affects interfacial bone modelling and remodelling. Int J Oral Maxillofac Implants 1994;9: 345–60.
[73] Isidor F. Loss of osseointegration caused by occlusal load of oral implants. A clinical and radiographic study in monkeys. Clin Oral Implants Res 1996;7:143–52.
[74] Isidor F. Histological evaluation of peri-implant bone at implant subjected to occlusal overload or plaque accumulation. Clin Oral Implants Res 1997;8:1–9.
[75] Duyck J, Rønold HJ, Van Oosterwyck H, Naert I, Vander Sloten J, Ellingsen JE. The influence of static and dynamic loading on marginal bone reactions around osseointegrated implants: an animal experimental study. Clin Oral Implants Res 2001;12:207–18.
[76] Chambrone L, Chambrone LA, Lima LA. Effects of occlusal overload on peri-implant tissue health: a systematic review of animal-model studies. J Periodontol 2010;81: 1367–78.
[77] Quirynen M, De Soete M, van Steenberghe D. Infectious risks for oral implants: a review of the literature. Clin Oral Implants Res 2002;13:1–19.
[78] Lang NP, Berglundh T. Periimplant diseases: where are we now? consensus of the seventh european workshop on periodontology. J Clin Periodontol 2011;38(Suppl. 11):178–81.
[79] Hürzeler MB, Quinones CR, Kohal RJ, Rohde M, Strub JR, Teuscher U, et al. Changes in peri-implant tissues subjected to orthodontic forces and ligature breakdown in monkeys. J Peridontol 1998;69:396–404.
[80] Gotfredsen K, Berglundh T, Lindhe J. Bone reactions adjacent to titanium implants subjected to static load. A study in the dog (I). Clin Oral Implants Res 2001;12:1–8.
[81] Gotfredsen K, Berglundh T, Lindhe J. Bone reactions adjacent to titanium implants with different surface characteristics subjected to static load. A study in the dog (II). Clin Oral Implants Res 2001;12:196–201.
[82] Gotfredsen K, Berglundh T, Lindhe J. Bone reactions adjacent to titanium implants subjected to static load of different duration. A study in the dog (III). Clin Oral Implants Res 2001;12:552–8.
[83] Kozlovsky A, Tal H, Laufer BZ, Leshem R, Rohrer MD, Weinreb M, et al. Impact of implant overloading on the peri-implant bone in inflamed and non-inflamed peri-implant mucosa. Clin Oral Implants Res 2007;18:601–10.
[84] Ikumi N, Suzawa T, Yoshimura K, Kamijo R. Bone response to static compressive stress at bone-implant interface: a pilot study of critical static compressive stress. Int J Oral Maxillofac Implants 2015 Jul–Aug;30(4):827–33. http://dx.doi.org/10.11607/jomi.3715.
[85] Mombelli A, van Oosten MA, Schurch Jr E, Land NP. The microbiota associated with successful or failing osseointegrated titanium implants. Oral Microbiol Immun 1987;2:145–51.
[86] De Smet E, Jaecques SV, Wevers M, Jansen JA, Jacobs R, Vander Sloten J, et al. Effect of controlled early implant loading on bone healing and bone mass in guinea pigs, as assessed by micro-CT and histology. Eur J Oral Sci 2006;114:232–42.
[87] Ko CC, Douglas WH, DeLong R, Rohrer MD, Swift JQ, Hodges JS, et al. Effects of implant healing time on crestal bone loss of a controlled-load dental implant. J Dent Res 2003;82:585–91.
[88] Leucht P, Kim JB, Wazen R, Currey JA, Nanci A, Brunski JB, et al. Effect of mechanical stimuli on skeletal regeneration around implants. Bone 2007;40:919–30.
[89] Kilkenny C, Browne WJ, Cuthill IC, Emerson M, Altman DG. Improving bioscience research reporting: the ARRIVE guidelines for reporting animal research. PLoS Biol 2010; 8:e1000412.

[90] Geris L, Andreykiv A, Van Oosterwyck H, Vandersloten JV, van Keulen F, Duyck J, et al. Numerical simulation of tissue differentiation around loaded titanium implants in a bone chamber. J Biomech 2004;37:763–9.

[91] Jaecques SV, Van Oosterwyck H, Muraru L, Van Cleynenbreugel T, De Smet E, Wevers M, et al. Individualised, micro CT-based finite element modelling as a tool for biomechanical analysis related to tissue engineering of bone. Biomaterials 2004;25: 1683–96.

[92] Mellal A, Wiskott HW, Botsis J, Scherrer SS, Belser UC. Stimulating effect of implant loading on surrounding bone. Comparison of three numerical models and validation by in vivo data. Clin Oral Implants Res 2004;15:239–48.

[93] Chvartsaid D, Koka S, Zarb G. Osseointegration failure. In: Zarb G, Albrektsson T, Baker G, et al., editors. Osseointegration: on continuing synergies in surgery, prosthodontics, biomaterials. Chicago: Quintessence; 2008. p. 157–64.

[94] Wennerberg A, Albrektsson T. Current challenges in successful rehabilitation with oral implants. J Oral Rehabil 2011;38:286–94.

[95] Duyck J, Vandamme K. The effect of loading on peri-implant bone: a critical review of the literature. J Oral Rehabil October 2014;41(10):783–94. http://dx.doi.org/10.1111/joor.12195. Epub 2014 Jun 3. Review.

[96] Laurell L, Lundgren D. Marginal bone level changes at dental implants after 5 years in function: a meta-analysis. Clin Implant Dent Relat Res 2011 Mar;13(1):19–28. http://dx.doi.org/10.1111/j.1708–8208.2009.00,182.x.

[97] Moraschini V, Poubel LA, Ferreira VF, Barboza Edos S. Evaluation of survival and success rates of dental implants reported in longitudinal studies with a follow-up period of at least 10 years: a systematic review. Int J Oral Maxillofac Surg 2015 Mar;44(3):377–88. http://dx.doi.org/10.1016/j.ijom.2014.10.023. Epub 2014 Nov 20.

Bone response to decontamination treatments for dental biomaterials

9

J. Diaz-Marcos
Scientific and Technological Centers of the University of Barcelona, Barcelona, Spain

9.1 Introduction

9.1.1 Dental implant materials

9.1.1.1 Brief history

The earliest chronologies of implant materials date back to two ancient civilizations, around 500 years ago when the Incas of Peru used gold and silver to repair trephination defects and in Egypt [1] where carved seashells and/or stones were placed into the human jaw bone to replace missing teeth. Other documented examples of early implants are those fabricated from noble metals and shaped to recreate natural roots. Petronius offered an early description of the use of alloplastic materials in 1565 when he described the closure of a cranial defect with a gold plate. Over the next 300 years, the use of implants was sporadic and often complicated by infection.

The use of man-made materials as bioimplants did not become widespread until the 1940s, when advances in biomaterial science led to the development of numerous materials suitable for implantation. Alloplastic implantation is indicated for the stabilization of fractures and for the reconstruction or augmentation of soft tissue defects or bony deformities. Searching for the ideal material was a challenge: it should not produce foreign body inflammatory response and it should discourage the growth of microorganisms. Besides, it should be sterilizable, nontoxic, nonallergenic, noncarcinogenic, and biologically compatible. Other criteria for the ideal implant material include resistance to strain and deformation, ease of removal, ease of shaping into the desired form, and, in certain circumstances, radiolucency [14].

Contemporary dental implant history starts during World War II. During his years in the army, Dr Norman Goldberg worked about dental restoration using metals that had been used to replace other parts of the body [2,3]. After a few years, in 1948, in partnership with Dr Aaron Gershkoff, they produced the first successful subperiosteal implant [2]. This success became the foundation of implant dentistry and they also became pioneers in teaching techniques in dental schools and dental societies around the world [2–4].

A milestone in dental implantology development occurred in 1957; Per-Ingvar Brånemark, while studying bone healing and regeneration, discovered that the bone could grow in proximity with the titanium (Ti) and that it could effectively be adhered to that metal without being rejected [5]. Therefore, Brånemark called this phenomenon

Bone Response to Dental Implant Materials. http://dx.doi.org/10.1016/B978-0-08-100287-2.00009-4

"osseointegration," and he carried out many further studies using both animal and human subjects. In 1965, he placed the first Ti dental implants into a 34-year-old human patient with missing teeth due to severe chin and jaw deformities. Brånemark inserted four Ti fixtures into the patient's mandible and several months later he used the fixtures as the foundation for a fixed set of prosthetic teeth [4]. The dental implants served for more than 40 years, until the end of the patient's life [2–7].

Brånemark published many studies on the use of Ti implants, and between 1978 and 1981 [8,9], he cofounded a company for the development and marketing of dental implants. Brånemark's discovery had such a profound impact in dentistry that, to the present day, over 7 million Brånemark System implants have been placed, even though hundreds of other companies produce dental implants [6,7].

Back to the early 1980s, Brånemark presented the results of his 15 years of human and animal research at the Toronto Conference on Osseointegration in Clinical Dentistry. After the conference, researchers from the United States were trained in Brånemark's methods in Sweden [4,10].

The 1980s showed new developments; US Food and Drug Administration approved the use of Ti dental implants and, in 1983, Dr Matts Andersson developed the Procera (Nobel Biocare, Zurich, Switzerland) computer-aided design and computer-aided manufacturing method of high precision, repeatable manufacturing of dental crowns [11]; the quality and anchorage of materials and techniques was improved [1]. During the mid-1980s, esthetic restorations became the main focus of important developments in dental implantology [4].

In the 1990s, the development of modern ceramics was also significant in setting new implant materials; during the same decade, dental implant companies incorporated ceramic surface treatments and ceramic-like elements to implants so as to enhance osseointegration [11–15].

Nowadays, tens of thousands of osseointegrated dental implants are placed every year, with an expectation of 95% success rate (in the case of single tooth replacement with an implant supported crown), with minimum risks and associated complications [4].

9.1.1.2 *Classification*

There are different types of dental implant and available materials, shapes, and surface characteristics. The most diverse designs and surface modifications have been developed to improve clinical outcomes, including a subperiosteal form, blade form, ramus frame, and endosseous form [16]. Several parameters in the design of endosseous implants affect their survival rate: body shape, size, chemical surface composition, and topographical features among others.

Typically, the most common implant materials include metals, calcium ceramics, polymers, and biologic materials. Nevertheless, the market is in constant transformation. The materials that promote biocompatibility, bioacceptance, and implant failures are a rare occurrence, provided that they are properly used and placed. For better understanding and better treatment we must know the materials and bone reaction toward them, as there is no single material that features all the desired properties of implant so far.

Pure Ti and Ti alloys are the most common material when it comes to dental implants because of their well-balanced combination of mechanical strength, chemical stability, and biocompatibility [17]. Basically, they are made out of grade 4 commercially pure Ti. However, Ti alloys, mainly Ti6Al4V, are also used since they are stronger, more fatigue resistant, and stronger than other grades of pure Ti [18,19]. Integration of titanium implants with the surrounding bone is critical for successful bone regeneration and healing of dental implant.

Alternative materials used in dental implants are 316L stainless steel and CoCR-Mo. PMMA (polymethyl methacrylate) and culture polystyrene and ceramic coatings such as hydroxyapatite and borosilicate glass seem to improve the ingrowth of bone, while promoting chemical integration of the implant with the bone.

9.1.2 Endosseous dental implants and osseointegration

The concept of osseointegration was discovered by Brånemark and his coworker [8] and it has had a pronounced impact on clinical treatment of oral implants. Osseointegration is the direct and stable anchorage of an implant due to the formation of bony tissue around the implant (Fig. 9.1). A number of systemic and local factors influence the production of an osseointegrated interface and therefore the stability of the implant.

The purpose of placement of endosseous dental implants is to achieve short- and long-term outcomes of osseointegration or biointegration of the bone with the implant, with faster and stronger bone formation. This will likely confer better stability during the healing process, which, preferentially, will improve the clinical performance in the area of poor bone quality and quantity while playing an important role in molecular interactions and cellular response. Initial events at the surface include the orientated adsorption of molecules from the surrounding fluid, creating a conditioned interface the cell responds to. Furthermore, such promotion may, in turn, accelerate bone healing, allowing immediate or early loading protocols.

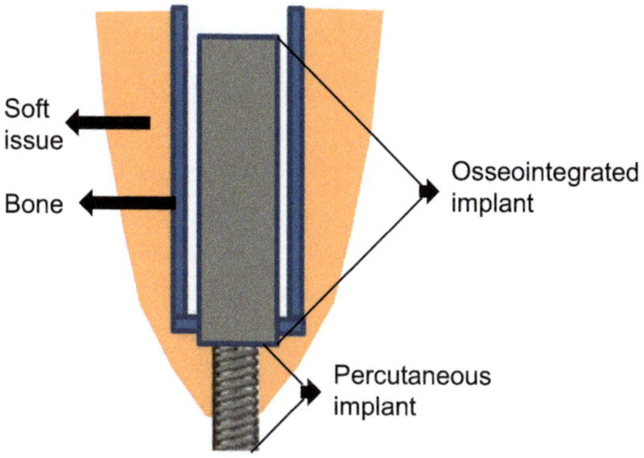

Figure 9.1 Osseointegrated implant for prosthetic attachment.

Therefore, one of the main objectives of the implant materials is to promote osseointegration. Only a few implant materials promote osseointegration and biointegration, as it is the case of Ti and Ti alloy (Ti6A14V). The long-term success of Ti alloy dental implants [20] largely depends on two factors; the first one is the rapid healing process and safe integration into the jaw bone (osseointegration) [21]. The surface topography of the Ti alloy is crucial for the long-term success of dental implants. The second key factor is the ability of surface titanium oxide to osseointegrate. In the last decade, treatments for Ti implant materials have been developed in a concentrated effort to improve the osseointegration process [22]. It has been recently shown that changes in the physicochemical properties of Ti alloy implants result in significant modulation of cell recruitment, adhesion, inflammation, and bone remodeling activities, in addition to regulation of the bone formation response [23]. The oxide limits dissolution of elements and promotion of the deposition of biological molecules that allow the bone to exist as close as 3 nm from the implant surface are two key factors of Ti success. However, two important details remain undefined, that is, the details of the ultrastructure of the gap between the implant and bone and the effect of elements that are released on the interface. These areas of investigation are particularly important in defining the differences between commercially pure titanium implants and those made of titanium, aluminum, and vanadium. Outstanding matters in dispute are the characteristics and mechanisms of these coatings, which are complex and affect the bone response and the degradation of the coatings [24].

Progress in dental implantology is likely to continue so as to clarify the nature of the interface between the material and bone and to develop biological molecules and artificial tissues. Scientists all over the world have deployed second-generation implants with engineered surfaces that can accelerate and improve implant osseointegration. This second wave of clinically used implants can feature surfaces that are mechanically blasted, acid etched, coated with bioactive molecules, anodized, and, more recently, laser modified [25–28]. These implants have been extensively documented in vivo, including long-term clinical studies and experimental histological and biomechanical evaluation in animal models. Additional information in clinical results of commercially available implants can be found [29–31].

9.1.3 Peri-implantitis and re-osseointegration

Peri-implantitis is an "inflammatory process around an implant, characterized by soft tissue inflammation and loss of supporting bone" [32] and peri-implant diseases are becoming a major health issue in dentistry [33]. Peri-implantitis is an opportunistic infection caused by bacteria (Fig. 9.2).

Biofilms form on all hard, nonshedding surfaces in an aqueous environment, such as implants in fluid systems. However, bone loss is a potential complication for dental implants once inflammation of the gum and dental tissue around the implant sets in due to bacterial infection. The advantageous dental implant surface properties, i.e., the high reactivity of the oxidized titanium that allows cellular adhesion, are altered by the presence of bacteria and the residues of their metabolic activity. Thus, the contaminated surface acts as a foreign body and can lead to more inflammation of the soft

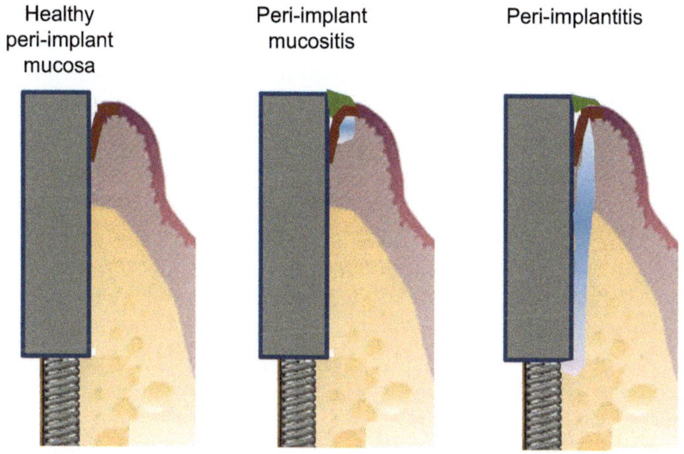

Figure 9.2 Peri-implantitis formation on dental implants.

tissue and bone loss surrounding the implant. Despite the magnitude of this problem and the potentially severe consequences, commonly acceptable treatment protocols are missing. Similarities in the etiology and pathogenesis of peri-implantitis and periodontitis suggest the utilization of similar treatment principles [34,35]. The treatment of peri-implantitis involves surface decontamination and cleaning, may include surgical and nonsurgical approaches, either individually or combined, and systemic antibiotics may also be incorporated. These different treatments for peri-implantitis could possibly be used in a strategic way to modify the implant surface and cause an improvement in the host-to-implant response [36]. The available literature is still lacking with large heterogeneity in the clinical response, thus suggesting possible underlying predisposing conditions that are not all clear to us. It is extremely important to understand the effect of the different dental treatments on the surface properties of the implant and whether these may accelerate the re-osseointegration of dental implants during healing after peri-implantitis. The osseointegration of dental implants is relatively long (3–6 months); therefore, surface modifications able to accelerate this phenomenon will lead to shorter healing times, lower failure rates, and minimization of discomfort for the patient [37]. In recent years, several treatment strategies (mechanical, chemical, physicochemical, etc.) have been proposed for the infection of the dental tissue around an implant (peri-implantitis) [38].

Peri-implantitis is becoming an ever growing oral health concern that is frequently encountered in the dental office. The number of dental implants that are currently placed annually is somewhat elusive; however, the best estimate available puts this figure at around 15 million new implants (worldwide) every year [39]. Of these, how many will eventually develop peri-implant diseases is also debatable [40–43] due to the different patient variables such as smoking [44,45], preexisting periodontal disease [46,47], oral hygiene [48,49], quality of prosthetic reconstruction [50,51], and some systemic conditions and medications [52,53]. Thus, with the current lack of universally accepted criteria for the definition of peri-implantitis, the use of different thresholds is likely to produce different prevalence rates. However, even with the more conservative estimates, the number of new implants that are likely to be affected by peri-implant diseases every year is in the high million range, of which seven to eight million are likely to develop peri-implant mucositis, whereas about three to four million will develop peri-implantitis. Nevertheless, despite the magnitude of this problem and the potentially severe consequences that may result from a nonresponsive peri-implantitis condition, commonly accepted protocols are yet to be agreed upon.

On the other hand, although considerable bone fill may occur following treatment of peri-implantitis, re-osseointegration appears to be limited and unpredictable. It is important to evaluate the effects of various decontamination techniques and implant surface configurations on re-osseointegration of contaminated dental implants. An additional consideration should be the fact that anti-infective therapy must precede any regenerative treatment. Anti-infective therapy may include good mechanical plaque removal such as the application of antiseptics and administration of antibiotics supported by an effective oral hygiene home care program, all of them being steps to reduce the number of pathogens. As a complement to this, a bone regenerative treatment may be indicated depending on the amount of bone lost, the defect morphology, and the patient's response and care.

Re-osseointegration is also influenced by rough surfaces [54], since it speeds up the osseointegration rate [55] and favors both bone-to-implant contact and biomechanical stability [18,56]. The quality of an implant surface can also influence both osseointegration and re-osseointegration. In this line, Parlar et al. [57] demonstrated that re-osseointegration failed to occur for implant surfaces exposed to bacterial contamination, but consistently occurred when a pristine implant component replaced the contaminated implant surface. However, the quality is not a key factor, since osseointegration can occur on implants that were contaminated and cleansed by different methods [58]. The cleansing of a previously plaque-contaminated implant is sufficient for re-osseointegration to occur.

9.2 Decontamination methods: description and applications

Dental personnel may be exposed to a broad range of microorganisms in the blood and saliva of patients they treat in the dental operatory. These include *Mycobacterium tuberculosis*, hepatitis B virus, staphylococci, streptococci, cytomegalovirus, herpes simplex virus types I and II, human T-lymphotropic virus type III/lymphadenopathy-associated virus, and a number of viruses that infect the upper respiratory tract. Infections may be transmitted in dental practice by blood or saliva through direct contact, droplets, or aerosols. Patients and dental health care workers have the potential of transmitting infections [59].

Oral infection, especially periodontitis, may affect the course and pathogenesis of a number of systemic diseases, such as cardiovascular disease, bacterial pneumonia, diabetes mellitus, and low birth weight. Three mechanisms or pathways linking oral infections to secondary systemic effects have been proposed: (i) metastatic spread of infection from the oral cavity as a result of transient bacteremia, (ii) metastatic injury from the effects of circulating oral microbial toxins, and (iii) metastatic inflammation caused by immunological injury induced by oral microorganisms. Periodontitis as a major oral infection that may affect the host's susceptibility to systemic disease in three ways: shared risk factors; subgingival biofilms acting as reservoirs of Gram-negative bacteria; and the periodontium acting as a reservoir of inflammatory mediators [60]. Bacteria from the oral biofilms may be aspirated into the respiratory tract to influence the initiation and progression of systemic infectious conditions such as pneumonia. Oral bacteria, poor oral hygiene, and periodontitis seem to influence the incidence of pulmonary infections, especially nosocomial pneumonia episodes in high-risk subjects [61].

It is recognized that infection-control strategies are important in preventing and controlling hepatitis B, acquired immunodeficiency syndrome, and other infectious diseases caused by blood-borne viruses [62–64]. The ability of hepatitis B virus to survive in the environment [65] and the high titers of virus in blood [66] make this virus a good model for infection-control practices devised to prevent transmission of a large number of other infectious agents by blood or saliva. Because all infected patients cannot be identified by history, physical examination, or readily available laboratory tests [63], an extremely precise technical protocol should be routinely used in the care of all patients in dental practices.

As mentioned earlier, the dental personnel suffer different pathologies because of the exposition to different microorganisms. Therefore, it is necessary to use and better understand the commonly exploited dental treatments to avoid and remove the microorganism and to improve the implants' ability to re-osseointegrate, or the tendency of bone to reintegrate into the implant material, during healing. The effects of various odontological treatments, such as ultrasonication, jet polishing, laser illumination, and chemical exposure on the implants' surface roughness and chemistry will be explained. When applied strategically, these dental methods may prove useful in improving the chances for re-osseointegration of implants after the successful treatment of peri-implantitis.

9.2.1 Methods

Several therapeutic approaches including mechanical, antiseptic, and air-abrasive treatment, photodynamic treatment, sonic, and ultrasonic scalers, lasers, air–powder abrasion, and various chemical solutions such as chlorhexidine digluconate (CHX), citric acid, hydrogen peroxide, and saline were applied and tested for implant surface decontamination (e.g., Schou et al. [67]). Although some of the above-mentioned interventions may be effective, no consensus has been reached about the most effective treatment for peri-implantitis [68,69].

The most relevant methods are shown below.

9.2.1.1 Mechanical means (dental curettes, ultrasonic scalers, air–powder abrasive)

Titanium brush and ultrasonic cleaning are the easiest to use under surgical conditions. Cotton pellets with saline solution may be adequate for the cleaning of microrough surfaces (Persson et al. [70]). Similarly, Schou et al. [67] demonstrated in their animal experiments that treatment of infected plasma-sprayed titanium surfaces with air–powder + citric acid, gauze soaked saline + citric acid or gauze soaked with CHX led to equal results.

9.2.1.2 Antiseptic and air-abrasive treatment

Air abrasives with sodium bicarbonate powder are capable of removing all viable cells but are the least convenient due to the grit and mess in a flapped surgical site. Soaked cotton pellets, air–powder abrasive, citric acid, delmopinol, chlorhexidine irrigation, and rotating brushes with pumice alone or in different combinations were used [71–74].

For decontamination of the infected implant surfaces, rinsing with saline (or cleaning with cotton pellets soaked with sterile saline) and air-abrasive treatments seem to work. Laser decontamination of the surface does not improve healing results. Nonsurgical therapy of implants with peri-implantitis does not lead to successful treatment outcomes.

9.2.1.3 Physicochemical methods

The most common physicochemical treatments are chemical surface reactions (e.g., oxidation, acid-etching), sand blasting, ion implantation, laser ablation, coating the surface with inorganic calcium phosphate, etc. These methods alter the energy, charge, and composition of the existing surface but they provide surfaces with modified roughness and morphology as well [75].

9.2.1.4 Ultrasound

Ultrasonic cleaning is a common technique of modern dentistry. It is used for both periodontal and peri-implant treatments. The ultrasonic tip is made of very thin hardened steel. Vibration induces a phenomenon called cavitation, which is the formation of cavities or bubbles in a liquid medium containing gas or vapor. In addition, the vibratory motion allows debridement, that is, the breakdown of microorganisms attached to the surface of the tooth or implant [19].

9.2.1.5 Laser application

The most important reasons for laser application in the treatment of peri-implantitis and for the oral implants success are the significant reduction in bacteria on the implant surface and the peri-implant tissues during irradiation and that it is a minimally invasive procedure to treat failing implants [76]. The laser decontamination of the surface caused by CO_2 laser irradiation has been reported to pose a risk because of the temperature increase of the implant surface. Then, it should be avoided for the removal of subgingival calculus since it causes melting and carbonization of the root cementum [77]. Using the LightWalker's Er:YAG 2940 nm wavelength, it is possible to clean the granulation tissues, both on the bone and implant surfaces, and thoroughly decontaminate the infected site. Er:YAG does not promote excessive heating [78] and is considered efficient for implant surface decontamination [77]. Nevertheless, it can produce temperature increase above the critical threshold to bone safety (10°C) after 10 s [79]. The erbium laser targets the water content to remove the granulation tissue selectively due to its ability to use long-pulse durations and low peak power, while ablating the microorganisms on the surface of the bone. The bactericidal effect of low-power Er:YAG on the surgical site is also effective against endotoxins and lipopolysaccharides, which provide the complete cleansing of the implant surface without chemicals or any surface modification on the implant. Er:YAG is also used with shorter pulse durations to activate bleeding and decorticating the bony wall of the defect.

On the contrary, Er,Cr:YSGG was reported [80] to be safe to titanium and zirconia material, but decontamination of the surface does not improve healing results. Er,Cr: YSGG laser irradiation used to decontaminate the implant surface is expected to have a different behavior in the oral cavity where the presence of water of the gingival fluid, saliva, and blood is different from the in vitro situation. The wavelength of Er,Cr:YSGG laser is highly specific to water and the behavior of the laser treatment to decontaminate superficial implants can be different depending on the clinical situation. Although there are few available studies, there is evidence of improved clinical results [81–82].

9.2.1.6 Photodynamic therapy

Photodynamic therapy (PDT) involves the use of light-activated dyes (photosensitizers). When the photosensitizers are activated in the presence of oxygen they produce cytotoxic species, which are known to be effective against viruses, bacteria, and fungi. Therefore, PDT can be used as a therapy for localized infections. PDT in dentistry involves the application of a photosensitizer gel. The photosensitizing gel produces free oxygen radicals, which are highly reactive when in contact with the cell walls of microorganisms and, thus, toxic to them. This therapy is often used for peri-implantitis treatment and several studies have demonstrated a high bactericidal effect of this process being a valuable alternative to conventional mechanical procedures [83–86]. To date the phenothiazine dyes (toluidine blue O and methylene blue) are the major photosensitizers that have been used clinically. Both are very effective photosensitizing agents for the inactivation of Gram-positive as well as Gram-negative periodontal pathogenic bacteria [87]. In this study, the Ti alloy implant samples were covered with a toluidine blue gel, then illuminated (Application FotoSan Lamp at 570 nm), left to stand for 1 min (100 μg/mL), then illuminated a second time (application of a soft laser 906 nm), and finally rinsed with plenty of physiological saline.

Also, in the treatment of periodontitis, PDT alone showed similar improvements when compared to deep scaling and root planning [84]. The application of antimicrobial PDT can effectively reduce the prevalence of pathogens on implant surfaces without causing any deleterious defects on the implant bone surfaces [88,89]. However, studies on patients are limited and clinically significant effects of antimicrobial PDT have not yet been demonstrated.

Currently, the clinically used dyes do not differentiate between bacteria and host cells. Thus, activation of PDT by lasers also causes damage to the host cells since it does not specifically react only with pathogens.

9.2.1.7 Biochemical methods

In addition to the physicochemical methods, biochemistry is generating a lot of excitement. Today we struggle to produce biomaterials that interact with specific targets within the body or mimic tissue architecture. It is well known that biological systems have a highly developed ability to recognize special features of the surface on the molecular scale. We look to nature when we design "biomimetic" materials to understand how cells interact with other cells, extracellular proteins, and tissues. This knowledge is then utilized to develop biomimetic strategies for functional, interactive biomaterials. These strategies include biodegradable and "smart" materials used in targeted drug delivery systems and tissue engineering, as well as biochemical modifications of biomaterial surfaces for implant or wound-healing applications [90,91]. The aim of biochemical methods applied to implants is to immobilize biomolecules (i.e., peptides, proteins, enzymes) on the surface to ensure specific cell and tissue responses (adhesion, signaling, stimulation) and to control the tissue–implant interface with molecules delivered directly there [92–95].

9.3 Implant surfaces and bone response after decontamination

9.3.1 Introduction to surface features

Surface roughness evaluation is very important for many fundamental problems such as friction, contact deformation, electrochemistry, heat and electric current conduction, tightness of contact joints, odontology, and positional accuracy. For this reason surface roughness has been the subject of experimental and theoretical investigations for many decades. The real surface geometry is so complicated that a finite number of parameters cannot provide a full description. If the number of parameters used is increased, a more accurate description can be obtained. Surface roughness parameters are normally categorized into four groups according to its functionality. These groups are defined as amplitude parameters, spacing parameters, hybrid parameters, and functional parameters.

Each component of surface texture has a different origin and effect in the interaction of the surface. Surface texture of any material can be separated in different component wavelength (Fig. 9.3).

Roughness parameters can be calculated in either two-dimensional (2D) or three-dimensional (3D) forms. 2D profile analysis has been widely used in science and engineering for more than half a century. In recent years, there was an increased need for 3D surface analysis.

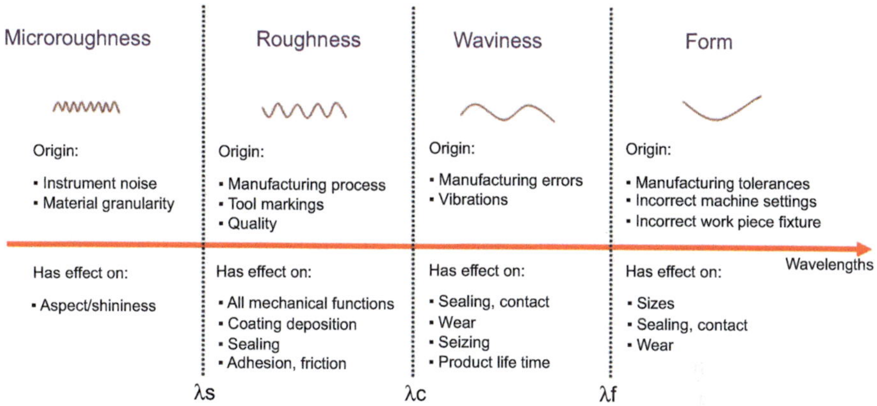

Figure 9.3 Surface texture components. Each component has a different effect depending on their interaction with the surface.

Smooth (polished, Ra < 0.5 μm) surfaces facilitate the epithelial cells attaching, cell growth, spreading, and the production of focal contacts on Ti surfaces [96]. There is a threshold surface roughness for bacterial retention (Ra = 0.2 μm) below which no further reduction in bacterial accumulation could be expected, whereas an increase in surface roughness above this threshold roughness resulted in a simultaneous increase in plaque accumulation, thereby increasing the risk for both caries and periodontal inflammation [97]. On the other hand, fibroblasts adhere as well to rough and even smooth surfaces [98]. In addition, the surface roughness and the oxide thickness affect the rate of bone adhesion in the early stages of implantation (1–7 weeks) [99,100].

Roughened surfaces may advantageously be applied to a variety of medical implants, including orthopedic implants, dental implants, cardiovascular implants, and so on. For orthopedic and dental implants, the rough surface facilitates interlocking of the implant with bone, tissue, or bone cement. This tends to minimize micromotion, a phenomenon that results in loosening of the implant. Roughened surfaces on cardiovascular implants promote desirable cell attachment, which has been linked with a reduction in thrombus response.

The growing of micro- and nanotechnologies is having a revolutionary and fundamental impact on surface engineering in implant dentistry and may represent a next generation of oral implant systems if possible to transfer to complex three-dimensional geometries.

Most implant systems are based on the fact that bone tissue can adapt to surface irregularities in the 1–100 μm range and that altering the surface topography of an implant can greatly improve its stability [101]. Textured implant, with a higher surface area, has the ability to achieve better bone-to-implant contact and is used to understand the effect of different types of textures and various methods of achieving the textured surfaces. The goal of various surface textures and techniques is to enhance the bone growth toward the implant surface. Surface treatments, such as titanium plasma-spraying, grit-blasting, acid-etching, anodization, or osteoconductive calcium phosphate coatings, promote bone healing and apposition, leading to the rapid biological fixation of implants thanks to the increasing surface roughness. Most of these surfaces are commercially available and have proven clinical efficacy (>95% over 5 years) [102]. Implant surfaces with microtopographies have shown a greater percentage of bone-to-implant contact when compared with machined or polished titanium surfaces. However, high surface roughness may result in an increase in ionic leakage as well as peri-implantitis [56].

The biological properties of titanium depend on its surface oxide film. Several methods have been employed to alter the surface topography and surface chemistry of the implant materials [103,104]. Elias et al. [105] show that if the surface morphology and properties of titanium dental implants are modified by mechanical and chemical treatments, the biological properties change since they depend on the Ti surface oxide film generated by the treatments that increase implants surface roughness and decrease the contact angle. It was found that (i) acid etching homogenized the surface roughness parameters; (ii) the anodized surface presented the smallest contact angle; (iii) the in vivo test suggested that, in similar conditions, the surface treatment had a beneficial effect on the implant biocompatibility measured through removal torque; and (iv) the anodized dental implant presented the highest removal torque.

Another parameter influenced by the roughness is bacterial plague retention since the primary aim of the surface texturing or treating is to enhance cellular activity and improve bone apposition [106,107]. Furthermore, microsurface roughness strives to enhance the osteoconduction through changes in surface topography and osteoinduction along the implant surface by utilizing the implant as a vehicle for local delivery of bioactive agents [108]. Plasma-etched surface also shows similar results; however, it is no better than surface topographies created by sand blasting or acid etching [109].

The precise role of surface chemistry and topography on the early events in dental implant osseointegration remains poorly understood. In addition, comparative clinical studies with different implant surfaces are rarely performed. The future of dental implantology should aim to develop surfaces with controlled and standardized topography or chemistry. This approach will be the only way to understand the interactions between proteins, cells, tissues, and implant surfaces. The local release of bone stimulating or resorptive drugs in the peri-implant region may also respond to difficult clinical situations with poor bone quality and quantity. These therapeutic strategies should ultimately enhance the osseointegration process of dental implants for their immediate loading and long-term success.

9.3.2 Microscopy techniques for analysis of surface roughness

The real surface geometry is so complicated that a finite number of parameters cannot provide a full description. If the number of parameters used is increased, a more accurate description can be obtained. Surface roughness parameters are normally categorized into four groups according to its functionality: amplitude, spacing, hybrid, and functional parameters. Each component of surface texture has a different origin and effect in the interaction of the surface.

The surface roughness of implants can be divided into macro-, micro-, and nanosized topologies [110]. Macrotopographic profiles of dental implants have a surface roughness in the range of millimeters to microns. Because the size of the topography is large (roughness more than 10 μm), it is directly related to implant geometry (e.g., threaded screw, solid body press-fit designs, and/or sintered bead technologies) [6,102,108]. Macrosized topographies with highly rough surfaces help in the initial implant stability and provide volumetric spaces for the growth of bone [56,108]. The microtopographic profiles of dental implants have a surface roughness in the range of 1–10 μm.

Different measuring instruments and techniques strongly influence the outcome of a topographic characterization. Furthermore, a screw-type design introduces problems for most measuring instruments. It is highly recommended to have a standard procedure to compare values from one study with another, that is, standards for topographic evaluation of oral implants in terms of measuring equipment, filtering process, and selection of parameters. It is suggested that the measuring instrument be able to measure all parts of a threaded implant if the investigation relates to such a design. Preferably, three-dimensional measurements should be performed. On screw-type implants, tops, valleys, and flanks should be evaluated. At least three samples in a batch should be evaluated, filter size must be specified, and at least one of each height, spatial, and hybrid parameter should be presented [102].

The following types of microscopy are highly recommended for use.

Confocal microscopy (CM) [110a]: Optical microscopy is in a state of explosive development. CM is one of the major metrological technologies used in the optical reconstruction. The confocal technique is able to measure surface topography precisely and reliably on the micrometric and nanometric scales. Confocal profilometers allow height measurement of surfaces with a wide range of textures (from very rough surfaces to very smooth ones) by scanning the sample vertically in steps so that each point on the surface passes through the focus. Since only one or a very small number of points on the surface are illuminated simultaneously, an in-plane scan must be carried out to build up the axial response, i.e., the confocal image, in each vertical step for all the points falling within the field of view of the lens used (Fig. 9.4). In the confocal mode, the profilometer can carry out measurements with an extraordinary lateral resolution.

Atomic force microscopy (AFM) [110b]: AFM is based on the contact between a microfabricated tip and the sample surface. As it is a scanning technique, the tip rasters the sample resolving its fine details down to the nanometric level thanks to a tip apex radius of ca. 5 nm. In a sense, it is the same principle used in a record player, where the needle rides on the grooves of the vinyl record. As the piezo stage proceeds with the scanning in the *XY* axis, the cantilever bends up or down (*Z* axis) and this finally becomes a change in the deflection position of a laser (Fig. 9.5).

Scanning electron microscopy (SEM) [110c]: The SEM consists mainly of a column, a specimen chamber, a display and an operating device. The interior of the column is kept under high vacuum and the electron beam produced by the electron gun is converted into a fine beam via electromagnetic lenses (condenser and objective lenses). By applying a scan signal to the deflection coils, the electron beam is scanned along the sample surface. As a result of electron–matter interaction, some signals are generated: secondary electrons, backscattered electrons, characteristic X-rays, cathodoluminescent light, and others. The SEM utilizes these signals to form images. Secondary

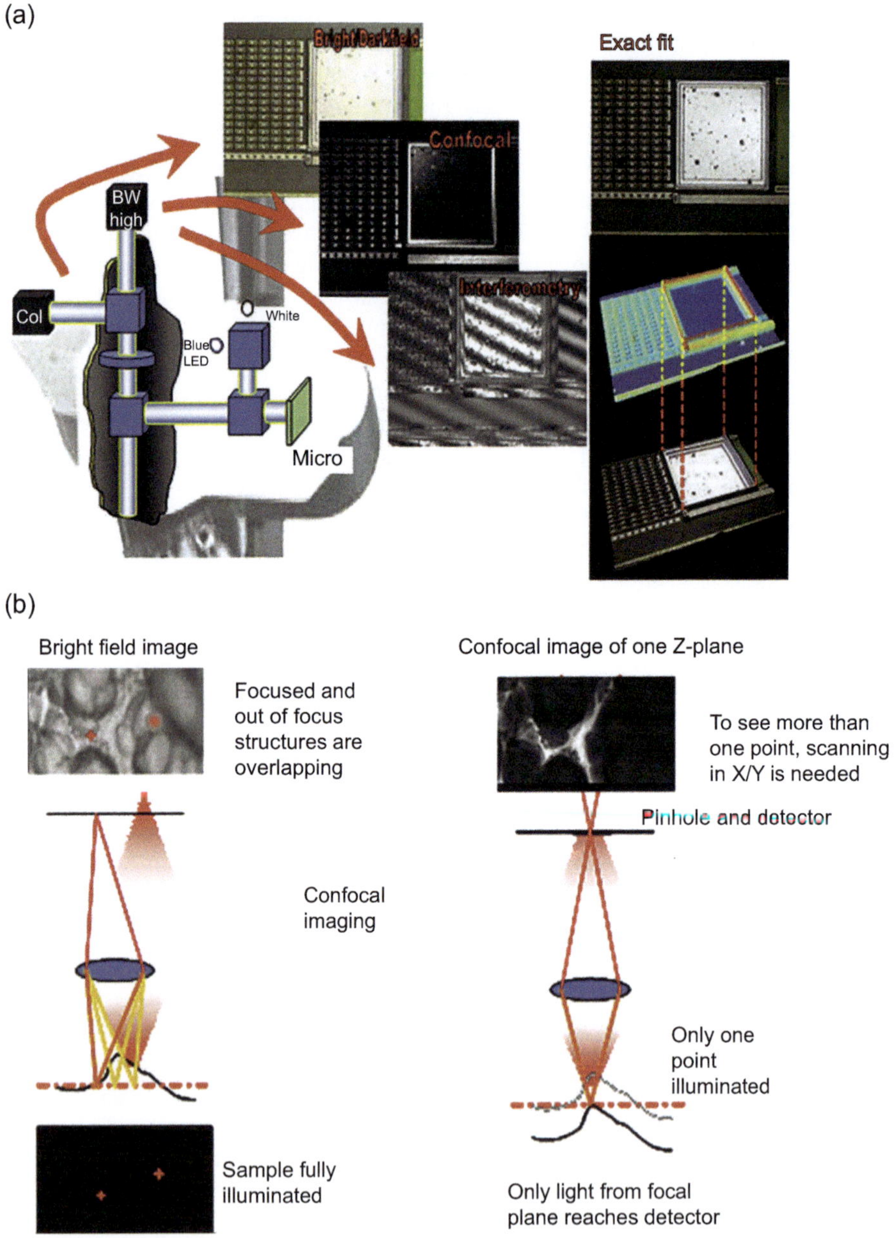

Figure 9.4 (a) Confocal (LEICA DCM3D; Leica Microsystems) scheme and (b) confocal image composition.

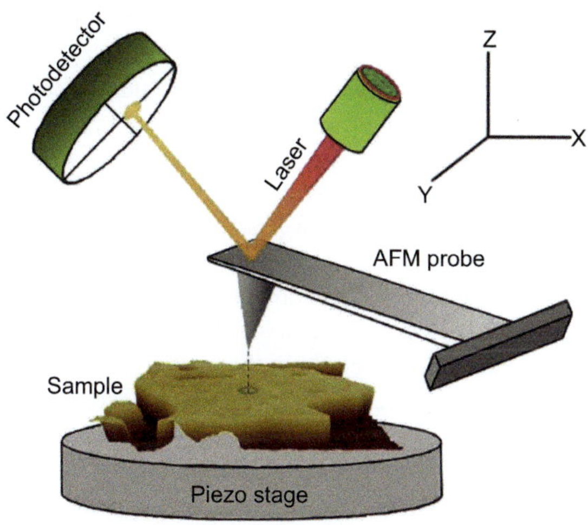

Figure 9.5 AFM schematics. The AFM probe tracks the sample surface, which is precisely moved in the XY axis by means of a piezo stage. The deflection of the AFM probe is tracked by a laser that reflects on a photodetector, which can detect probe movements in the subnanometric range.

electrons are produced near the sample surface and reflect the fine topographical structure of the sample. Backscattered electrons are those reflected upon striking the atoms composing the sample, and the number of these electrons depends on the composition (average atomic number, crystal orientation, etc.) of the sample. The primary (exciting) electrons may also be scattered inelastically by the atoms of the sample, ejecting electrons of the inner-atomic shells and originating characteristic X-rays.

9.4 Summary and conclusions

This chapter attempted to explore the literature on dental implants materials, designs, decontamination treatments, and the influence of surface topographies and roughness of endosseous dental implant on the bone response after decontamination treatments.

Endosseous dental implants are available with various surface characteristics ranging from relatively smooth machined surfaces to more roughened surfaces created by coatings, blasting by various substances, acid treatments, or combinations of the treatments.

The purpose of placement of endosseous dental implants is to achieve short- and long-term outcomes of osseointegration or biointegration of the bone with the implant, with faster and stronger bone formation. A wide variety of materials has been used for these implants, but only a few promote osseointegration and biointegration.

Titanium and titanium alloy (TJ6A14V) have been the most widely used for the fabrication of oral implants, showing a wide variety of surface characteristics both in terms of structural and chemical properties. The drive toward ceramic implants to satisfy the increasing esthetic demands and metal-free request of some patients is fraught with compromise.

Peri-implantitis is becoming an ever-growing oral health concern that is frequently encountered in the dental office. Re-osseointegration is possible to obtain on a previously contaminated implant surface and can occur in experimentally induced peri-implantitis defects following therapy.

The surface modifications outlined above retain the key physical properties of the implants and modify only their outermost surfaces with the ultimate goal of achieving the desired biological response and may influence the degree of re-osseointegration. Surface treatments are normally carried out to modify and yet maintain desirable properties of the substrate materials, especially in the dental implant industry.

Physicochemical, physical, and chemical surface decontamination techniques should be applied alongside regenerative surgical procedures to obtain optimum re-osseointegration and successfully treat peri-implantitis. These methods will help us in understanding better how implant material surface modification affects the bone–implant interface and the development of a method, which optimizes the implant's re-osseointegration properties during healing after the successful treatment of peri-implantitis, the infection of the dental tissue surrounding the implant. It is not completely clear the degree of influence of the surface roughness and chemistry on osseointegration. The ideal degree of roughness for an optimal clinical performance still remains unknown. The quality of dental implant depends on the properties of the surface. To have good osseointegration, material roughness of the surface played an important role.

Different measuring instruments and techniques strongly influence the outcome of a topographic and roughness characterization. It is highly recommended to have a standard procedure to compare values from one study with another, that is, standards for topographic evaluation of oral implants in terms of measuring equipment, filtering process, and selection of parameters. It is suggested that the measuring instrument be able to measure all parts of a threaded implant if the investigation relates to such a design. Preferably, three-dimensional measurements should be performed. CM, AFM, and SEM are highly recommended to be used to analyze topographic and roughness parameters.

References

[1] Gaviria L, Salcido JP, Guda T, Ong JL. Current trends in dental implants. J Korean Assoc Oral Maxillofac Surg 2014;40(2):50–60.

[2] Rethman MP. Introduction & historical perspectives on dental implants. Chic Hu-Friedy 2010:1–4.

[3] Garber D. The esthetic dental implant: letting restoration be the guide. J Am Dent Assoc 1995;126(3):319–25.

[4] Sullivan RM. Implant dentistry and the concept of osseointegration: a historical perspective. J Calif Dent Assoc 2001;29:737–45.

[5] Find out who was responsible for starting dental implant history [Internet] [place unknown]: Dental-Health-Advice. Available from: http://www.dental-health-advice.com/dental-implant-history.html.
[6] Searson LJ. History and development of dental implants. In: Narim L, Wilson HF, editors. Implantology in general dental practice. Chicago: Quintessence Publishing Co; 2005. p. 19–41.
[7] Dental implant history [Internet] Albufeira: Cris Piessens Clinic. Available from: http://www.crispiessensclinic.com/implant_history.html.
[8] Brånemark PI. Osseointegration and its experimental background. J Prosthet Dent 1983;50(3):399–410.
[9] Brånemark PI, Zarb G, Albrektsson T. Tissue-integrated prostheses: osseointegration in clinical dentistry. Chicago: Quintessence; 1985.
[10] Kawahara H, Kawahara D. The history and concept of implant. Tokyo: AQB Implant System; 2014.
[11] Nobel Biocare has a 40-year heritage of scientific research and innovation [Internet] Zürich-Flughafen: Nobel Biocare. Available from: http://corporate.nobelbiocare.com/en/our-company/history-and-innovations/.
[12] Di Giallorenzo D. History of dental implants. Collegeville (PA): Lanap & Implant Center of Pennsylvania. Available from: http://perioimplants.us/history-of-dental-implants.
[13] Osman RB, Swain MV. A critical review of dental implant materials with an emphasis on titanium versus zirconia. Materials 2015;8:932–58.
[14] Lacefield WR. Current status of ceramic coatings for dental implants. Implant Dent 1998;7:315–22.
[15] Barrere F, van der Valk CM, Meijer G, Dalmeijer RA, de Groot K, Layrolle P. Osteointegration of biomimetic apatite coating applied onto dense and porous metal implants in femurs of goats. J Biomed Mater Res 2003;67:655–65.
[16] Han HS. Design of new root-form endosseous dental implant and evaluation of fatigue strength using finite element analysis [Master's thesis]. Iowa: The University of Iowa; 2009.
[17] Brunette DM, Tengvall P, Textor M, Thomsen P. Titanium in medicine: material science, surface science, engineering, biological responses, and medical applications. Berlin (Germany): Springer; 2001.
[18] Specifications book. 4th ed. International Titanium Association; 2005.
[19] Ballo AM, Omar O, Xia W, Palmquist A. In: Turkyilmaz I, editor. Dental implant surfaces—physicochemical properties, biological performance, and trends. Implant dentistry—a rapidly evolving practice; 2011.
[20] Diaz-Marcos J, Vilana J, Espías AF, Sánchez LA, Parahy F. The effects of peri-implantitis decontamination treatments on the surface roughness and chemistry of a titanium alloy used for dental implants: implications for bone reintegration. Leica Science Lab; 2014.
[21] Anil S, Anand PS, Alghamdi H, Jansen JA. In: Turkyilmaz I, editor. Dental implant surface enhancement and osseointegration. Implant dentistry–a rapidly evolving practice; 2011.
[22] Le Guéhennec L, Soueidan A, Layrolle P, Amouriq Y. Surface treatments of titanium dental implants for rapid osseointegration. Dent Mater 2007;23:844–54.
[23] Wennerberg A, Albrektsson T. Effects of titanium surface topography on bone integration: a systematic review. Clin Oral Implants Res 2009;20:172–84.
[24] Wataha JC. Materials for endosseous dental implants. J Oral Rehabil 1996;23(2):79–90.

[25] Cochran DL, Schenk RK, Lussi A, Higginbottom FL, Buser D. Bone response to unloaded and loaded titanium implants with a sandblasted and acid-etched surface: a histomorphometric study in the canine mandible. J Biomed Mater Res 1998;40: 1–11.
[26] Jansen JA, Wolke JGC, Swann S, van der Waerden JPCM, de Groot K. Application of magnetron-sputtering for producing ceramic coatings on implant materials. Clin Oral Implants Res 1993;4:28–34.
[27] Palmquist A, Lindberg F, Emanuelsson L, Branemark R, Engqvist H, Thomsen P. Biomechanical, histological, and ultrastructural analyses of laser micro- and nano-structured titanium alloy implants: a study in rabbit. J Biomed Mater Res A 2010;92: 1476–86.
[28] Brånemark R, Emanuelsson L, Palmquist A, Thomsen P. Bone response to laser-induced micro- and nano-size titanium surface features. Nanomedicine 2011;92(4): 1476–86.
[29] Esposito M, Coulthard P, Thomsen P, Worthington HV. The role of implant surface modifications, shape and material on the success of osseointegrated dental implants. A Cochrane systematic review. Eur J Prosthodont Restor Dent 2005;13:15–31.
[30] Esposito M, Worthington HV, Thomsen P, Coulthard P. Interventions for replacing missing teeth: different types of dental implants. Cochrane Database Syst Rev 2005;1:CD003815.
[31] Albrektsson T, Wennerberg A. Oral implant surfaces: Part 1–review focusing on topographic and chemical properties of different surfaces and in vivo responses to them. Int J Prosthodont 2004;17:536–43.
[32] Berglundh T, Gotfredsen K, Zitzmann NU, Lang NP, Lindhe J. Spontaneous progression of ligature induced peri-implantitis at implants with different surface roughness: an experimental study in dogs. Clin Oral Implants Res 2007;18:655–61.
[33] Machtei EE. Treatment alternatives to negotiate peri-implantitis. Adv Med 2014.
[34] Meffert RM. Periodontitis vs. peri-implantitis: the same disease? the same treatment? Crit Rev Oral Biol Med 1996;7:278–91.
[35] Lang NP, Berglundh T, Heitz-Mayfield LJ, Pjetursson BE, Salvid GE, Sanz M. Consensus statements and recommended clinical procedures regarding implant survival and complications. Int J Oral Maxillofac Implants 2004;19(Suppl.):150–4.
[36] Omar O, Lenneras M, Svensson S, Suska F, Emanuelsson L, Hall J, et al. Integrin and chemokine receptor gene expression in implant-adherent cells during early osseointegration. J Mater Sci Mater Med 2010;21:969–80.
[37] Turzo K. Surface aspects of titanium dental implants. In: Sammour RH, editor. Book chapter: molecular studies and novel applications for improved quality of human life; 2012.
[38] Zablotsky MH, Diedrich DL, Meffert RM. Detoxification of endotoxin-contaminated titanium and hydroxyapatite-coated surfaces utilizing various chemotherapeutic and mechanical modalities. Implant Dent 1992;1:154–8.
[39] http://www.idataresearch.com/research-categories/dental/dental-implants-market-research-reports/.
[40] Berglundh T, Persson L, Klinge B. A systematic review of the incidence of biological and technical complications in implant dentistry reported in prospective longitudinal studies of at least 5 years. J Clin Periodontol 2002;29(Suppl. 3):197–212.
[41] Zitzmann NU, Berglundh T. Definition and prevalence of peri-implant diseases. J Clin Periodontol 2008;35(Suppl. 8):286–91.
[42] Mombelli A, Muller N, Cionca N. The epidemiology of peri-implantitis. Clin Oral Implants Res 2012;23(Suppl. 6):67–76.

[43] Atieh MA, Alsabeeha NH, Faggion Jr CM, Duncan WJ. The frequency of peri-implant diseases: a systematic review and meta-analysis. J Periodontol 2013;84(11):1586–98.
[44] Rinke S, Ohl S, Ziebolz D, Lange K, Eickholz P. Prevalence of periimplant disease in partially edentulous patients: a practice-based cross-sectional study. Clin Oral Implants Res 2011;22(8):826–33.
[45] Rodriguez-Argueta OF, Figueiredo R, Valmaseda-Castellon E, Gay-Escoda C. Postoperative complications in smoking patients treated with implants: a retrospective study. J Oral Maxillofac Surg 2011;69(8):2152–7.
[46] Cho-Yan Lee J, Mattheos N, Nixon KC, Ivanovski S. Residual periodontal pockets are a risk indicator for periimplantitis in patients treated for periodontitis. Clin Oral Implants Res 2012;23(3):325–33.
[47] Roccuzzo M, Bonino F, Aglietta M, Dalmasso P. Ten year results of a three arms prospective cohort study on implants in periodontally compromised patients—Part 2: clinical results. Clin Oral Implants Res 2012;23(4):389–95.
[48] Carcuac O, Jansson L. Peri-implantitis in a specialist clinic of periodontology. Clinical Features and risk indicators. Swed Dent J 2010;34(2):53–61.
[49] Serino G, Strom C. Peri-implantitis in partially edentulous patients: association with inadequate plaque control. Clin Oral Implants Res 2009;20(2):169–74.
[50] Wadhwani C, Rapoport D, la Rosa S, Hess T, Kretschmar S. Radiographic detection and characteristic patterns of residual excess cement associated with cement-retained implant restorations: a clinical report. J Prosthet Dent 2012;107(3):151–7.
[51] Balevi B. Implant-supported cantilevered fixed partial dentures. Evid Based Dent 2010; 11(2):48–9.
[52] Renvert S, Aghazadeh A, Hallstrom H, Persson GR. Factors related to peri-implantitis—a retrospective study. Clin Oral Implants Res 2014;25(4):522–9.
[53] Lindhe J, Meyle J. Peri-implant diseases: consensus report of the Sixth European Workshop on Periodontology. J Clin Periodontol 2008;35(Suppl. 8):282–5.
[54] Renvert S, Polyzois I, Maguire R. Re-osseointegration on previously contaminated surfaces: a systematic review. Clin Oral Implants Res 2009;20(Suppl. 4):216–27.
[55] Abrahamsson I, Berglundh T, Linder E, Lang NP, Lindhe J. Early bone formation adjacent to rough and turned endosseous implant surfaces. An experimental study in the dog. Clin Oral Implants Res 2004;15:381–92.
[56] Shalabi MM, Gortemaker A, Van't Hof MA, Jansen JA, Creugers NHJ. Implant surface roughness and bone healing: a systematic review. J Dent Res 2006;85:496–500.
[57] Parlar A, Bosshardt DD, Cetiner D, Schafroth D, Unsal B, Haytaç C, et al. Effects of decontamination and implant surface characteristics on re-osseointegration following treatment of peri-implantitis. Clin Oral Implants Res 2009;20:391–9.
[58] Kolonidis SG, Renvert S, Hammerle CHF, Lang NP, Harris D, Claffey N. Osseointegration on implant surfaces previously contaminated with plaque. An experimental study in the dog. Clin Oral Implants Res 2003;14:373–80.
[59] Ahtone J, Goodman RA. Hepatitis B and dental personnel: transmission to patients and prevention issues. J Am Dent Assoc 1983;106:219–22.
[60] Li X, Kolltveit KM, Tronstad L, Olsen I. Systemic diseases caused by oral infection. Clin Microbiol Rev 2000;13(4):547–58.
[61] Paju S, Scannapieco FA. Oral Dis 2007;13(6):508–12.
[62] Crawford JJ. State-of-the-art practical infection control in dentistry. J Am Dent Assoc 1985;110:629–33.
[63] Cottone JA, Mitchell EW, Baker CH, et al. Proceedings of the national symposium on hepatitis B and the dental profession. J Am Dent Assoc 1985;110:614–49.

[64] Cundy KR, Hinks E, Kleger B, Miller LA. Acquired immunodeficiency syndrome (AIDS): precautions for health-care workers and allied professionals. MMWR Morb Mortal Wkly Rep 1983;32:450−1.
[65] Bond WW, Favero MS, Petersen NJ, Gravelle CR, Ebert JW, Maynard JE. Survival of hepatitis B virus after drying and storage for one week. Lancet 1981:550−1 [Letter].
[66] Shikata T, Karasawa T, Abe K, Uzawa T, Suzuki H, Oda T, et al. Hepatitis B e antigen and infectivity of hepatitis B virus. J Infect Dis 1977;136:571−6.
[67] Schou S, Holmstrup P, Skovgaard LT, Stoltze K, Hjørting H. Implant surface preparation in the surgical treatment of experimental periimplantitis with autogenous bone graft and ePTFE membrane in cynomolgus monkeys. Clin Oral Implants Res 2003;14:412−22.
[68] Klinge B, Hultin M, Berglundh T. Periimplantitis. Dent Clin North Am 2005;49:661−76.
[69] Esposito M, Grusovin MG, Coulthard P, Worthington HV. Interventions for replacing missing teeth: treatment of periimplantitis. Cochrane Database Syst Rev 2006;19: CD004970.
[70] Persson LG, Ericsson I, Berglundh T, Lindhe J. J Clin Periodontol 2001;28(3):258−63.
[71] Klinge B, Gustafsson A, Berglundh T. A systematic review of the effect of anti-infective therapy in the treatment of periimplantitis. J Clin Periodontol 2002; 29(Suppl. 3):213−25.
[72] Roos-Jansaker A, Renvert S, Egelberg J. Treatment of peri-implant infections: a literature review. J Clin Periodontol 2003;30:467−85.
[73] Renvert S, Roos-Jansaker A, Claffey N. Nonsurgical treatment of periimplant mucositisand periimplantitis. J Clin Periodontol 2008;35:305−15.
[74] Kotsovilis S, Karoussis IK, Fourmousis I. Therapy of peri-implantitis: a systematic review. J Clin Periodontol 2008;35:621−9.
[75] Ratner BD, Shoen FJ, Lemons JE, Hoffman AS. Thin films, grafts, and coatings. In: Ratner BD, Hoffman AS, Schoen FJ, Lemons JE, editors. Biomaterials science: an introduction to materials in medicine. San Diego (California, USA): Academic Press; 1996. p. 309−12.
[76] Romanos GE, Gutknecht N, Dieter S, Schwarz F, Crespi R, Sculean A. Laser wavelengths and oral implantology. Lasers Med Sci 2009;24(6):961−70.
[77] Meyle J. Mechanical, chemical and laser treatments of the implant surface in the presence of marginal bone loss around implants. Eur J Oral Implantol 2012;5(Suppl.):71−81.
[78] Kreisler M, Al Haj H, d'Hoedt B. Temperature changes at the implant-bone interface during simulated surface decontamination with Er:YAG laser. Int J Prosthodont 2002; 15(6):582−7.
[79] Geminiani A, Caton JG, Romanos GE. Temperature increase during CO(2) and Er:YAG irradiation on implant surfaces. Implant Dent 2011;20(5):379−82.
[80] Hauser-Gerspach I, Stübinger S, Meyer J. Bactericidal effects of different laser systems on bacteria adhered to dental implant surfaces: an in vitro study comparing zirconia with titanium. Clin Oral Implants Res Mar 2010;21(3):277−83.
[81] Azzeh MM. Er,Cr:YSGG laser-assisted surgical treatment of peri-implantitis with 1-year reentry and 18-month follow-up. J Periodontol 2008;79(10):2000−5.
[82] Cassoni A, Miranda PV, Rodrigues JA, Coelho de Lacerda S, Blay A, Awad J. Thermal effects on zirconia substrate after Er,Cr:YSGG irradiation. Rev Odontol UNESP 2013;42: 6 [Araraquara].
[83] Meisel P, Kocher T. Photodynamic therapy for periodontal diseases: state of the art. J Photochem Photobiol B 2005;79(2):159−70.
[84] Oliveira RR, Schwartz-Fo HO, Novaes Jr AB, Garlet GP, Taba Jr M. Antimicrobial photodynamic therapy in the non-surgical. J Periodontol 2007;78:965−73.

[85] Pfitzner A, Sigusch BW, Albrecht V, Glockmann E. Killing of period-ontopathogenic bacteria by photodynamic therapy. J Periodontol 2004;75:1343.
[86] Ishikawa I, Baehni P. Nonsurgical periodontal therapy—where do we stand now? Periodontol 2000 2004;36:9—13.
[87] Kömerik N, Nakanishi H, MacRobert AJ, Henderson B, Speight P, Wilson M. Antimicrob Agents Chemother 2003;47(3):932—40.
[88] Haas R, Baron M, Dortbudak O, Watzek G. Lethal photosensitization, autogenous bone, and e-PTFE membrane for the treatment of peri-implantitis: preliminary results. Int J Oral Maxillofac Implants 2000;15:374—82.
[89] Dortbudak O, Haas R, Bernhart T, Mailath-Porkomy G. Lethal photosensitilization for decontamination of implant surfaces in the treatment of peri-implantitis. Clin Oral Implants Res 2001;12(2):104—8.
[90] Dillow AK, Lowman AM. Biomimetic materials and design. New York, Basel: Marcel Dekker; 2002. p. 507—31.
[91] de Jonge LT, Leeuwenburgh SCG, Wolke JGC, Jansen JA. Organic-inorganic surface modifications for titanium implant surfaces. Pharm Res 2008;25(10):2357—69.
[92] Hoffman AS. Biologically functional materials. In: Biomaterials science: an introduction to materials in medicine; 1996.
[93] Ratner BD, Hoffman AS, Schoen FJ, Lemons JE. Engineering 1998;26(2):338 [San Diego, California, USA].
[94] Ito Y, Kajihara M, Imanishi Y. Materials for enhancing cell adhesion by immobilization of cell-adhesive peptide. J Biomed Mater Res 1991;25:1325—37.
[95] Puleo DA, Nanci A. Understanding and controlling the bone-implant interface. Biomaterials 1999;20(23—24):2311—21.
[96] Baharloo B, Textor M, Brunette DM. Substratum roughness alters the growth, area, and focal adhesions of epithelial cells, and their proximity to titanium surfaces. J Biomed Mater Res A 2005;74(1):12—22.
[97] Bollen CM, Lambrechts P, Quirynen M. Comparison of surface roughness of oral hard materials to the threshold surface roughness for bacterial plaque retention: a review of the literature. Dent Mater 1997;13(4):258—69.
[98] Klinge B, Meyle J. Soft-tissue integration of implants. Consensus report of Working Group 2. Clin Oral Implants Res 2006;17(Suppl. 2):93—6.
[99] Larsson C, Thomsen P, Lausmaa J, Rodahl M, Kasemo B, Ericson LE. Bone response to surface modified titanium implants: studies on electropolished implants with different oxide thickness and morphology. Biomaterials 1994;15:1062—74.
[100] Larsson C, Thomsen P, Aronsson BO, Rodahl M, Lausmaa J, Kasemo B, et al. Bone response to surface modified titanium implants: studies on the early tissue response to machined and electropolished implants with different oxide thicknesses. Biomaterials 1996;17:605—61.
[101] Albrektsson T, Berglundh T, Lindhe J. Osseointegration: Historic background and current concepts. In: Clinical periodontology and implant dentistry. 4th ed. Oxford: Blackwell Munksgaard; 2003. p. 809—20.
[102] Mustafa K, Wennerberg A, Wroblewski J, Hultenby K, Lopez BS, Arvidson K. Determining optimal surface roughness of TiO(2) blasted titanium implant material for attachment, proliferation and differentiation of cells derived from human mandibular alveolar bone. Clin Oral Implants Res 2001;12(5):515—25.
[103] Stanford CM. Advancements in implant surface technology for predictable long-term results — Report. US Dentistry. 2006. p. 30—2.

[104] Alla RK, Ginjupalli K, Upadhya N, Shammas M, Ravi RK, Sekhar R. Surface roughness of implants: a review. Trends Biomater Artif Organs 2011;25(3):112–8.
[105] Elias CN, Oshida Y, Lima JH, Muller CA. Relationship between surface properties (roughness, wettability and morphology) of titanium and dental implant removal torque. J Mech Behav Biomed Mater 2008;1(3):234–42.
[106] Kohles SS, Clark MB, Brown CA, Kennedy JN. Direct assessment of profilometric roughness variability from typical implant surface types. Int J Oral Maxillofac Implants 2004;19(4):510–6.
[107] De Monserrat I, Risa I, Hiroki K, ken-Ichiro T, Naoko Y, Toshi-Ichiro T, et al. Dental implant surface roughness and topography: a review of the literature. J Gifu Dent Soc 2009;35(3):89–95.
[108] Stanford CM. Surface modifications of dental implants. Aus Dent J 2008;53(Suppl. 1): 26–33.
[109] Pieles U, Bühler T, von Rechenberg B, Voelter K, Snetiv D, Schlottig F. Investigation of a unique nanostructured dental implant surface. Eur Cells Mater 2007;14(Suppl. 3):95.
[110] [a] Diaz-Marcos J, Pinna F, Oncins G. Advanced optical microscopies for materials: new trends. In: Seoane JR, Llovet Ximenes X, editors. Handbook of instrumental techniques for materials, chemical and biosciences research, vol. 1. Barcelona (Spain): Universitat de Barcelona. Centres Científics i Tecnològics; 2011, ISBN 9788461553730. p. 64–74. M.T. 6.
[b] Oncins G, Díaz-Marcos J. Atomic Force microscopy: probing the nanoworld. In: Seoane JR, Llovet Ximenes X, editors. 9788461553730, editor. Handbook of instrumental techniques for materials, chemical and biosciences research, vol. 1. Barcelona (Spain): Universitat de Barcelona. Centres Científics i Tecnològics; 2011. p. 75–84. M.T. 7.
[c] García-Veigas J, Prats E, Domínguez A, Villuendas A. Advanced applications of scanning electron microscopy in geology. In: Seoane JR, Llovet Ximenes X, editors. Handbook of instrumental techniques for materials, chemical and biosciences research, vol. 1. Barcelona (Spain): Universitat de Barcelona. Centres Científics i Tecnològics; 2011, ISBN 9788461553730. p. 55–63. M.T. 5.

Anti-resorptive treatment in osteoporosis and their deleterious effects on maxillary bone metabolism in clinical dentistry

10

D. Soto-Peñazola, M. Peñarrocha-Diago, J.V. Bagán-Sebastián, L. Bagán-Debon
University of Valencia, Valencia, Spain

10.1 Introduction

Osteoporosis is defined as a metabolic skeletal disease characterized by decreased bone mass showing a deleterious effect that induces a degradation of the microarchitecture of the bone tissue, caused by increase of the marrow spaces, resulting in fragility of the bone tissue with subsequent greater risk of fractures [1]. The World Health Organization defines it as a generalized disease of the skeleton characterized by a decrease of 25% of bone mass; also osteopenia is a term that characterizes the physiological bone mineral density decrease between 10% and 25% from the standard condition as a precursor to osteoporosis [1].

Although it is defined by several factors such as calcium and vitamin D deficiency, sedentary and genetic factors, the postmenopausal estrogen deficiency is the major known etiology since estrogen regulates bone remodeling and the cessation of estrogen production induces a bone remodeling imbalance with bone resorption exceeding bone formation, leading to bone fragility and increasing the risk of fracture [2].

Osteoporosis and the fractures associated with it are a major public health concern, because of related morbidity and disability, diminished quality of life, and mortality. The condition is responsible for about 1700 fractures a day (about 650,000 a year) in the European Union [3], implying significant costs to public health systems mainly due to the complications associated with it.

To attempt to prevent an increase in the rates of bone loss in osteoporotic patients, the antiresorptive therapy is frequently indicated [4]. However, in recent clinical reports adverse events have been described such as complications in the jawbones, mainly associated with bisphosphonates (BPs) [5]. This pathology was defined as osteonecrosis of the jaws (ONJ), being an interesting and relevant topic in oral medicine [6], oral surgery [7], and implant dentistry [8,9], as well as the relationship with other systemic diseases such as sclerosis [10] and diabetes mellitus [11].

Bone Response to Dental Implant Materials. http://dx.doi.org/10.1016/B978-0-08-100287-2.00010-0

The present chapter aims to offer the most relevant information related to this topic, in this manner helping clinicians, in the attempt to upgrade their knowledge baggage. We will update the concept, diagnosis, and classification of ONJ due to BPs.

10.2 Concept, diagnosis and classification of BP-associated ONJ

10.2.1 Background

BPs are stable pyrophosphate analogs that modulate bone metabolism and are generally used to treat certain diseases involving bone resorption, such as osteoporosis or Paget's disease (usually administered via the oral route), or hypercalcemia associated to different malignancies such as multiple myeloma and bone metastases secondary to solid tumors of the breast or other locations (via the intravenous route). BPs fundamentally act by inhibiting bone resorption, with the limitation of osteoclast activity, although they also exert an antiangiogenic effect [12,13].

Other antiresorptive drugs apart from BPs are also used to treat osteoporosis, multiple myeloma, and bone metastases. In this regard, denosumab an inhibitor of the receptor activator of nuclear factor kappa-B ligand (RANKL), a type II membrane protein and member of the tumor necrosis factor (TNF) superfamily, it is know to affects the inmune response and modulates the bone remodeling and regeneration, has been included in the treatment guides as an option for preventing bone problems (e.g., hip or vertebral fractures), and is administered via a subcutaneous route every 6 months for the management of osteoporosis [12,14].

However, the use of both BPs and other antiresorptive drugs can produce adverse effects in the form of gastrointestinal disorders or ONJ. The latter is defined as an area of exposed or necrotic bone that fails to heal within 8 weeks in patients who have received or are receiving BPs in the absence of radiotherapy in the cervicofacial area [15]. The pathogenesis of ONJ remains unclear, although the suppression of osteoclast mediated bone remodeling with consequent bone sclerosis has been suggested as the likely causal mechanism. There is an increased risk of ONJ when BPs are administered in combination with antiangiogenic agents such as bevacizumab or sunitinib [16].

10.2.2 Prevalence and incidence

10.2.2.1 BPs for the treatment of osteoporosis

The prevalence of ONJ is far greater in patients treated with intravenous BPs than in those who receive oral BPs; indeed, some authors consider the association between oral BPs and ONJ to be insignificant [17]. As a result, the recommendations regarding dental treatment (e.g., surgery or dental implant placement) in such patients can be vague and lack supporting evidence [17].

10.2.2.2 Oral BPs

The prevalence of ONJ varies greatly (0.001−0.10%), depending on the literature source [18,19]. With a treatment duration of 4 years or more, the reported prevalence is 0.21%, whereas the prevalence drops to 0.04% with shorter duration [18]. In a European multicenter study involving 470 cases of ONJ due to BPs, a total of 37 (7.8%) were attributed to oral BPs prescribed for the treatment of osteoporosis [17]. The clinical significance of the oral route, therefore, should not be underestimated. The incidence ranges from 1.04 to 69 cases per 100,000 patients/year [19]. Kühl et al. [20] recorded a mean incidence of 0.12%, whereas other authors [21] have described incidences of between 0.0009% and 0.034%.

10.2.2.3 Intravenous BPs for the treatment of cancer

The prevalence of ONJ is greater in cancer patients treated with intravenous BPs, being between 0% and 0.348% [19]. The incidence ranges from 0 to 90 cases per 100,000 patients/year [8]. The prevalence of ONJ in cancer patients treated with intravenous BPs varies between 0.52% and 7.4%, depending on the source [14,16,22]. The incidence in turn ranges from 0.8% to 12% [20,21].

On comparing denosumab with BPs in cancer patients, the former drug has been found to offer lower bone events and it has superior safety in patients with kidney disease. However, the associated ONJ rate is similar to that observed with BPs and hypocalcemia is comparatively more frequent [23,24].

The systemic risk factors for ONJ are the type of BP used, the administration route, the duration of treatment, the cumulative dose, the background disease for which the medication is prescribed, concomitant therapies (e.g., chemotherapy, corticosteroids, antiangiogenic agents, etc.), patient habits (smoking, alcohol, etc.), gender, age, genetic factors, and other disease conditions such as diabetes mellitus, rheumatoid arthritis, hemodialysis, and so on [16,25].

The local risk factors in turn include dentoalveolar surgery (especially extractions)—this being the leading risk factor for ONJ in cancer patients subjected to antiresorptive treatment—as well as dental and periodontal infection, and removable dentures. Anatomical factors (mandible, torus) also play a role [16,22,25].

10.2.3 Concept and diagnosis

A number of terms have been used in reference to the ONJ due to BP, including BP-associated ONJ (BAONJ), BP-related ONJ (BRONJ), BP-induced ONJ (BIONJ), BP-related ON (BRON), or simply BP osteonecrosis (BON) [26].

In 2003, the first cases of ONJ due to BPs were published by Marx [27] and since then there has been a growing number of articles on this subject [28]. Since the year 2006, different societies and expert panels have proposed a number of clinical descriptions for defining this new disease entity [29]. As an example, in 2006, the American Dental Association considered the typical clinical presentation of ONJ to include pain, swelling of the soft tissues, infection, tooth mobility, suppuration, and bone exposure. Likewise, in 2006, the Australia and New Zealand ONJ work group [30] underscored the lack of a clear definition of the disease.

At the beginning, ONJ was described as an "area of exposed bone persisting for over 6 weeks." The condition was to be suspected in patients with bone exposure in the maxillofacial region following oral surgery. Other symptoms such as pain and infection could also be present. In 2006, the American College of Rheumatology reported that ONJ typically manifests as an intraoral lesion with the exposure of white-yellowish bone, sometimes associated to the presence of an intra- or extraoral fistula.

Likewise, in 2006, the American Association of Endodontists indicated that patients with ONJ present at least one of the following characteristics: ulceration of the mucosa with bone exposure in the upper maxilla or mandible, pain or swelling, infection and suppuration, or sensory alterations [29]. It is thus clear that no agreement has been reached regarding the definition of this adverse drug event. In 2007, the American Association of Oral and Maxillofacial Surgeons (AAOMS), in its position document on BRONJ, defined the latter as the exposure of necrotic bone in the maxillofacial region persisting for more than 8 weeks, in patients with current or past BP therapy and no antecedents of radiotherapy of the maxillary region [31].

In the same year, the American Society for Bone and Mineral Research (ASBMR) defined a "confirmed case" of BRONJ as the presence of an area of exposed bone in the maxillofacial region failing to heal within 8 weeks after having been identified by a health professional in a patient with current or past treatment with BPs and no antecedents of radiotherapy of the maxillary region. A "suspected case" in turn was defined as an area of exposed bone in the maxillofacial region, present for less than 8 weeks, and identified by a health professional in a patient with the same characteristics as described above [32].

In 2008, the Canadian Association of Oral and Maxillofacial Surgeons published a consensus document with management guidelines referred to BRONJ in which the "confirmed case" and "suspected case" definitions introduced by the ASBMR were maintained [33]. In 2009, this same work group published a review on the subject in which the same definitions were maintained without changes [19].

The AAOMS, likewise in 2009, published an update on the subject without modifying the definition, which they had proposed 2 years earlier and has been maintained up until 2014 [15]. However, the AAOMS did introduce a new stage (referred to as stage 0) corresponding to patients with symptoms but no exposed bone. Colella et al. and Bedogni et al., among others, considered that the term BRONJ should be redefined to include patients in stage 0 [34,35].

Based on cases published by other authors and on the habitual clinical findings, they suggested that the definition of BRONJ should include not only cases with exposed bone but also those with necrotic bone in which bone exposure has not yet occurred [34]. Furthermore, they considered that the diagnosis and classification should be based not only on the clinical picture but also on the radiological findings [34,35]. Other investigators such as Bagan et al., Junquera and Gallego, and Mawardi et al. [28,36,37] suggested that ONJ may manifest in the absence of bone exposure, particularly in the early stages, with fistulas, pain, and radiographic alterations. On the other hand, cases have been published in which ONJ has been associated to other antiresorptive agents such as denosumab or cancer drugs with antiangiogenic effects such as sunitinib, sorafenib, bevacizumab, or sirolimus. As a result, some authors have proposed other terms such as drug-induced ONJ or ONJ associated to antiresorptive agents, in reference to this disorder [21,26].

In 2014, the AAOMS proposed a change in nomenclature in favor of the term medication-related osteonecrosis of the jaws (MRONJ) [25]. In addition, the AAOMS update of 2014 criteria and modified its definition. In this regard, a patient is considered to have MRONJ if all of the following conditions are met [25]:

- Current or past treatment with antiresorptive or antiangiogenic drugs.
- Exposed bone or intra or extraoral fistulization in the maxillofacial region communicating with the bone and persisting for more than 8 weeks.
- No history of maxillary radiotherapy or clear maxillary metastatic disease.

However, in 2015 the International Task Force on Osteonecrosis of the Jaw defined ONJ as follows [38]:

- Exposed bone in the maxillofacial region that fails to heal in 8 weeks after identification by a health professional.
- Exposure to an antiresorptive agent.
- No history of craniofacial radiotherapy.

The diagnosis is essentially clinical [39]. On the other hand, it must be taken into account that there may be one or more sites of bone exposure [40]. Furthermore, these sites may remain asymptomatic for prolonged periods of time (weeks, months, or even years), or some clinical signs and symptoms may manifest before ONJ is clinically detectable and develops. Such signs and symptoms consist of pain, bone and/or gingival swelling, erythema, suppuration, soft tissue ulceration, intra- or extraoral fistular trajectories, tooth mobility, paresthesia, and even anesthesia, in the absence of any apparent dental/periodontal cause. The radiographic findings range from variable radiotransparency or radio-opacity to the absence of any radiological signs. In the absence of bone exposure, these findings alone were not regarded as sufficient to diagnose BRONJ [32].

At present, the latest update of the AAOMS corresponding to 2014 [25] considers that the presence of these manifestations, even in the absence of bone exposure (equivalent to stage 0 of the 2009 classification), is indicative of prodromal BRONJ, and that over time up to 50% of these patients will progress toward disease stages 1, 2, or 3.

Clinically, the exposure of necrotic bone mostly occurs after dentoalveolar surgery (extractions or the placement of dental implants), although it can also be spontaneous. The most frequent location is the mandible (62−82% of the cases), maxilla (8−18%), or both (up to 20% of the cases), with a predominance of the molar and premolar regions. The exposed bone is generally colonized by oral bacteria, giving rise to secondary infections [22,39].

The differential diagnosis of ONJ should be made with other conditions such as alveolar osteitis, sinusitis, osteomyelitis, periodontitis/gingivitis, periapical disease caused by caries, mucositis, osteoradionecrosis, temporomandibular joint disease, and certain forms of cement bone dysplasia with secondary sequestration phenomena [32,38]. Accordingly, the patient case history and the clinical examination remain the most sensitive tools for diagnosing ONJ [38,41].

The two most controversial aspects in the diagnosis of ONJ since the publication of the first case series have been: (1) the diagnosis of ONJ in the absence of bone exposure; and (2) the need for radiological or imaging confirmation of the diagnosis. These two aspects will be examined in greater detail below.

10.2.3.1 Diagnosis of ONJ in the absence of exposed bone

Most authors have accepted the definition of ONJ proposed by the AAOMS in 2007, i.e., an area of exposed bone in the maxillofacial region that fails to heal within 6–8 weeks, in a patient with current or past treatment with BPs but without head and neck radiotherapy. However, as has been commented above, some investigators have suggested that ONJ may manifest without bone exposure, particularly in the early stages of the disease. As an example, Junquera and Gallego [36] described two patients with bone sequestration that could be clinically and radiographically classified as corresponding to stage 3 ONJ, but without bone exposure. In these cases, pain and swelling were the main symptoms. The authors suggested that there is a variant of ONJ without bone exposure.

Based on their clinical experience, Bagan et al. [28] proposed that the three stages of the 2006 classification of Ruggiero et al. [42] should include patients with intraoral fistulas but no bone exposure, since these patients otherwise could not be assigned to any stage. Mawardi et al. [37] described five patients subjected to treatment with BPs who developed deep periodontal pockets, tooth mobility or intraoral fistulas with or without suppuration, with swelling in some cases, and with radiographic alterations (sequestration, sclerosis, lack of postextraction socket healing), but without exposure of necrotic bone.

After several months, bone exposure occurred in the same zone. The authors considered these cases as corresponding to early stage BAONJ and proposed to modify the definition of BONJ to include a new category: "suspected BONJ" or stage 0s, since in the same way as Bagan et al. [28], they were unable to assign the patients to any of the three established ONJ stages.

On the other hand, Fedele et al. [41] studied 332 patients with ONJ and found that 28.9% of the subjects have clinical manifestations consistent with the purported ONJ variant without bone exposure. The clinical manifestations in decreasing order of frequency were maxillary pain, fistulization, bone expansion, and gingival swelling. In addition, the symptoms developed spontaneously without previous extractions or surgery, and in 29.1% of the cases no radiological alterations were observed in the panoramic X-ray or computed tomography (CT) explorations.

Manifest bone exposure was seen over time (up to 2 years of follow-up) in 53.1% of these patients. According to the authors, these findings may have a significant impact upon the existing epidemiological data and on the design of future studies. According to Patel et al. [21], the absence of exposed bone in patients with ONJ can produce a delay in diagnosis, prolong the disease, and cause it to become refractory to treatment. They proposed a diagnostic and therapeutic approach to cases of ONJ, without bone exposure based on the symptoms, assessment of the risk factors, the radiographic evidence, and patient refractoriness to medical treatment. The authors suggested a modification of the AAOMS staging or classification system, as will be seen below.

Schiodt et al. [43] indicated that the proportion of ONJ without bone exposure may be high (29–45% of all cases of ONJ) and that this fact could result in potential underreporting of the disease in epidemiological studies. The authors evaluated 102 patients with ONJ, with and without bone exposure, and established comparisons between the two groups to determine whether they corresponded to the same disease condition or not. No significant differences were found between the two groups in terms of the demographic data, symptoms, clinical, and radiological characteristics, histopathological findings, or survival. As a result, they concluded that both presentations are part of the same disease and proposed a new ONJ classification including patients without bone exposure, as will be described below. Last, as we have seen, the AAOMS update of the year 2014 [25] modifies the definition of ONJ, with the inclusion of cases of ONJ without bone exposure, although the classification does not contemplate such presentations.

10.2.3.2 Need for radiological or imaging confirmation of the diagnosis

Ruggiero et al. [42], in an article presenting guidelines for the diagnosis, staging, and treatment of ONJ, described the existence of both early and late radiographic maxillary changes that could simulate other disorders (periapical disease, osteomyelitis, myeloma, or metastatic disease). In the case of important bone involvement, regions with a mottled appearance (similar to the pattern seen in osteomyelitis) could be found. Likewise, widening of the periodontal ligament and bone osteosclerosis could be observed, particularly in the region of the lamina dura.

However, according to these authors, the radiographic changes were not evident until important bone alteration had developed. They consequently suggested that the panoramic and periapical X-ray studies might not reveal significant changes in the early stages of ONJ. According to Khosla et al. [32], in the presence of well-established disease, imaging techniques are not needed for diagnostic purposes since the presence of exposed bone and other clinical signs and symptoms suffice to identify ONJ. Nevertheless, they recognized that such techniques may be of importance in the early identification of ONJ.

Other authors have used imaging techniques in patients of this kind, including CT, magnetic resonance imaging (MRI), scintigraphy, and panoramic and periapical X-rays. As an example, Bianchi et al. [44] studied 32 patients with ONJ, comparing the alterations found in panoramic X-rays versus CT. The latter technique was found to be far superior, with the detection of lesions in almost twice as many patients. In all cases, CT detected structural alterations of the trabecular bone and cortical erosion.

In comparison, the panoramic X-rays failed to detect bone sequestration in almost half of the cases. Intense periosteal reaction was a common finding, and oroantral communications could also be observed. Bedogni et al. [35] proposed a new classification of ONJ, as will be seen below based particularly on the CT findings. Likewise, Bedogni et al. [45] conducted a large retrospective multicenter study of the CT findings in

799 patients with ONJ. They found that the severity (extension) of the lesions can be identified and measured with CT much more accurately than with panoramic X-rays or clinical inspection, as proposed by some classifications—including that of the AAOMS of 2009.

The authors attempted to correlate the findings with the stages proposed by the AAOMS in 2009 and concluded that these stages are unable to correctly identify disease extent or involvement, except in stage 3. On the other hand, Arce et al. [46] conducted a review of the findings in ONJ with different imaging techniques.

According to these authors, the radiographic findings are not specific. Intraoral and panoramic X-rays may show widening of the lamina dura and of the periodontal ligament, osteolysis, diffuse sclerosis, and a lack of postextraction socket healing. The more advanced the disease, the greater the sclerosis and narrowing of the mandibular canal. Zones of ONJ can be identified in areas without exposed bone. CT offers a three-dimensional view of the extent of the lesion and can detect minor sequestrations.

Focal sclerosis with a disorganized trabecular pattern is present in the early stages of the disease, and neck adenopathies and masticatory muscle thickening simulating a tumor mass can be detected. MRI in turn can detect bone marrow and soft tissue involvement, nerve bundles, and adenopathies. Bone scintigraphy with technetium-99 shows enhanced radionuclide uptake between 10 and 14 days before bone mineral loss becomes significant enough to be detectable on X-rays.

The problem with scintigraphy is its lack of specificity and low resolution [46,47]. Bagan et al. [10] analyzed the degree of sclerosis in different ONJ stages using CT and investigated the relationship between the degree of sclerosis, the clinical symptoms, and the extent of the radiotransparencies in 43 cases—establishing comparisons with a group of 40 controls without bone lesions. The patients with ONJ had more intense sclerosis than the controls ($p < .01$). Furthermore, the degree of sclerosis increased with the clinical stage of ONJ and was correlated to the extent of the radiotransparency. Morphological analysis of the necrotic bone (sequestrations) using micro-CT has been unable to demonstrate the existence of unique distinguishing features in patients with ONJ in different stages [48].

10.2.4 Classification

Ruggiero et al. proposed an ONJ classification comprising three stages [42]: stage 1 = bone exposure but without signs or symptoms of infection; stage 2 = bone exposure/necrosis with clinical evidence of infection; stage 3 = the above manifestations and also alterations such as pathological fractures, extraoral fistulas, or osteolysis extending to the inferior mandibular margin.

In 2007, the AAOMS adopted this classification [31], although in addition to the group of patients with BRONJ (with its three stages), they included another group of patients comprising individuals at risk. These patients were defined as subjects without evident exposed or necrotic bone or symptoms but who have been treated with oral or intravenous BPs. In the year 2009, the AAOMS added a stage 0 to its classification, involving alterations (pain, tooth mobility, fistulas, radiographic changes, etc.) that may have been due to treatment with BPs, but without exposed bone.

The risk of progression toward more advanced stages of the disease was not known at that time [15].

Other classifications have also introduced the idea that ONJ may be present despite the absence of bone exposure. As an example, McMahon et al. [49] considered that an early stage of ONJ with or without symptoms may exist in which bone exposure has not yet occurred, since the first bone changes are found at marrow level, not in cortical bone, and that early detection of this stage could improve the patient strategy of treatment.

They also considered that imaging techniques and histological studies are needed to more precisely categorize the different ONJ stages. The authors proposed six stages (Table 10.1) but also considered that a stage 0 could be useful for identifying patients at risk. Mawardi et al. suggested the inclusion of a stage 0s as corresponding to "suspected BRONJ." This stage in turn would comprise two subcategories: 0ss in the presence of symptoms, and 0sa in the absence of symptoms [37].

Bagan et al. in turn included fistulas in stages 1, 2, and 3, although without bone exposure, and subdivided stage 2 into stages 2a and 2b according to whether the condition responded to conservative management or not [28]. Yoneda et al. accepted the definition of ONJ of the AAOMS, but proposed the introduction of four stages in accordance with the situation of the disease in Japan at that time [50].

This classification is basically the same as that of the AAOMS of 2009, but stage 0 moreover includes hypoesthesia or anesthesia of the lower lip as symptom and the presence of deep periodontal pockets as a clinical sign (Table 10.2). Other authors such as Bagan et al., in 2012, aimed to validate the classification of the AAOMS of 2009 with a retrospective study of 126 cases of ONJ due to intravenous and oral BPs, comparing both groups and determining whether all the cases could be assigned to one or other of the proposed stages [7].

More cases of ONJ without exposed bone were observed in the oral BP group, with a larger number of advanced cases (stages 2 or 3) in the intravenous oral BP group. In addition, six cases could not be assigned to any of the stages, for despite the presence of extraoral fistulas and mandibular fracture, no exposed bone was identified. The authors consequently proposed a new modification of the classification of Ruggiero et al. [15], with the inclusion in stage 3 of the term "exposed and necrotic bone or oral fistula without exposed bone" (Table 10.1).

10.2.4.1 Other classification proposals

Bedogni et al. proposed a new classification with three stages [35] as follows: stage 1 = focal ONJ, stage 2 = diffuse ONJ, and 3 = complicated ONJ. In addition to clinical findings, this classification includes CT imaging findings and eliminates stage 0. According to these authors, the clinical manifestations of pain and suppuration should not be used to differentiate between stages, since they only define symptomatic or asymptomatic forms of BRONJ within one same stage. This contributes to avoid patient migration from stage 1 to stage 2 or vice versa (ping-pong effect). These authors fundamentally used the CT findings to classify the patients. The presence of bone sequestration was not considered as a sign of complex BRONJ (Table 10.2).

Table 10.1 Proposals for modification of the ONJ classification of the AAOMS [15,31] by McMahon et al. [49], Bagan et al. [7,28], Mawardi et al. [37], and Yoneda et al. [50]

McMahon et al. [49]	Bagán et al. [28]	Mawardi et al. [37]	Yoneda et al. [50]	Bagan et al. [7]
Stage 1: No exposed/necrotic bone; Moderate and intermittent maxillary pain; Normal dental/mucosal and radiographic findings Scintigraphy, CT and MRI reveal osteoblastic activity but no evident infection.	**Stage 1**: Presence of exposed necrotic bone or small oral fistula without exposure of necrotic bone—asymptomatic.	Proposed modification the classification of the AAOMS of 2007 [31], introducing a new stage called 0s.	Same specifications as the AAOMS in its classification of 2009 except: **Stage 0:** Includes hypoesthesia or anesthesia of the lower lip and/or deep periodontal pockets.	The same stages as in the 2009 classification, but also:
Stage 2: No exposed/necrotic bone; Moderate and constant maxillary pain; Normal dental/mucosal findings, but Rx reveal sclerotic changes and radiotransparencies; Scintigraphy, CT and MRI show alterations; No evidence of infection.	**Stage 2a**: Presence of exposed necrotic bone or small oral fistula without exposure of necrotic bone. Patient with symptoms controlled by medical treatment.	**Stage 0s**: "Suspected ONJ"; Absence of exposed bone, presence of fistulas, severe tooth mobility, deep periodontal pockets, positive radiographic findings		**Stage 3**: Exposed necrotic bone or oral fistula without exposed bone, in patients with pain, infection and one or more of the following: radiographic evidence of bone necrosis extending beyond the alveolar bone, pathological fracture, extraoral fistula, oroantral oronasal communication, osteolysis extending to the inferior mandibular margin or sinus floor.

Stage 3: No apparent exposed/necrotic bone, constant and severe maxillary pain requiring analgesia, mucosal edema, erythema with severe pain of the alveolar bone, dental Rx, scintigraphy, CT and MRI show alterations, there may be infection, although not of dental origin. **Stage 4**: <2 cm exposed/necrotic bone without cortical fenestration Important and constant maxillary pain requiring potent analgesia. The mucosa surrounding the exposed bone is red and swollen. Moderate swelling of the surrounding tissues, without clear evidence of infection, dental Rx, scintigraphy, CT, and MRI show alterations, dental disease discarded. **Stage 5**: >2 cm exposed/necrotic bone with or without cortical fenestration, constant and severe maxillary pain requiring analgesia, the mucosa surrounding the exposed bone is red and swollen, mild to moderate swelling of the peripheral tissues with or without purulent suppuration, dental Rx, scintigraphy, CT and MRI show alterations, dental disease discarded.	**Stage2b**: Presence of exposed necrotic bone or small oral fistula without exposure of necrotic bone Patient with symptoms not controlled by medical treatment. **Stage 3**: Pathological fracture, extraoral fistula, osteolysis extending to the inferior mandibular margin.	Two subcategories: **Stage 0ss**: "Suspected" and symptomatic **Stage 0sa**: "Suspected" and asymptomatic.		

Continued

Table 10.1 Continued

McMahon et al. [49]	Bagán et al. [28]	Mawardi et al. [37]	Yoneda et al. [50]	Bagan et al. [7]
Stage 6: >4 cm exposed/necrotic bone with cortical fenestration and infection important and constant maxillary pain requiring potent analgesia fetidness. Dental Rx, scintigraphy, CT and MRI show alterations the mucosa surrounding the exposed bone is red and swollen, one or more of the following: pathological fracture, extraoral fistula, oroantral fistula, osteolysis extending to the inferior mandibular margin, dental disease discarded.				

CT, computed tomography; *MRI*, magnetic resonance imaging; *ONJ*, osteonecrosis of the jaws; *Rx*, X-ray.
Adapted from Gavalda C, Bagan JV. Concept, diagnosis and classification of bisphosphonate-associated osteonecrosis of the jaws. A review of the literature. Med Oral Patol Oral Cir Bucal May 1, 2016;21(3):e260–70.

Table 10.2 Proposals for the classification of ONJ according to Bedogni et al. [35] and Franco et al. [52]

Bedogni et al. [35]	Franco et al. [52]
Stage 1 Focal ONJ *Clinical signs and symptoms*: bone exposure, sudden tooth mobility, no postextraction socket healing, mucosal fistula, inflammation, abscess formation, trismus, important mandibular deformity, and/or lip hypoesthesia/paresthesia *CT findings*: Increased bone density limited to alveolar bone (trabecular thickening and/or focal osteosclerosis), with or without the following signs: Sclerotic and markedly thickened hard lamina, persistent socket space, and/or cortical disruption **1a.** Asymptomatic **1b.** Symptomatic (pain and purulent secretion)	**Clinical and radiological findings** **Stage 0** No exposed bone, with nonspecific radiographic findings such as osteosclerosis and periosteal hyperplasia, and nonspecific symptoms such as pain **Stage I** Exposed bone and/or radiographic evidence of necrotic bone[a], or persistent socket space <2 cm in greater diameter, with or without pain
Stage 2 Diffuse ONJ *Clinical signs and symptoms*: The same as in stage 1 *CT findings*: Increased bone density extending to the basal layer (diffuse osteosclerosis), with or without the following signs: Inferior dental nerve canal prominence, periosteal reaction, sinusitis, bone sequestration and/or oroantral fistula **2a.** Asymptomatic **2b.** Symptomatic (pain and purulent secretion)	**Stage II** Exposed bone and/or radiographic evidence of necrotic bone[a], between 2 and 4 cm in major diameter, with pain responsive to NSAIDs, and possible abscesses
Stage 3 Complicated ONJ As in stage 2, with one or more of the following: *Clinical signs and symptoms*: Extraoral fistula, mandibular stump displacement, nasal fluid drainage *CT findings*: Osteosclerosis of adjacent bone (zygoma, hard palate), pathological mandibular fracture, and/or osteolysis extending to the sinus floor	**Stage III** Exposed bone and/or radiographic evidence of necrotic bone[a], >4 cm in greater diameter, with intense pain that responds or does not respond to NSAIDs, abscesses, orocutaneous and/or maxillary sinus fistulization, with mandibular nerve involvement

CT, computed tomography; *NSAIDs*, nonsteroidal antiinflammatory drugs.
[a]Radiographic evidence of necrotic bone: irregular areas of hypo- and hypercalcification and/or bone sequestration.
Adapted from Gavalda C, Bagan JV. Concept, diagnosis and classification of bisphosphonate-associated osteonecrosis of the jaws. A review of the literature. Med Oral Patol Oral Cir Bucal May 1, 2016;21(3):e260–70.

According to Franco et al., most of the existing classifications are useful from the clinical and diagnostic perspective but none of them offer a surgical orientation to the surgeon [52]. They proposed a new dimensional staging system, classifying the lesions by size following panoramic X-ray and CT evaluation, with a view to making treatment decisions easier (Table 10.2).

Patel et al. modified the classification of the AAOMS of 2009 with the purpose of incorporating patients without bone exposure and of guiding treatment [21]. They distinguished between patients with and without bone exposure and in the latter group those individuals without symptoms were classified as corresponding to stage 1, whereas those with symptoms were assigned to stages 2 or 3 (Table 10.3).

As it has been commented before, Schiodt et al. considered ONJ with and without bone exposure to correspond to the same disease entity [43]. Accordingly, they modified the classification of Patel et al. [21], eliminating stage 0 and classifying patients both with and without bone exposure in stages 1, 2, or 3 (Table 10.3).

10.2.4.2 Actual classification and staging system proposed by the AAOMS

The classification or staging system proposed by the AAOMS [25], and the therapeutic strategies for each stage, is described below:

- At risk: Patients on antiresorptive or antiangiogenic treatment via the oral or intravenous route, and with no symptoms or apparent bone necrosis.
- Stage 0 (disease variant without bone exposure): No clinical evidence of necrotic bone, although with clinical findings, radiographic changes, and nonspecific symptoms.

  Among the symptoms:
  - Tooth pain in the absence of a dental cause.
  - Maxillary bone pain that may irradiate to the region of the temporomandibular joint.
  - Pain of the maxillary sinuses that may be associated to inflammation and thickening of the sinus walls.
  - Altered neurosensory function.

  Among the clinical findings:
  - Tooth mobility that cannot be explained by periodontitis.
  - Periapical or periodontal fistulas not associated to pulp necrosis secondary to trauma, caries, or restorations.

  Among the radiographic findings:
  - Loss or resorption of alveolar bone that cannot be explained by periodontitis.
  - Changes in trabecular-dense bone pattern, with no formation of new bone in extraction sockets.
  - Zones of osteosclerosis in alveolar bone or around the basal layer.
  - Thickening or opacification of the periodontal ligament (thickening of the lamina dura, sclerosis, and reduction of the periodontal ligament space).
- Stage 1: Exposed bone or intra or extraoral fistulization in the maxillofacial region penetrating to the bone, in asymptomatic patients without evidence of infection. In addition, radiographic findings such as those described in stage 0 may be observed in the alveolar bone.
- Stage 2: Exposed bone or intra- or extraoral fistulization in the maxillofacial region penetrating to the bone, with infection evidenced by pain and erythema in the region or exposed

Table 10.3 Proposals for the staging of ONJ according to Patel et al. [21] and Schiodt et al. [43]

Patel et al. [21]		Schiodt et al. [43]	
Clinical bone exposure Same stages as AAOMS 2009 [15]	**Absence of bone exposure asymptomatic** *Stage 1 NE* No clinical evidence of infection; there may be radiographic findings[a] **Symptomatic** *Stage 2 NE* No exposed necrotic bone; clinical evidence of infection, presence of intraoral fistulas, swelling, pain, paresthesia/dysesthesia, and radiographic evidence of bone necrosis *Stage 3 NE* As in stage 2 NE, with one or more of the following: • Radiographic evidence of bone necrosis extending beyond alveolar bone • Pathological fracture • Extraoral fistula • Oroantral, oronasal communication • Osteolysis extending to the inferior mandibular margin or sinus floor	**Bone exposure** Asymptomatic *Name: E-ONJ, stage 1* **Bone exposure** Symptoms of infection *Name: E-ONJ, stage 2* As in stage 3 of the AAOMS *Name: E-ONJ, stage 3*	**No bone exposure** Asymptomatic *Name: NE-ONJ, stage 1* **No bone exposure** Symptoms of infection *Name: NE-ONJ, stage 2* **No bone exposure, with** **Necrosis** in patients with pain, infection, and one or more of the following: Necrotic bone without exposure, as evidenced by imaging techniques, extending beyond alveolar bone, i.e., inferior margin or ramus of the mandible, maxillary sinus and zygoma, pathological fracture, extraoral fistula, oroantral or oronasal communication, osteolysis extending to the inferior mandibular margin or sinus floor *Name: NE-ONJ, stage 3*

E-ONJ, osteonecrosis of the jaws with exposure; *NE-ONJ*, osteonecrosis of the jaws with no exposure; *ONJ*, osteonecrosis of the jaws.
[a]Osteosclerosis, cortical rupture, osteolysis, subperiosteal bone deposit, thickening of the lamina dura, and widening of the periodontal ligament space.
Adapted from Gavalda C, Bagan JV. Concept, diagnosis and classification of bisphosphonate-associated osteonecrosis of the jaws. A review of the literature. Med Oral Patol Oral Cir Bucal May 1, 2016;21(3):e260–70.

bone with suppuration. In addition, radiographic findings such as those described in stage 0 may be observed in alveolar bone.

- Stage 3: Exposed bone or intra- or extraoral fistulization in the maxillofacial region penetrating to the bone, with pain, infection, and at least one of the following signs:
  - Necrotic bone extending beyond the alveolar bone (inferior margin or ramus of the mandible, maxillary sinus, and zygoma).
  - Pathological fracture
  - Extraoral fistula
  - Oroantral or oronasal communication
  - Osteolysis extending to the inferior margin of the mandible or sinus floor

As can be seen, no unified classification or staging system has yet been established for use by all professionals—although most studies are based on the classification of the AAOMS. In coincidence with other authors such as Bedogni et al. [35], Patel et al. [21], and Schiodt et al. [43], we consider that stage 0 should be suppressed and that ONJ should be classified into three stages regardless of whether or not there is bone exposure. Furthermore, it would be advisable to establish the diagnosis not only on the basis of the clinical data but also on the findings of the CT scan, since the latter technique offers greater information on the extent and severity of the disorder. Further studies and consensus are therefore needed with a view to adopting a single international classification allowing the conduction and comparison of epidemiological studies, and contributing to the treatment decision-making process.

10.3 BPs, osteonecrosis, and implant dentistry

BIONJ is characterized by the exposure for over 8 weeks of necrotic bone in the maxillofacial region, BP therapy, in the absence of prior maxillary radiotherapy [15,53,54]. Although the condition is typically confined to the maxillofacial region, there have been reports of cases in the hip, tibia, and femur [55]. The reason for such exclusive involvement of the jaws is subject to controversy.

In this sense, many factors could be implicated, including the anatomical characteristics of alveolar bone, its fine overlying epithelial layer, the mechanical stress caused by chewing, inflammatory processes (periodontitis), and a complex oral microbiota involving the presence of bacteria such as *Fusobacterium*, *Bacillus*, *Actinomyces*, *Staphylococcus*, *Streptococcus*, *Selenomonas* and *Treponema* [56,57]. The appearance of osteonecrosis is a serious complication that affects patient quality of life and causes important morbidity [15,58].

10.3.1 Etiopathogenesis

A number of factors have been related to the etiopathogenesis of ONJ, such as immune disorders and alterations of the reparatory mechanisms, since 95% of all patients with ONJ present tumors as background disease. Although vascular impairment has been postulated as one of the key elements in the etiopathogenesis of ONJ, the latter has also been erroneously linked to avascular necrosis in other locations such as the hip, since there are no clinical or physiopathological parallelisms between the two disorders. Diminished bone turnover and toxicity at both bone level and in the soft tissues have also been cited as etiopathogenic factors [59].

BPs have been reported to act directly upon keratinocytes and fibroblasts, inhibiting their activities through aging processes and apoptosis. This in turn affects cell proliferation and migration, resulting in a lack of reepithelization of the oral mucosa [60]. Although the physiopathology of ONJ remains to be fully clarified, the inhibition of bone remodeling has been suggested to play a significant role. The best evidence in support of this hypothesis comes from patients not treated with BPs. There have been reports of ONJ in patients treated with drugs such as denosumab that inhibit bone remodeling by acting upon the RANKL receptor [61]. There have also been descriptions of ONJ without previous BP treatment in patients with herpes-zoster infections and HIV-positive individuals [62].

The half-life of the BPs in blood is short (between 30 min and 2 h), although once bound to bone these drugs can persist within the body for years [63]. Although the presence of bacteria has been demonstrated in patients with BIONJ, it is not clear whether infection is a primary or a secondary cause of the disorder [15,50]. Many patients present antecedents of local trauma, particularly dental extractions (70%), with a lesser incidence of other surgical procedures. ONJ has been reported to develop spontaneously in 30–50% of the cases [64], particularly in locations where the gingival mucosa is thinner [15,50]. In a review of 468 dental implants in 115 patients subjected to oral BP therapy, no cases of ONJ were observed, and only two implants failed.

The success rate was therefore similar to that recorded in patients without BP treatment. In the absence of other diseases or medications, the placement of implants and their osseointegration during the first 3 years of treatment with oral BPs can be regarded as safe [65]. In another retrospective study [66], involving implant placement in 61 patients treated with oral BPs for an average of 3.3 years, no cases of ONJ were recorded during follow-up (12–24 months), and the implant success rate was 100%. Neverthcless, it must be taken into account that a number of authors [57,58,64,67,68] have described cases of BIONJ in patients with dental implants.

10.3.2 Risk factors

A number of studies [15,53,54] have analyzed the risk factors underlying of BIONJ. Treatment with potent intravenous BPs such as zolendronate or pamidronate, and tooth extractions, are the most important factors, with an estimated risk of between 6.7% and 9.1% after extraction [54]. Other potentially influencing factors are periodontal or periapical surgical procedures, the presence of dental abscesses, anatomical factors such as the presence of a torus, the duration of BP treatment, the number of treatment cycles, diabetes, deficient oral hygiene, and the concomitant administration of corticosteroids or thalidomide [15,28,56,69]. A genetic influence has also been postulated in the development of the disease through the cytochrome P450-2C enzyme system (CYP2C8), since the latter is implicated in the arachidonic acid metabolism and cholesterol biosynthesis, and can modulate angiogenesis and osteoblast differentiation in bone [50,53].

Recently, it was described a potential role of diabetes mellitus (DM) in the pathogenesis of MRONJ and the mechanisms by which DM may increase the risk for MRONJ. Factors related to DM pathogenesis and treatment may contribute to poor bone quality through multiple damaged pathways, including microvascular ischemia, endothelial cell dysfunction, reduced remodeling of bone, and increased apoptosis of osteoblasts and osteocytes [11].

In addition, DM induces changes in immune cell function and promotes inflammation. This increases the risk for chronic infection in the settings of cancer and its treatment, as well as antiresorptive medication exposure, thus raising the risk of developing MRONJ. A genetic predisposition for MRONJ, coupled with *CYP 450* gene alterations, has been suggested to affect the degradation of medications for DM such as thiazolidinediones and may further increase the risk for MRONJ [11].

10.3.3 Diagnosis and treatment

Several authors [42,64] consider that suspension of oral BP treatment for a period of 6–12 months results in clinical improvement and even spontaneous resolution of the condition. Suspension is therefore advisable, provided the systemic clinical conditions of the patient allow the interruption of BP therapy. Since 25% of trabecular bone and 3% of cortical bone are renewed each year, the interruption of BP treatment theoretically could have a beneficial effect, since the newly formed bone is unable to absorb BP [70].

However, in a study involving 25 patients, BP suspension was not seen to exert an effect [58]. Corticosteroid discontinuation also should be considered in patients concomitantly receiving these drugs as maintenance therapy [71]. It has been suggested that these patients should receive conservative management, since the mucosal disruptions resolve in at least 23–53% of the cases after following a series of recommendations: administration of topical chlorhexidine and systemic antibiotics in cases of pain and infection, the suppression of BP treatment, or hyperbaric oxygen therapy [28,68].

A preliminary study [69] of 10 patients has described a conservative treatment option based on direct ozone (O_3) application in gel form, thereby facilitating ozone release over the necrotic bone. Beneficial results were obtained, since in two patients (20%) the radiological controls showed disappearance of the lesions and complete regeneration of the oral tissues. The shedding of bone sequestration was recorded in eight patients (80%), with complete reepithelization of the lesions in two cases. There were no cases of ONJ relapse after 8 months of follow-up. Such therapy therefore should be regarded as an effective, safe, and simple treatment option in application to BIONJ measuring $\leq$2.5 cm in size. Another described treatment option is the administration of isoprenoid geranyl diphosphate (metabolic form of geraniol), which reverts inhibition of the mevalonate pathway induced by nitrogenated BPs [72].

Bocanegra-Pérez et al. [73] recommend treating these patients on a conservative basis, administering oral antibiotics such as amoxicillin—clavulanic acid 1000/62.5 mg two tablets/day/30 days, or metronidazole 250 mg two tablets/8 h/10–20 days, and 0.12% chlorhexidine rinses three to four times a day. The fistulas in turn can be treated with an intravenous perfusion of ciprofloxacin 2 mg/mL. In a case series published by Marx et al. [27], 90% of the patients in stages 1 and 2 were stabilized with conservative treatment in the form of oral rinses and systemic antibiotics.

Another study [25] found 3–10% of the patients fail to respond to conservative treatment or suffer pathological fractures—surgery being needed, with resection of the necrotic bone. The importance of aggressive treatment has been underscored in a study [74] in which conservative management was not effective. A surgical technique has been described, based on fluorescence-guided bone resection of 20 ONJ zones in 15 patients—the success rate being 85% after 4 weeks of follow-up [75]. The treatment response has been reported to be variable, with a poorer response in patients with maxillary sinusitis associated to ONJ [76]. The treatment guidelines proposed by Bagan et al. [28] are described in Table 10.4.

10.3.4 Prevention

It has long been reported that the determination of CTX (C-terminal telopeptide of type 1 collagen) in the serum of patients treated with BP could be of use in predicting ONJ in patients subjected to oral surgery. Patients with CTX $\geq$ 150 pg/mL can undergo any

Table 10.4 Proposed staging classification and treatment of BIONJ

Staging		Treatment
Stage 1	Exposure of necrotic bone or small oral ulceration without exposure of necrotic bone, with no symptoms.	Daily rinse with 0.12% chlorhexidine and follow-up.
Stage 2	**2a.** Exposure of necrotic bone or small oral fistula without exposure of necrotic bone, with symptoms controlled by medical treatment.	Daily rinse with 0.12% chlorhexidine, antibiotics, analgesics and follow-up.
	2b. Exposure of necrotic bone or small oral fistula without exposure of necrotic bone, with symptoms not controlled by medical treatment.	Daily rinse with 0.12% chlorhexidine, antibiotics, analgesics and surgery with elimination of bone necrosis.
Stage 3	Mandibular fracture, cutaneous fistula, osteolysis extending to lower margin.	Daily rinse with 0.12% chlorhexidine, antibiotics, analgesics, and extensive surgery with bone resection.

Adapted from Bagan JV, Jimenez Y, Diaz JM, Murillo J, Sanchis JM, Poveda R, et al. Osteonecrosis of the jaws in intravenous bisphosphonate use: proposal for a modification of the clinical classification. Oral Oncol July 2009;45(7): 645–46.

type of surgery with only minimum risks and without the need to suspend the medication; however, in the presence of CTX < 150 pg/mL the risks increase [64]. In contrast, other authors [77,78] have not found CTX to offer any true predictive value. Additionally, in the same manner Flychy-Fernández et al. [79], established that no relationship between oral dose administered was observed BP (total dose or expressed in mg/kg b.w.) and serum CTX concentration and suspension of the medication did not influence the serum CTX levels.

As a result, its use must be viewed with caution, and the CTX values cannot be used as a definitive indicator of the risk of suffering BIONJ. Serum osteocalcin is another marker that could be of use in predicting the risk of ONJ. In this sense, concentrations below the normal limits could indicate problems with the bone formation process and may be regarded as a risk factor [78]. Periapical X-rays can also be important, revealing sclerotic areas and loss of the inferior alveolar nerve contour caused by progressive sclerosis [47].

It has been shown that the adoption of preventive measures before and during intravenous BP therapy in cancer patients with bone metastases and in individuals with multiple myeloma is accompanied by a 75% reduction in the incidence of ONJ. Whenever possible, such preventive measures should include adequate oral hygiene before administering BP treatment, together with the extraction of teeth showing a poor prognosis, caries control, and monitorization of the correct fitting of removable dentures [15]. All patients treated with BPs are at risk of developing osteonecrosis as a result of such medication. This potential complication therefore should be explained to the patient by both the prescribing physician and the dental surgeon in charge of oral treatment, with the obtainment of informed consent in all cases.

Finally, a recent systematic review with meta-analyses performed to assess the impact of BP therapy upon dental implant survival, demonstrates that dental implant placement in patients receiving BPs does not reduce the dental implant success rate. On the other hand, such patients are not without complications, and risk evaluation therefore must be established on an individualized basis, as one of the most serious although infrequent complications of BP therapy is BP-related ONJ. The authors suggest that further prospective studies involving larger sample sizes and longer durations of follow-up are required to confirm the results obtained [80].

References

[1] Consensus development conference: diagnosis, prophylaxis, and treatment of osteoporosis. Am J Med June 1993;94(6):646−50.

[2] Friedlander AH. The physiology, medical management and oral implications of menopause. J Am Dent Assoc January 2002;133(1):73−81.

[3] WHO/Europe. Evidence-informed policy-making − what evidence is there for the prevention and screening of osteoporosis?. 2016. Available at: http://www.euro.who.int/en/data-and-evidence/evidence-informed-policy-making/publications/pre2009/what-evidence-is-there-for-the-prevention-and-screening-of-osteoporosis.

[4] Chen L, Wang G, Zheng F, Zhao H, Li H. Efficacy of bisphosphonates against osteoporosis in adult men: a meta-analysis of randomized controlled trials. Osteoporos Int September 2015;26(9):2355–63.
[5] Flichy-Fernandez AJ, Balaguer-Martinez J, Penarrocha-Diago M, Bagan JV. Bisphosphonates and dental implants: current problems. Med Oral Patol Oral Cir Bucal July 1, 2009; 14(7):E355–60.
[6] Ata-Ali F, Ata-Ali J, Flichy-Fernandez AJ, Bagan JV. Osteonecrosis of the jaws in patients treated with bisphosphonates. J Clin Exp Dent February 1, 2012;4(1):e60–5.
[7] Bagan JV, Hens-Aumente E, Leopoldo-Rodado M, Poveda-Roda R, Bagan L. Bisphosphonate-related osteonecrosis of the jaws: study of the staging system in a series of clinical cases. Oral Oncol August 2012;48(8):753–7.
[8] Flichy-Fernandez AJ, Gonzalez-Lemonnier S, Balaguer-Martinez J, Penarrocha-Oltra D, Penarrocha-Diago MA, Bagan-Sebastian JV. Bone necrosis around dental implants: a patient treated with oral bisphosphonates, drug holiday and no risk according to serum CTX. J Clin Exp Dent February 1, 2012;4(1):e82–5.
[9] Lopez-Cedrun JL, Sanroman JF, Garcia A, Penarrocha M, Feijoo JF, Limeres J, et al. Oral bisphosphonate-related osteonecrosis of the jaws in dental implant patients: a case series. Br J Oral Maxillofac Surg December 2013;51(8):874–9.
[10] Bagan JV, Cibrian RM, Lopez J, Leopoldo-Rodado M, Carbonell E, Bagan L, et al. Sclerosis in bisphosphonate-related osteonecrosis of the jaws and its correlation with the clinical stages: study of 43 cases. Br J Oral Maxillofac Surg March 2015;53(3):257–62.
[11] Peer A, Khamaisi M. Diabetes as a risk factor for medication-related osteonecrosis of the jaw. J Dent Res February 2015;94(2):252–60.
[12] Pichardo SE, van Merkesteyn JP. Bisphosphonate related osteonecrosis of the jaws: spontaneous or dental origin? Oral Surg Oral Med Oral Pathol Oral Radiol September 2013;116(3):287–92.
[13] Kumar V, Shahi AK. Nitrogen containing bisphosphonates associated osteonecrosis of the jaws: a review for past 10 year literature. Dent Res J (Isfahan) March 2014;11(2):147–53.
[14] Qi WX, Tang LN, He AN, Yao Y, Shen Z. Risk of osteonecrosis of the jaw in cancer patients receiving denosumab: a meta-analysis of seven randomized controlled trials. Int J Clin Oncol April 2014;19(2):403–10.
[15] Ruggiero SL, Dodson TB, Assael LA, Landesberg R, Marx RE, Mehrotra B, et al. American Association of Oral and Maxillofacial Surgeons position paper on bisphosphonate-related osteonecrosis of the jaws—2009 update. J Oral Maxillofac Surg May 2009;67(5 Suppl.):2–12.
[16] Campisi G, Fedele S, Fusco V, Pizzo G, Di Fede O, Bedogni A. Epidemiology, clinical manifestations, risk reduction and treatment strategies of jaw osteonecrosis in cancer patients exposed to antiresorptive agents. Future Oncol February 2014;10(2): 257–75.
[17] Otto S, Abu-Id MH, Fedele S, Warnke PH, Becker ST, Kolk A, et al. Osteoporosis and bisphosphonates-related osteonecrosis of the jaw: not just a sporadic coincidence—a multi-centre study. J Craniomaxillofac Surg June 2011;39(4):272–7.
[18] Lo JC, O'Ryan FS, Gordon NP, Yang J, Hui RL, Martin D, et al. Prevalence of osteonecrosis of the jaw in patients with oral bisphosphonate exposure. J Oral Maxillofac Surg February 2010;68(2):243–53.
[19] Khan AA, Sandor GK, Dore E, Morrison AD, Alsahli M, Amin F, et al. Bisphosphonate associated osteonecrosis of the jaw. J Rheumatol March 2009;36(3):478–90.
[20] Kuhl S, Walter C, Acham S, Pfeffer R, Lambrecht JT. Bisphosphonate-related osteonecrosis of the jaws—a review. Oral Oncol October 2012;48(10):938–47.

[21] Patel S, Choyee S, Uyanne J, Nguyen AL, Lee P, Sedghizadeh PP, et al. Non-exposed bisphosphonate-related osteonecrosis of the jaw: a critical assessment of current definition, staging, and treatment guidelines. Oral Dis October 2012;18(7):625–32.
[22] Thumbigere-Math V, Tu L, Huckabay S, Dudek AZ, Lunos S, Basi DL, et al. A retrospective study evaluating frequency and risk factors of osteonecrosis of the jaw in 576 cancer patients receiving intravenous bisphosphonates. Am J Clin Oncol August 2012; 35(4):386–92.
[23] Lipton A, Fizazi K, Stopeck AT, Henry DH, Brown JE, Yardley DA, et al. Superiority of denosumab to zoledronic acid for prevention of skeletal-related events: a combined analysis of 3 pivotal, randomised, phase 3 trials. Eur J Cancer November 2012;48(16): 3082–92.
[24] Peddi P, Lopez-Olivo MA, Pratt GF, Suarez-Almazor ME. Denosumab in patients with cancer and skeletal metastases: a systematic review and meta-analysis. Cancer Treat Rev February 2013;39(1):97–104.
[25] Ruggiero SL, Dodson TB, Fantasia J, Goodday R, Aghaloo T, Mehrotra B, et al. American Association of Oral and Maxillofacial Surgeons position paper on medication-related osteonecrosis of the jaw–2014 update. J Oral Maxillofac Surg October 2014;72(10): 1938–56.
[26] Ruggiero SL. Emerging concepts in the management and treatment of osteonecrosis of the jaw. Oral Maxillofac Surg Clin North Am February 2013;25(1):11–20. v.
[27] Marx RE, Sawatari Y, Fortin M, Broumand V. Bisphosphonate-induced exposed bone (osteonecrosis/osteopetrosis) of the jaws: risk factors, recognition, prevention, and treatment. J Oral Maxillofac Surg November 2005;63(11):1567–75.
[28] Bagan JV, Jimenez Y, Diaz JM, Murillo J, Sanchis JM, Poveda R, et al. Osteonecrosis of the jaws in intravenous bisphosphonate use: proposal for a modification of the clinical classification. Oral Oncol July 2009;45(7):645–6.
[29] Silverman SL, Landesberg R. Osteonecrosis of the jaw and the role of bisphosphonates: a critical review. Am J Med February 2009;122(2 Suppl.):S33–45.
[30] Sambrook P, Olver I, Goss A. Bisphosphonates and osteonecrosis of the jaw. Aust Fam Physician October 2006;35(10):801–3.
[31] Advisory Task Force on Bisphosphonate-Related Ostenonecrosis of the Jaws. American association of oral and maxillofacial surgeons. American association of oral and maxillofacial surgeons position paper on bisphosphonate-related osteonecrosis of the jaws. J Oral Maxillofac Surg March 2007;65(3):369–76.
[32] Khosla S, Burr D, Cauley J, Dempster DW, Ebeling PR, Felsenberg D, et al. Bisphosphonate-associated osteonecrosis of the jaw: report of a task force of the American Society for Bone and Mineral Research. J Bone Min Res October 2007;22(10):1479–91.
[33] Khan AA, Sandor GK, Dore E, Morrison AD, Alsahli M, Amin F, et al. Canadian consensus practice guidelines for bisphosphonate associated osteonecrosis of the jaw. J Rheumatol July 2008;35(7):1391–7.
[34] Colella G, Campisi G, Fusco V. American association of oral and maxillofacial surgeons position paper: bisphosphonate-related osteonecrosis of the Jaws-2009 update: the need to refine the BRONJ definition. J Oral Maxillofac Surg December 2009;67(12): 2698–9.
[35] Bedogni A, Fusco V, Agrillo A, Campisi G. Learning from experience. Proposal of a refined definition and staging system for bisphosphonate-related osteonecrosis of the jaw (BRONJ). Oral Dis September 2012;18(6):621–3.
[36] Junquera L, Gallego L. Nonexposed bisphosphonate-related osteonecrosis of the jaws: another clinical variant? J Oral Maxillofac Surg July 2008;66(7):1516–7.

[37] Mawardi H, Treister N, Richardson P, Anderson K, Munshi N, Faiella RA, et al. Sinus tracts—an early sign of bisphosphonate-associated osteonecrosis of the jaws? J Oral Maxillofac Surg March 2009;67(3):593—601.
[38] Khan AA, Morrison A, Hanley DA, Felsenberg D, McCauley LK, O'Ryan F, et al. Diagnosis and management of osteonecrosis of the jaw: a systematic review and international consensus. J Bone Min Res January 2015;30(1):3—23.
[39] Tubiana-Hulin M, Spielmann M, Roux C, Campone M, Zelek L, Gligorov J, et al. Physiopathology and management of osteonecrosis of the jaws related to bisphosphonate therapy for malignant bone lesions. A French expert panel analysis. Crit Rev Oncol Hematol July 2009;71(1):12—21.
[40] Margaix-Munoz M, Bagan J, Poveda-Roda R. Intravenous bisphosphonate-related osteonecrosis of the jaws: influence of coadjuvant antineoplastic treatment and study of buccodental condition. Med Oral Patol Oral Cir Bucal March 1, 2013;18(2):e194—200.
[41] Fedele S, Porter SR, D'Aiuto F, Aljohani S, Vescovi P, Manfredi M, et al. Nonexposed variant of bisphosphonate-associated osteonecrosis of the jaw: a case series. Am J Med November 2010;123(11):1060—4.
[42] Ruggiero SL, Fantasia J, Carlson E. Bisphosphonate-related osteonecrosis of the jaw: background and guidelines for diagnosis, staging and management. Oral Surg Oral Med Oral Pathol Oral Radiol Endod October 2006;102(4):433—41.
[43] Schiodt M, Reibel J, Oturai P, Kofod T. Comparison of nonexposed and exposed bisphosphonate-induced osteonecrosis of the jaws: a retrospective analysis from the Copenhagen cohort and a proposal for an updated classification system. Oral Surg Oral Med Oral Pathol Oral Radiol February 2014;117(2):204—13.
[44] Bianchi SD, Scoletta M, Cassione FB, Migliaretti G, Mozzati M. Computerized tomographic findings in bisphosphonate-associated osteonecrosis of the jaw in patients with cancer. Oral Surg Oral Med Oral Pathol Oral Radiol Endod August 2007;104(2):249—58.
[45] Bedogni A, Fedele S, Bedogni G, Scoletta M, Favia G, Colella G, et al. Staging of osteonecrosis of the jaw requires computed tomography for accurate definition of the extent of bony disease. Br J Oral Maxillofac Surg September 2014;52(7):603—8.
[46] Arce K, Assael LA, Weissman JL, Markiewicz MR. Imaging findings in bisphosphonate-related osteonecrosis of jaws. J Oral Maxillofac Surg May 2009;67(5 Suppl.):75—84.
[47] Morag Y, Morag-Hezroni M, Jamadar DA, Ward BB, Jacobson JA, Zwetchkenbaum SR, et al. Bisphosphonate-related osteonecrosis of the jaw: a pictorial review. Radiographics November 2009;29(7):1971—84.
[48] Allen MR, Pandya B, Ruggiero SL. Lack of correlation between duration of osteonecrosis of the jaw and sequestra tissue morphology: what it tells us about the condition and what it means for future studies. J Oral Maxillofac Surg November 2010;68(11):2730—4.
[49] McMahon RE, Bouquot JE, Glueck CJ, Griep JA, Adams WR, Spolnik KJ, et al. Staging bisphosphonate-related osteonecrosis of the jaw should include early stages of disease. J Oral Maxillofac Surg September 2007;65(9):1899—900.
[50] Yoneda T, Hagino H, Sugimoto T, Ohta H, Takahashi S, Soen S, et al. Bisphosphonate-related osteonecrosis of the jaw: position paper from the Allied Task Force Committee of Japanese Society for Bone and Mineral Research, Japan Osteoporosis Society, Japanese Society of Periodontology, Japanese Society for Oral and Maxillofacial Radiology, and Japanese Society of Oral and Maxillofacial Surgeons. J Bone Min Metab July 2010;28(4): 365—83.
[51] Gavalda C, Bagan JV. Concept, diagnosis and classification of bisphosphonate-associated osteonecrosis of the jaws. A review of the literature. Med Oral Patol Oral Cir Bucal May 1, 2016;21(3):e260—70.

[52] Franco S, Miccoli S, Limongelli L, Tempesta A, Favia G, Maiorano E, et al. New dimensional staging of bisphosphonate-related osteonecrosis of the jaw allowing a guided surgical treatment protocol: long-term follow-up of 266 lesions in neoplastic and osteoporotic patients from the university of bari. Int J Dent 2014;2014:935657.
[53] Bittner T, Lorbeer N, Reuther T, Bohm H, Kubler AC, Muller-Richter UD, et al. Hemimandibulectomy after bisphosphonate treatment for complex regional pain syndrome: a case report and review on the prevention and treatment of bisphosphonate-related osteonecrosis of the jaw. Oral Surg Oral Med Oral Pathol Oral Radiol January 2012; 113(1):41–7.
[54] Borromeo GL, Tsao CE, Darby IB, Ebeling PR. A review of the clinical implications of bisphosphonates in dentistry. Aust Dent J March 2011;56(1):2–9.
[55] Gupta S, Jain P, Kumar P, Parikh PM. Zoledronic acid induced osteonecrosis of tibia and femur. Indian J Cancer July–September, 2009;46(3):249–50.
[56] Landesberg R, Woo V, Cremers S, Cozin M, Marolt D, Vunjak-Novakovic G, et al. Potential pathophysiological mechanisms in osteonecrosis of the jaw. Ann N Y Acad Sci February 2011;1218:62–79.
[57] Hoefert S, Eufinger H. Relevance of a prolonged preoperative antibiotic regime in the treatment of bisphosphonate-related osteonecrosis of the jaw. J Oral Maxillofac Surg February 2011;69(2):362–80.
[58] Manfredi M, Merigo E, Guidotti R, Meleti M, Vescovi P. Bisphosphonate-related osteonecrosis of the jaws: a case series of 25 patients affected by osteoporosis. Int J Oral Maxillofac Surg March 2011;40(3):277–84.
[59] Reid IR, Cundy T. Osteonecrosis of the jaw. Skelet Radiol January 2009;38(1):5–9.
[60] Kim RH, Lee RS, Williams D, Bae S, Woo J, Lieberman M, et al. Bisphosphonates induce senescence in normal human oral keratinocytes. J Dent Res June 2011;90(6): 810–6.
[61] Aghaloo TL, Felsenfeld AL, Tetradis S. Osteonecrosis of the jaw in a patient on Denosumab. J Oral Maxillofac Surg May 2010;68(5):959–63.
[62] Feller L, Wood NH, Raubenheimer EJ, Meyerov R, Lemmer J. Alveolar bone necrosis and spontaneous tooth exfoliation in an HIV-seropositive subject with herpes zoster. SADJ March 2008;63(2):106–10.
[63] Marx RE. Pamidronate (Aredia) and zoledronate (Zometa) induced avascular necrosis of the jaws: a growing epidemic. J Oral Maxillofac Surg September 2003;61(9):1115–7.
[64] Marx RE, Cillo Jr JE, Ulloa JJ. Oral bisphosphonate-induced osteonecrosis: risk factors, prediction of risk using serum CTX testing, prevention, and treatment. J Oral Maxillofac Surg December 2007;65(12):2397–410.
[65] Grant BT, Amenedo C, Freeman K, Kraut RA. Outcomes of placing dental implants in patients taking oral bisphosphonates: a review of 115 cases. J Oral Maxillofac Surg February 2008;66(2):223–30.
[66] Fugazzotto PA, Lightfoot WS, Jaffin R, Kumar A. Implant placement with or without simultaneous tooth extraction in patients taking oral bisphosphonates: postoperative healing, early follow-up, and the incidence of complications in two private practices. J Periodontol September 2007;78(9):1664–9.
[67] Narongroeknawin P, Danila MI, Humphreys Jr LG, Barasch A, Curtis JR. Bisphosphonate-associated osteonecrosis of the jaw, with healing after teriparatide: a review of the literature and a case report. Spec Care Dent March–April 2010;30(2):77–82.
[68] Shirota T, Nakamura A, Matsui Y, Hatori M, Nakamura M, Shintani S. Bisphosphonate-related osteonecrosis of the jaw around dental implants in the maxilla: report of a case. Clin Oral Implants Res December 2009;20(12):1402–8.

[69] Ripamonti CI, Cislaghi E, Mariani L, Maniezzo M. Efficacy and safety of medical ozone (O(3)) delivered in oil suspension applications for the treatment of osteonecrosis of the jaw in patients with bone metastases treated with bisphosphonates: preliminary results of a phase I-II study. Oral Oncol March 2011;47(3):185–90.
[70] Wutzl A, Pohl S, Sulzbacher I, Seemann R, Lauer G, Ewers R, et al. Factors influencing surgical treatment of bisphosphonate-related osteonecrosis of the jaws. Head Neck February 2012;34(2):194–200.
[71] Bagan J, Blade J, Cozar JM, Constela M, Garcia Sanz R, Gomez Veiga F, et al. Recommendations for the prevention, diagnosis, and treatment of osteonecrosis of the jaw (ONJ) in cancer patients treated with bisphosphonates. Med Oral Patol Oral Cir Bucal August 1, 2007;12(4):E336–40.
[72] Marcuzzi A, Zanin V, Crovella S, Pontillo A. Comments on "Geranylgeraniol–a new potential therapeutic approach to bisphosphonate associated osteonecrosis of the jaw" by Ziebart T et al. (2011). Oral Oncol May 2011;47(5):436–7. author reply 438.
[73] Perez SB, Barrero MV, Hernandez MS, Knezevic M, Navarro JM, Millares JR. Bisphosphonate-associated osteonecrosis of the jaw. A proposal for conservative treatment. Med Oral Patol Oral Cir Bucal December 1, 2008;13(12):E770–3.
[74] Tirelli G, Biasotto M, Chiandussi S, Dore F, De Nardi E, Di Lenarda R. Bisphosphonate-associated osteonecrosis of the jaws: the limits of a conservative approach. Head Neck September 2009;31(9):1249–54.
[75] Pautke C, Bauer F, Otto S, Tischer T, Steiner T, Weitz J, et al. Fluorescence-guided bone resection in bisphosphonate-related osteonecrosis of the jaws: first clinical results of a prospective pilot study. J Oral Maxillofac Surg January 2011;69(1):84–91.
[76] Maurer P, Sandulescu T, Kriwalsky MS, Rashad A, Hollstein S, Stricker I, et al. Bisphosphonate-related osteonecrosis of the maxilla and sinusitis maxillaris. Int J Oral Maxillofac Surg March 2011;40(3):285–91.
[77] Bagan JV, Jimenez Y, Gomez D, Sirera R, Poveda R, Scully C. Collagen telopeptide (serum CTX) and its relationship with the size and number of lesions in osteonecrosis of the jaws in cancer patients on intravenous bisphosphonates. Oral Oncol November 2008; 44(11):1088–9.
[78] Kwon YD, Ohe JY, Kim DY, Chung DJ, Park YD. Retrospective study of two biochemical markers for the risk assessment of oral bisphosphonate-related osteonecrosis of the jaws: can they be utilized as risk markers? Clin Oral Implants Res January 2011;22(1):100–5.
[79] Flichy-Fernandez AJ, Alegre-Domingo T, Gonzalez-Lemonnier S, Balaguer-Martinez J, Penarrocha-Diago M, Jimenez-Soriano Y, et al. Study of serum CTX in 50 oral surgical patients treated with oral bisphosphonates. Med Oral Patol Oral Cir Bucal May 1, 2012; 17(3):e367–70.
[80] Ata-Ali J, Ata-Ali F, Penarrocha-Oltra D, Galindo-Moreno P. What is the impact of bisphosphonate therapy upon dental implant survival? A systematic review and meta-analysis. Clin Oral Implants Res February 2016;27(2):e38–46.

Biocompatibility and cellular response to dental implant materials

11

B. Zavan
University of Padova, Padova, Italy

11.1 Introduction

A medical device, such as dental implants are, is a scaffold that coming in contact with the patient's body and is expected to perform its intended function without resulting in any adverse effect to the patient. Potential adverse effects could occur, both short term (acute) and long term (chronic), to the body [1].

For this reason, medical devices are typically subject to biocompatibility tests and biological evaluation to assess the interaction with tissue, cells, or body fluids according to their classification. The primary aim of a device biocompatibility assessment is indeed to protect the patient from potential biological risks. To this aim, specific international rules define standard procedures that must be followed to test the biocompatibility and the safety of medical devices.

The main source of guidance on the essential requirements for biological safety is ISO 10993:2003 Biological evaluation of medical devices [2].

This standard defines devices in terms of their invasiveness and duration of patient contact and subsequently determines what level of safety testing manufacturer's need to successfully complete prior to putting their product on the market.

The document reports specific tests that depend on the following:

- the type of medical device;
- its intended use;
- the nature;
- duration of contact between the medical device and the body.

The test that can be performed can include testing such as:

- cytotoxicity;
- sensitization;
- irritation;
- intracutaneous reactivity;
- systemic toxicity;
- subchronic toxicity;
- genotoxicity;
- implantation;
- hemocompatibility.

Bone Response to Dental Implant Materials. http://dx.doi.org/10.1016/B978-0-08-100287-2.00011-2

Moreover, to be put on market medical devices need to respond to the minimum testing requirements for both community european (CE) marking (for Europe market) and US Food and Drug Administration (FDA) (for US market) submissions. All the medical device biocompatibility testing must be carried out under rigorous laboratory control working in good laboratory practice.

Prior to 2012, Japan had its own written guidelines, different from those laid out within ISO 10993 in several important ways. Because of this, medical devices intended for use in the Japan market were generally tested using different study protocols to meet these Japanese-specific guidelines. With the global harmonization efforts in the last decade, the recent revisions to the ISO guidelines have adopted or referenced the Japanese study protocols. In 2012, Japan's Ministry of Health, Labour, and Welfare released the revised guidelines of biocompatibility assessment that are largely harmonized with the ISO standards. In 2013, FDA released a draft biocompatibility guidance that also reflects the recent revisions of the ISO standards.

Components of ISO 10993 relevant to medical device manufacturers are composed of several parts:

- ISO 10993-1: Part 1: Evaluation and testing
- ISO 10993-3: Part 3: Tests for genotoxicity, carcinogenicity, and reproductive toxicity
- ISO 10993-4: Part 4: Selection of tests for interactions with blood
- ISO 10993-5: Part 5: Tests for in vitro cytotoxicity
- ISO 10993-6: Part 6: Tests for local effects after implantation
- ISO 10993-9: Part 9: Framework for identification and quantification of potential degradation products
- ISO 10993-10: Part 10: Tests for irritation and delayed-type hypersensitivity
- ISO 10993-11: Part 11: Tests for systemic toxicity
- ISO 10993-13: Part 13: Identification and quantification of degradation products from polymeric medical devices
- ISO 10993-14: Part 14: Identification and quantification of degradation products from ceramics
- ISO 10993-15: Part 15: Identification and quantification of degradation products from metals and alloys
- ISO 10993-16: Part 16: Toxicokinetic study design for degradation products and leachables
- ISO 10993-17: Part 17: Establishment of allowable limits for leachable substances
- ISO 10993-18: Part 18: Chemical characterization of materials
- ISO/TS 10993-19: Part 19: Physicochemical, morphological and topographical characterization of materials
- ISO/TS 10993-20: Part 20: Principles and methods for immunotoxicology testing of medical devices

11.2 Cell lines

For the in vitro testing, established cell lines are preferred and obtained from recognized repositories. ISO, namely, indicates to use BALB/c 3T3 cells, clone 31, and JCRB 9005, prepared from CCL-163 (ATCC). Where specific sensitivity is required, primary cell cultures, cell lines, and organotypic cultures obtained directly from living tissues should only be used if reproducibility and accuracy of the response can be demonstrated. If a stock culture of a cell line is stored, storage should be at −80°C or below in the corresponding culture medium but containing a cryoprotectant, e.g., dimethyl sulfoxide or glycerol. Long-term storage (several months up to many years) is only possible at −130°C or below. After thawing from stock, passage the cells two to three times before using them in the test [3].

Only cells free from *mycoplasma* shall be used for the test. Before use, stock cultures should be tested for the absence of *mycoplasma*. It is important to check cells regularly (e.g., morphology, doubling time, modal chromosome number) because sensitivity in tests can vary with passage number.

11.3 Determination of cytotoxicity

Determination of cytotoxic effects could be either qualitative or quantitative. Quantitative evaluation of cytotoxicity is preferable. Qualitative means are appropriate for screening purposes.

11.3.1 Qualitative evaluation

An example of qualitative evaluation can be represented by the microscopical examination of the cells using cytochemical staining to assess changes in morphology, vacuolization, detachment, cell lysis, and membrane integrity.

The change from normal morphology shall be recorded in the test report descriptively or numerically [4].

The analyses can be performed on plastic cultures or in agar support.

An example of a way to grade test samples in monolayer cultures can be represented by the follow scheme:

- 0 (None): when we observe discrete intracytoplasmatic granules, no cell lysis, and no reduction of cell growth;
- 1 (Slight): when not more than 20% of the cells are round, loosely attached, and without intracytoplasmatic granules, or show changes in morphology; occasional lysed cells are present; and only slight growth inhibition is observable;
- 2 (Mild): when not more than 50% of the cells are round, devoid of intracytoplasmatic granules, no extensive cell lysis and not more than 50% growth inhibition is observable;
- 3 (Moderate): when not more than 70% of the cell layers contain rounded cells or are lysed; cell layers are not completely destroyed, but more than 50% of growth inhibition is observable;
- 4 (Severe): when nearly complete or complete destruction of the cell layers (Fig. 11.1).

If the test is conducted on agar supports, the reactivity grades for agar [5] and filter diffusion test and direct contact test can be one of the following:

- 0 (None): no detectable zone around or under specimen;
- 1 (Slight): some malformed or degenerated cells under specimen;
- 2 (Mild): zone limited to area under specimen;
- 3 (Moderate): zone extending specimen size up to 1.0 cm;
- 4 (Severe): zone extending farther than 1.0 cm beyond specimen (Fig. 11.2).

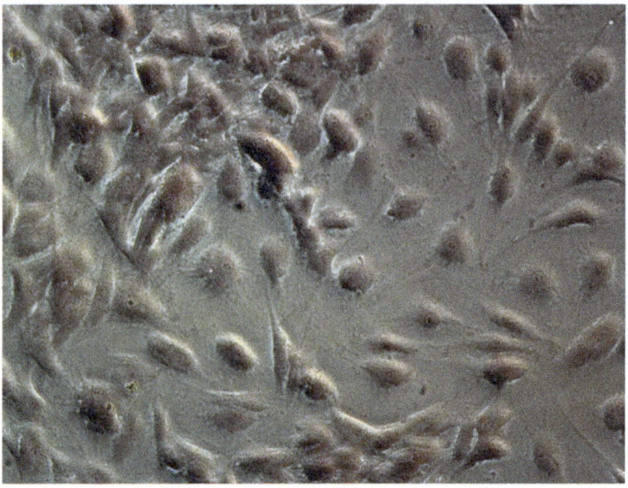

Figure 11.1 Monolayer of cells in the presence of an extract of titanium surfaces. Cells have been stained with ematoxillin eosin and show a fused shape morphology with no intracytoplasmatic granules.

11.3.2 Quantitative evaluation

Quantitative evaluation is related to the measure of cell death, inhibition of cell growth, cell proliferation, or colony formation. The number of cells, amount of protein, release of enzymes, release of vital dye, reduction of vital dye, or any other measurable parameter may be quantified by objective means.

Reduction of cell viability by more than 30% is considered a cytotoxic effect.

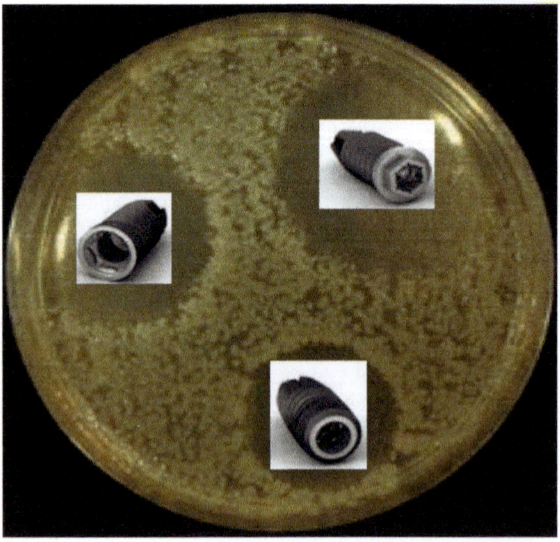

Figure 11.2 Agar diffusion assay allows migration tracking for a prolonged period of time.

The basic procedure requires the use of specific cells lines such as BALB/c 3T3 cells that must be seeded into 96-well plates and maintained in culture for 24 h to form a semiconfluent monolayer. They are then exposed to the test compound over a range of concentrations. After 24 h exposure, neutral red uptake (NRU) is determined for each treatment concentration and compared to that determined in control cultures. For each treatment, the inhibition of growth percentage is calculated, if the extract exhibits a cytotoxic effect on the cells. The concentration inhibiting plating efficiency to 50% (IC50) (i.e. the concentration producing 50% reduction of NRU) is calculated from the concentration–response and expressed as a dilution percentage of the extract. The neat extract is designated as 100% extract [6].

11.4 Colony formation cytotoxicity test

In this test, V79 cells (recommended because they make large and clear colonies) need to be seeded into six-well plates and maintained in culture for 24 h to start growing in a logarithmic phase. They are then exposed to the test compound and incubated for 6 days to make colonies large enough to count. Colonies are fixed with methanol, stained with Giemsa solution, and counted. If the extract obtained from the dental implant exhibits a cytotoxic effect on the cells, the IC50 is calculated and expressed as a percentage of the extract.

Positive and negative controls should be included in every cytotoxicity test [7]. Positive and negative reference materials are recommended: Zinc diethyldithiocarbamate (ZDEC) and Zinc dibutyl dithiocarbamate (ZDBC).

The acceptance criteria that need to be used for ZDEC and ZDBC are:

a. IC50 for ZDEC should not exceed 7%.
b. IC50 for ZDBC should not exceed 80% (Fig. 11.3).

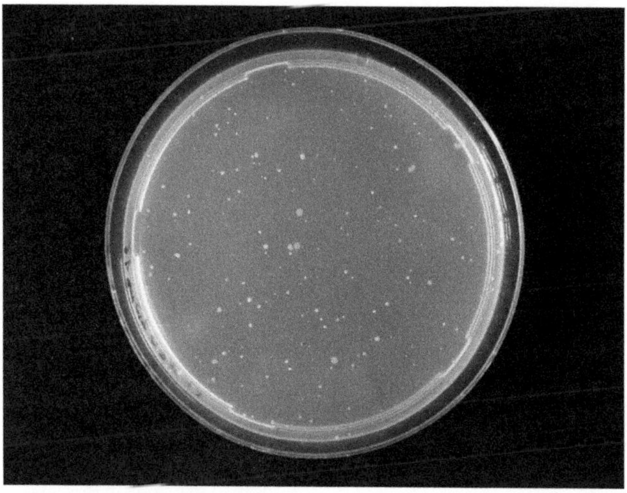

Figure 11.3 Colony formation on agar support.

11.5 MTT cytotoxicity test

Yellow water-soluble MTT (3-(4,5-dimethylthiazol-2-yl)-2,5-diphenyltetrazoliumbromid) is metabolically reduced in viable cells to a blue-violet insoluble formazan. Briefly, the supernatant of cell cocultures is gently harvested from the multiwell tissue culture plate and 1 mL of MTT solution [0.8 mg/mL in phosphate buffered saline (PBS)] is added. Cultures are returned to the incubator, and, after 3 h, the supernatant is harvested again. Each cell culture is then transferred and the viable cells, correlating to the color intensity, are determined by photometric measurements using Eppendorf microtube and 1 mL of extraction solution (0.01 N of HCl in isopropanol). The Eppendorf microtubes are vortexed vigorously for 5 min to enable total color release from the scaffolds, then centrifuged at 14,000 rpm for 5 min, and the supernatants read at 534 nm.

The absolute value of optical density, OD570, obtained in the untreated blank indicates whether the 1×10^4 cells seeded per well have grown exponentially with normal doubling time during 2 days of the assay.

A test meets the acceptance criteria if the mean OD570 of blank, *W*, is 0.2.

To check for systematic cell seeding errors, blanks are placed both at the left side (row 2) and the right side (row 11) of the 96-well plate. A test meets acceptance criteria if the left and the right mean of the blanks do not differ by more than 15% from the mean of all blanks.

Checks for cell seeding errors may also be performed by examining each plate under a phase contrast microscope to ensure that cell quantity is consistent. Microscopic evaluation obviates the need for two rows of blanks.

A decrease in number of living cells results in a decrease in the metabolic activity in the sample. This decrease directly correlates to the amount of blue-violet formazan formed, as monitored by the optical density at 570 nm.

The lower the Viab.% value, the higher is the cytotoxic potential of the test item.

If viability is reduced to <70% of the blank, it has a cytotoxic potential. The 50% extract of the test sample should have at least the same or a higher viability than the 100% extract; otherwise the test should be repeated (Fig. 11.4).

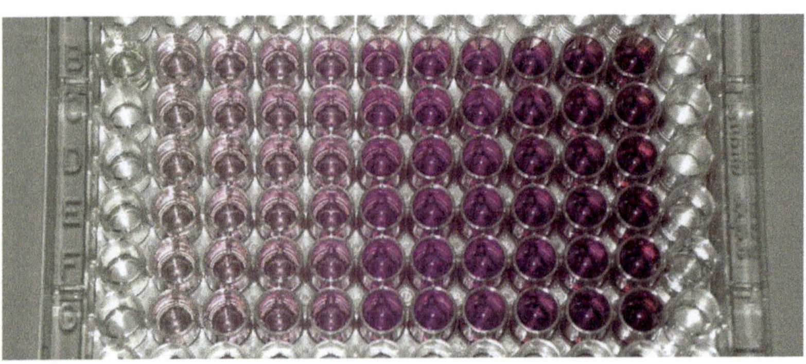

Figure 11.4 MTT test.

11.6 XTT cytotoxicity test

This test protocol is based on the measurement of the viability of cells via mitochondrial dehydrogenases, see Ref. [8]. XTT (2,3-*bis*(2-methoxy-4-nitro-5-sulfophenyl)-5-[(phenylamino)carbonyl]-2*H*-tetrazolium hydroxide) is metabolically reduced in viable cells to a water-soluble formazan product. The number of viable cells correlates to the color intensity determined by photometric measurements.

L929 cells are seeded into 96-well plates and maintained in culture for 24 h to form a semiconfluent monolayer. They are then exposed to the test compound over a range of concentrations. After 24 h exposure, the formazan formation is determined for each treatment concentration and compared to that determined in control cultures. For each treatment, the percentage inhibition of growth is calculated.

XTT is stocked fresh in 56–60°C medium eagle, without phenol red, at a concentration of 1 mg/mL with the aid of a shaker. Solution is sterilized by sterile filtration using syringe filters (pore size of 0.22 μm). Phenazine metosulfate (PMS) is made as a solution of 5 mM in PBS buffer and sterile filtered through a 0.22-μm sterile filter. PMS solution is added to the XTT solution shortly before usage in a concentration of 25 μM (5 μL of a 5 mM PMS/mL XTT solution). The XTT/PMS solution is then immediately added to the test wells.

The absolute value of optical density (OD450) obtained in the untreated blank indicates whether the 1×10^4 cells seeded per well have grown exponentially with normal doubling time during the 2 days of the assay. A test meets the acceptance criteria if the mean OD450 of blanks, *W*, is 0.2.

To check for systematic cell seeding errors, blanks are placed both at the left side (row 2) and the right side (row 11) of the 96-well plate (row 1 and row 12 shall not be used).

A test meets the acceptance criteria if the left and the right mean of the blanks do not differ by more than 15% from the mean of all blanks.

Checks for cell seeding errors may also be performed by examining each plate under a phase contrast microscope to ensure that cell quantity is consistent. Microscopic evaluation obviates the need for two rows of blanks.

11.7 Ames test

The mutagenic potential of Ti implants is evaluated by the Ames test performed with the Salmonella Mutagenicity Complete Test Kit (Moltox, Molecular toxicology Inc., Boone, NC, USA). Nutrient broth (blank) is used as the extraction vehicle; aluminum oxide ceramic rod (VITA In-Ceram Alumina CA-12, CE 0124, lot 15320) is used as negative control; ICR 191 Acridine (Moltox, 60–101) and sodium azide (Moltox, 60–103) were used as positive controls. Extraction conditions were (24 ± 2)h at (37 ± 1)°C. Three replicates are performed for each sample. The bacteria plates are incubated with the different extracts for 48 h at 37°C, and the number of revertant colonies per plate was counted. Interpretation of results: negative (not mutagenic) if the number of reverted colonies is equivalent to those observed with blank and negative controls; positive (mutagenic) if the number of reverted colonies is equivalent to those observed with positive controls [9] (Fig. 11.5).

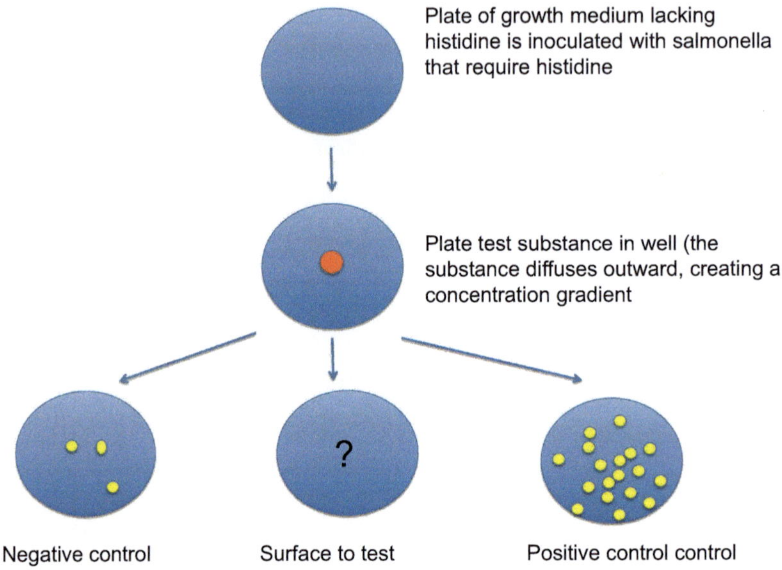

Figure 11.5 Representation of Ames test.

11.8 Hemolysis assay

The blood compatibility of Ti implants could be evaluated by the hemolysis assay performed following standard practices set forth in ASTM F756. Blood is obtained from three healthy New Zealand rabbits, pooled, then diluted in PBS to a total hemoglobin concentration of 10 ± 1 mg/mL. One milliliter of diluted rabbit blood is added to 7 mL of the following PBS extracts. For the extraction of the test material, triplicate 2 g portions of Ti implants are covered with 10 mL PBS. For the negative control, triplicate 30 cm^2 portions of high-density polyethylene are covered with 10 mL of PBS. For the positive control, triplicate 10 mL portions of sterile water for injection are used. Extraction conditions were 50°C for 72 h for all samples. Each tube is incubated for 3 h at 37°C with periodic inversions. Following incubation, the tubes were centrifuged for 15 min at $800 \times g$. A 1 mL aliquot of the resulting supernatant from test materials, negative and positive controls was added to 1 mL of Drabkin's reagent (Sigma-Aldrich) and incubated at room temperature for 15 min. The reaction product between hemoglobin and Drabkin's reagent is a cyanoderivative that was quantified by measuring absorbance at 540 nm with a multilabel plate reader (Victor 3 Perkin Elmer, Milano, Italy) [10–21]. The hemolysis index (HI) is then calculated using the mean absorbance value (OD) for each group as follows:

$$\text{HI (\%)} = \text{OD (test material)} - \text{OD (negative control)/OD (positive control)} - \text{OD (negative control)} \times 100.$$

Interpretation of results: nonhemolytic if the HI was 2% or less; hemolytic if HI was higher than 2% (Fig. 11.6).

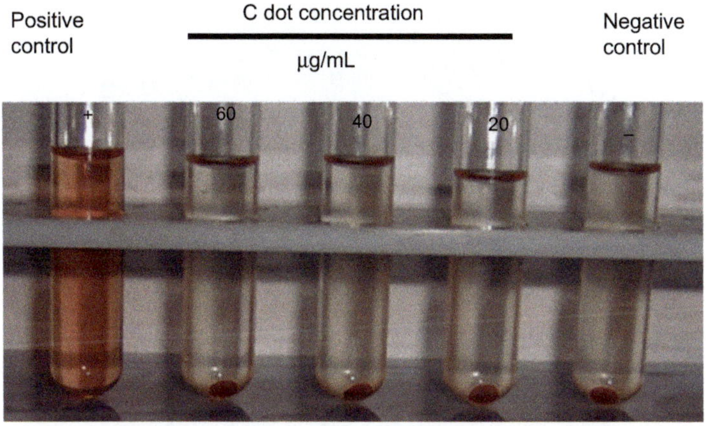

Figure 11.6 Visual representation of hemolitic process.

11.9 Karyotype analysis

After 30 days of culture on Ti implants, cells are exposed to colchicine (Sigma-Aldrich, St. Louis, MO, USA) for 6 h, washed in PBS, dissociated with trypsin (Lonza S.r.l), and centrifuged at 300 g for 5 min. The pellet is carefully suspended again and incubated in 1% sodium citrate for 15 min at 37°C, then fixed and spread onto −20°C cold glass slides. Metaphases of cells are Q-banded and karyotyped in accordance with the International System for Human Cytogenetic Nomenclature recommendations. At least five metaphases need to be analyzed for three expansions (Fig. 11.7).

11.10 Alternatives in animal testing

There is no doubt that the best test species for humans are humans.

To predict toxicity, corrosivity, and other safety variables as well as the effectiveness of a new product for humans such dental implants have involved the use of animals. But today, scientists have developed and validated alternative methods shown to lead to safer and more effective products for humans than animal testing.

For example, skin corrosivity and irritation can be easily measured using three-dimensional human skin equivalent systems such as EpiDerm and SkinEthic. Additional alternatives include EpiSkin (a model of reconstructed human epithelium) and a variety of sophisticated, computer-based quantitative structure activity relationship models that predict skin corrosivity and irritation by means of correlating a new drug or chemical with its likely activity, properties, and effects with classification accuracy between 90% and 95%.

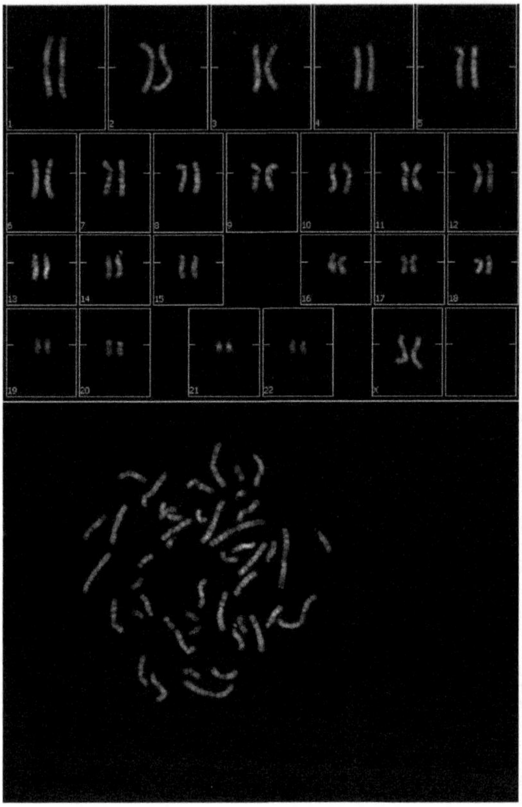

Figure 11.7 Karyotype analysis of adipose derived stem cells (ADSCs) seeded on the Ti implants for 30 days. No chromosomal alterations are present.

Often these are based on tissue engineering (TE). TE is "an interdisciplinary field that applies the principles of engineering and life sciences toward the development of biological substitutes that restore, maintain, or improve tissue function or a whole organ." TE has also been defined as "understanding the principles of tissue growth, and applying this to produce functional replacement tissue for clinical use." Powerful recent developments in the multidisciplinary field of TE have yielded a novel set of tissue replacement parts and implementation strategies. Scientific advances in biomaterials, stem cells, growth and differentiation factors, and biomimetic environments have created unique opportunities to fabricate tissues in the laboratory from combinations of engineered extracellular matrices ("scaffolds"), cells, and biologically active molecules [22]. Among the major challenges now facing TE there is the need for more complex functionality with biomechanical stability in laboratory-grown tissues destined for transplantation. So it has been possible, starting from a 2 × 2 cm skin human biopsy, to realize completely autologous cutaneous substitutes not only composed of two structures of the skin, dermis and epidermis, but also containing other important components: microvascular network, micronervous network, skin immonocompetent system, and melanocyte system [23]. The final goal is to develop effective and easy handling of skin substitutes that can be used to reproduce human skin anatomy and physiology, introducing new advantages linked to successful grafting or for in vitro testing.

Technique:

Human dermal fibroblasts are prepared according to a modified version of the Rheinwald & Green protocol. After epithelial sheet dispase removal, dermis was cut into small pieces (2–3 mm^2) and fibroblasts were isolated by sequential trypsin (0.05%) and collagenase type I digestion. Cells are isolated and then cultured with Dulbecco's Modified Eagle's Medium supplemented with 10% fetal bovine serum. At confluence, fibroblasts are harvested and seeded at a density of $3 \times 10^5/cm^2$ on squares of biomaterials (1.5 × 1.5 cm) in the above-mentioned medium containing sodium ascorbate (50 mg/mL) (step 5). The nonwoven squares could be fixed on culture plates either by means of stainless steel rings or through a fibrin clot.

Cocultures of fibroblasts and keratinocytes (bilayer substitutes): After these first attempts, given that fibroblasts are the main constituent of the dermis and are normally used to grow keratinocytes, the concept of a coculture was introduced to produce in vitro a composite skin replacement composed of an epithelial layer overlaid onto a dermal substitute. The presence of fibroblasts within the grafted region is thus a major advantage. Several lines of research are being pursued to define the best conditions of use [24]. These include studies of allogenic fibroblast persistence in humans. Such fibroblasts persist in animals, but in humans, even if allogenic fibroblasts give similar results to autologous fibroblasts, their ultimate fate is unknown. Definition of fibroblast populations within the dermis has been undertaken. There is clear evidence that, depending on the anatomical region or the depth within the dermis, fibroblasts can be distinguished on the basis of functional criteria. It would be useful to have markers to select those cells that would be most efficient within dermal substitutes. At present despite active research in this field there is still no commercially available fibroblast marker [25]. Last, the possibility of using mesenchymal stem cells collected from bone marrow or peripheral blood, which seem to participate in wound healing, is being evaluated. In addition to skin substitutes for permanent skin replacement, other applications can help to rapidly cover patients' wounds (despite eventual rejection of allogenic cells) or accelerate healing. It is already known that allogenic epidermal cell cultures promote external ulcer healing [26], probably by secreting factors (matrix metalloproteinases, growth factors, etc.) that promote wound cleansing and stimulate the activity of cells present at the wound site. At the end, the importance of the scaffold for a dermal-like tissue must be stressed.

In fact, the design of a dermal-like tissue critically depends on the use of an ideal scaffold, which must allow the dermis to develop into a three-dimensional architecture. One of the most important features of the scaffold is its porosity, which has to fit the neovessel ingrowth from the host tissue (angiogenesis) during the wound healing process. In addition, the biomaterial should be fully biocompatible and totally degradable being substituted by a full functional extracellular matrix in the long term.

In Europe one of the most important advances in regulatory toxicology has been the implementation of the Globally Harmonized System for the identification, classification, and labeling of substances, mixtures, and preparations (United Nations—Economic Commission for Europe, 2009). The hazard associated with a single chemical substance or a mixture of two or more substances refers to their intrinsic property to cause a particular effect, in this case, acute skin irritation and corrosion. In regulatory terms, skin corrosion represents irreversible damage to the skin, whereas skin irritation is characterized by clinical evidence of inflammation, which is entirely reversible.

In the past, the potential of a substance or preparation to cause skin irritation or corrosion has been assessed using a rabbit skin test. However, in vitro alternatives have now taken the place of the rabbit test and in a similar manner aim at a basic hazard identification of chemicals, which can cause burns or a significant level of acute skin irritation. These efforts in regulatory toxicology are directed toward the characterization of the intrinsic properties of substances, with subsequent application of that knowledge to mixtures and formulations. Hazard information from human studies is unfortunately not available, since due to ethical reasons, testing in humans for classification and labeling purposes is not accepted.

To obtain controlled human acute skin irritation information, an alternative strategy involving a protocol for the use of human volunteers, the 4 h human patch test (4 h HPT) to characterize skin irritation hazard has been developed and described extensively in the literature [27–29].

The 4 h HPT provides the opportunity to identify substances with significant skin irritation potential without recourse to the use of animals. It can be applied for the evaluation of skin effects of single substances as well as mixtures and formulations. The human skin irritation test is very similar to the regulatory accepted in vivo rabbit skin irritation test, but it is designed to limit the intensity of skin reactions in human volunteers. The value of the method is in (1) providing data for the identification of those substances or formulation, which should or should not be classified as irritant, and (2) providing "gold standard" data for future validations of alternative/in vitro methods replacing the in vivo rabbit test for classification and labeling purposes in regulatory toxicology.

In the material that follows, the literature has been surveyed to permit the assembly of an extended catalog of substances to which human subjects have been exposed using the 4 h HPT protocol. Only on very few occasions, substances appeared to possess a greater ability to generate irritant skin reactions than had been expected. More importantly, many more substances had only a very limited effect on the skin. Consequently, it is essential that new in vitro toxicology tests are calibrated and whenever possible validated against human data rather than use information from in vivo rabbit assays obtained usually from outdated databases.

11.11 The 4 h human patch test—protocol

The human 4-h patch test procedure involves the application of 0.2 mL (0.2 g for solid test materials) on a 25-mm plain Hill Top Chamber containing a Webril pad (Hill Top Companies, Cincinnati, OH, USA), moistened for solid test materials, to the skin of the upper outer arm of 30 human volunteers for up to 4 h. To avoid the production of unacceptably strong reactions, test materials are applied progressively from 15 to 30 min through 1, 2, 3, and 4 h. Each progressive application is at a new skin site. The shorter exposure periods can be omitted if the study directors are satisfied that excessive reactions will not occur following longer exposure. Treatment sites are assessed for the presence of irritation at 24, 48, and 72 h after patch removal. A volunteer with a reaction at any of the assessments is considered to have demonstrated a "positive" irritant reaction and treatment with the causative substance does not proceed on that person. For panelists with a "+" or greater response at application times of less than 4 h, it is assumed that they would present a stronger irritant reaction if exposed for 4 h. However, once a "+" or greater response is obtained, there is no need to subject these panelists to further treatment with that substance. In evaluating the results, what is measured is the number of panelists who had a positive "irritant" reaction after a 4-h exposure. If irritation reactions to the undiluted test substance are significantly greater than or not significantly different (using Fisher's exact test) from the level of reaction in that same panel of volunteers to 20% sodium dodecyl sulfate (SDS), the substance should be classified as irritant to skin (I); where the level of reaction is substantially and statistically significantly lower than the response to SDS, the substance is not classified (NC). Very occasionally, where the response is significantly stronger (and faster to occur), e.g., to 0.5% NaOH, then the substance is suggested to be a potential corrosive (C).

11.12 Alternative method for dental implant osteointegration

The use of dental implants has become widespread as prosthetic therapy for patients with missing teeth. The success of an implant relies on the presence of adequate bone quantity and quality at the placement site because the implant needs to undergo "osseointegration." By definition, osseointegration is seen as the close contact between bone and implant. The bone response is related to implant surface properties. Various surfaces have been studied and applied to improve biological properties of the implant, which favors the mechanism of osseointegration. This strategy aims at promoting the mechanism of osseointegration with faster and stronger bone formation to confer better stability during the healing process, thus allowing more rapid loading of the implant. In this context, an increased interest in the improvement of osseointegration through topographic and chemical dental implant surface modifications was observed over the last years. To date, dental implant osseointegration is current studied in various animal models.

In this view, Sivolella et al. [30] proposed a novel in vitro method to predict the in vivo dental implant osseointegration. Starting from the experience on stem cell biology and TE strategy available in the laboratory, the authors developed and confirmed a method to evaluate in vitro the osteointegrative properties of implants. This method requires the in vitro generation of a lived bone scaffold combined with an implant, followed by mechanical and biological test.

Their results demonstrated that if the implants are inserted in a live scaffold, a significantly higher force to extract the implants will be needed compared with the controls, which are scaffolds on which the cells are not present, and these results are strongly correlated with the biological properties of the surfaces. These are the results that are determined by the vivo test.

This method is conducted in three phases:

Phase 1: In vitro generation of a scaffold combined with an implant.

Customized cylindrical implants are be inserted in the bone blocks by means of two customized drilling guides with a twist drill and dedicated drill stops.

Phase 2: In vitro reconstruction of a three-dimensional bone like tissue.

Mesenchymal stem cells are seeded into a scaffold combined with the implant prepared in the previous phase and their commitment into osteogenic line.

Phase 3: Analyses of osseointegration.

Histological and molecular analyses will be performed to evaluate the quality and quantity of bone production, analyses of cell population, protein production, cell differentiation, and bone-to-implant contact (bic).

Mechanical test: pull-out test

The pull-out test will be performed to measure the force needed to extract an embedded insert from a concrete mass.

Phase 4: Correlation of our in vitro results with data present in the literature. Their pull-out test will be correlated with bone-to-implant contact previously obtained in vivo with the same surfaces.

11.13 Benefits of non-animal testing

1 Alternative scientific tests are often more reliable than animal tests.
2 The use of human tissue in toxicity testing is more accurate than the animal models.

The "lethal dose 50" (LD50) test forces animals to ingest toxic and lethal substances to the endpoint where 50% of the animals in the study die—and those that do not are later killed. The late Dr. Björn Ekwall (Cytotoxicology Laboratory in Sweden) developed a replacement for the LD50 test that measured toxicity at a precision rate of up to 85% accuracy compared to the LD50 rate of 61–65%. This test, far more accurate than the animal models, uses donated human tissue rather than animal tissue. Furthermore, the test is conducted to study the toxic effects on specific human organs, whether or not the toxic substance permeates the blood barrier. The test is useful to conduct highly sophisticated and precise experiments, the results of which will help to reveal information that the agonizing death of an animal of a different species would not reveal.

3 Nonanimal tests are more cost-effective, practical, and expedient.
4 Cruelty-free products are more environmentally friendly.

In toxicity testing, researchers breed, test, and ultimately dispose of millions of animals as pathogenic or hazardous waste. Cruelty-free testing is less harmful to the environment or creates less waste.

The need for alternatives to the traditional use of animals in toxicity testing was officially recognized by the US government in 1993 with the passage of the National Institutes of Health Reauthorization Act. Requirements under the Act led to the establishment of an ad hoc committee called the Interagency Coordinating Committee for the Validation of Alternative Methods (ICCVAM). ICCVAM was made a permanent committee under the ICCVAM Authorization Act of 2000 and is composed of representatives from 15 US federal regulatory and research agencies.

Under the National Toxicology Program's Interagency Center for the Evaluation of Alternative Toxicological Methods, ICCVAM's mission is "to promote the development, validation, and regulatory acceptance of new, revised, and alternative regulatory safety testing methods." Emphasis is on alternative methods that will reduce, refine (less pain and distress), and replace the use of animals in testing while maintaining and promoting scientific quality and the protection of human health, animal health, and the environment.

References

[1] Directive 93/42/EEC.

[2] ISO 10993. Biological evaluation of medical devices. 2003.

[3] Brown A, Zaky S, Ray Jr H, Sfeir C. Porous magnesium/PLGA composite scaffolds for enhanced bone regeneration following tooth extraction. Acta Biomater January 2015;11: 543–53.

[4] Miller F, Hinze U, Chichkov B, Leibold W, Lenarz T, Paasche G. Validation of eGFP fluorescence intensity for testing in vitro cytotoxicity according to ISO 10993-5. J Biomed Mater Res B Appl Biomater December 24, 2015.

[5] Pusnik M, Imeri M, Deppierraz G, Bruinink A, Zinn M. The agar diffusion scratch assay – A novel method to assess the bioactive and cytotoxic potential of new materials and compounds. Sci Rep February 10, 2016;6:20854. http://dx.doi.org/10.1038/srep20854.

[6] Bang SM, Moon HJ, Kwon YD, Yoo JY, Pae A, Kwon IK. Osteoblastic and osteoclastic differentiation on SLA and hydrophilic modified SLA titanium surfaces. Clin Oral Implants Res July 2014;25(7):831–7.

[7] Gardin C, Ricci S, Ferroni L, Guazzo R, Sbricoli L, De Benedictis G, et al. Decellularization and delipidation protocols of bovine bone and pericardium for bone grafting and guided bone regeneration procedures. PLoS One July 20, 2015;10(7):e0132344.

[8] Klinger A, Tadir A, Halabi A, Shapira L. The effect of surface processing of titanium implants on the behavior of human osteoblast-like Saos-2 cells. Clin Implant Dent Relat Res March 2011;13(1):64–70.
[9] Ferroni L, Gardin C, Bressan E, Calvo-Guirado JL, Isola M, Piattelli A, et al. Ionized Ti surfaces increase cell adhesion properties of mesenchymal stem cells. J Biomater Tissue Eng 2015;5:1–9.
[10] Gardin C, Ferroni L, Bressan E, Calvo-Guirado JL, Degidi M, Piattelli A, et al. Adult stem cells properties in terms of commitment, aging and biological safety of grit-blasted and Acid-etched ti dental implants surfaces. Int J Mol Cell Med 2014 Fall; 3(4):225–36.
[11] ISO 10993–1. Part 1: evaluation and testing.
[12] ISO 10993–3. Part 3: tests for genotoxicity, carcinogenicity and reproductive toxicity.
[13] ISO 10993–4. Part 4: selection of tests for interactions with blood.
[14] ISO 10993–5. Part 5: tests for in vitro cytotoxicity.
[15] ISO 10993–6. Part 6: tests for local effects after implantation.
[16] ISO 10993–9. Part 9: framework for identification and quantification of potential degradation products.
[17] ISO 10993–10. Part 10: tests for irritation and delayed-type hypersensitivity.
[18] ISO 10993–11. Part 11: tests for systemic toxicity.
[19] ISO 10993–13. Part 13: identification and quantification of degradation products from polymeric medical devices.
[20] ISO 10993–14. Part 14: identification and quantification of degradation products from ceramics.
[21] ISO 10993–15. Part 15: identification and quantification of degradation products from metals and alloys.
[22] Ferroni L, Bellin G, Emer V, Rizzuto R, Isola M, Gardin C, et al. Treatment by Therapeutic Magnetic Resonance (TMR™) increases fibroblastic activity and keratinocyte differentiation in an in vitro model of 3D artificial skin. J Tissue Eng Regen Med June 5, 2015. http://dx.doi.org/10.1002/term.2031.
[23] Tonello C, Zavan B, Cortivo R, Brun P, Panfilo S, Abatangelo G. In vitro reconstruction of human dermal equivalent enriched with endothelial cells. Biomaterials March 2003;24(7): 1205–11.
[24] Tonello C, Vindigni V, Zavan B, Abatangelo S, Abatangelo G, Brun P, et al. In vitro reconstruction of an endothelialized skin substitute provided with a microcapillary network using biopolymer scaffolds. FASEB J September 2005;19(11):1546–8.
[25] Figallo E, Flaibani M, Zavan B, Abatangelo G, Elvassore N. Micropatterned biopolymer 3D scaffold for static and dynamic culture of human fibroblasts. Biotechnol Prog January-February;23(1):210–6.
[26] Zavan B, Vindigni V, Vezzù K, Zorzato G, Luni C, Abatangelo G, et al. Hyaluronan based porous nano-particles enriched with growth factors for the treatment of ulcers: a placebo-controlled study. J Mater Sci Mater Med January 2009;20(1):235–47. http://dx.doi.org/10.1007/s10856-008-3566-3.
[27] Basketter D, Jírova D, Kandárová H. Review of skin irritation/corrosion hazards on the basis of human data: a regulatory perspective. Interdiscip Toxicol June 2012;5(2):98–104.
[28] Robinson MK, Perkins MA, Basketter DA. Application of a 4-h human patch test method for comparative and investigative assessment of skin irritation. Contact Dermatitis April 1998;38(4):194–202.

[29] Basketter DA, Griffiths HA, Wang XM, Wilhelm KP, McFadden J. Individual, ethnic and seasonal variability in irritant susceptibility of skin: the implications for a predictive human patch test. Contact Dermatitis October 1996;35(4):208–13.
[30] Sivolella S, Brunello G, Ferroni L, Berengo M, Meneghello R, Savio G, et al. A novel in vitro technique for assessing dental implant osseointegration. Tissue Eng Part C Methods November 19, 2015.

Analysis of bone response to dental bone grafts by advanced physical techniques

12

A. Giuliani
Università Politecnica delle Marche, Ancona, Italy

12.1 Introduction: bone response to dental grafts and the problem of conventional investigating techniques

The choice of a natural or a synthetized scaffold represents a key issue in bone tissue engineering because it is going to act as a template for cell interactions and bone extracellular matrix formation, providing structural support to the newly formed tissue [1]. In fact, an optimal scaffold has several characteristics, including a three-dimensional (3D) aspect, highly interconnected porosity, and biocompatibility. Furthermore, it needs to be preferably bioresorbable (with a controllable resorption rate) and favor cell adhesion, proliferation, and differentiation. Finally, the mechanical properties of the scaffold should be similar to those of the tissues at the site of grafting [1–4].

Regarding biomaterials for bone grafts, several approaches have been shown to be effective in stimulating bone regeneration, and ceramics perhaps showed the best results [5,6]. Indeed ceramic materials, due to their inorganic nature and ionic composition, are adequate for bone applications. Examples of ceramic materials are calcium phosphates, such as hydroxyapatite, tricalcium phosphate, and coralline-derived calcium phosphate, known for their ability to bond and stimulate bone regeneration [7,8].

Although the stimulatory effect of ceramics on bone tissue formation was proved, innovative alternative solutions are actually under investigation to find ideal constructs for bone tissue engineering, with special reference to dental districts.

One possible alternative is given by the heterologous natural bone. It is constituted by collagenized bone-substitute biomaterials of porcine origin [9,10] composed of carbonated nanocrystalline hydroxyapatite (HA), containing organic material. Another possible alternative is given by the anorganic bovine bone (ABB), which is a high-porosity deproteinized bovine bone constituted by calcium-deficient carbonate apatite with a structure similar to the human bone (from a chemical and physical perspective) [11,12].

Although these natural biomaterials are characterized by useful properties such as osteoconduction, osteoinduction, no adverse reactions, and no inflammatory infiltration, they also exhibit some limitations: in particular, the porcine bone particles present

Bone Response to Dental Implant Materials. http://dx.doi.org/10.1016/B978-0-08-100287-2.00012-4

marked staining differences from the host bone and have a lower affinity for the stains, whereas ABB undergoes no or limited resorption and a limited vascularization. For these reasons, some results are controversial and need further investigations.

Furthermore, in the recent years, dental bone grafts are oriented toward constructs where materials, cells, and biologically active molecules are combined. This is a crucial issue, since cells and growth factors are the two key elements when discussing bone biology/healing, their interaction being fundamental for an effective regeneration process.

Thus, there is evidence that, although continuous progress is being made in understanding osseous healing process, the recent research approaches combining biomaterials, cells, and biologically active molecules need to be further investigated before they will find their way into effective use in clinical practice.

In this direction, the bone response to dental bone grafts is conventionally investigated by microscopy techniques, such as light, fluorescence, scanning, and transmission electron microscopy. In Fig. 12.1, a microcomputed tomography (micro-CT) volumetric reconstruction of a biphasic calcium phosphate scaffold after grafting in a maxillary sinus defect of a sheep animal model is shown. In the table on the right, a partial morphometric analysis of the newly formed bone is reported, considering the bone volume-to-total volume ratio and the mean bone thickness after 3 months from grafting. The high variability of these parameters, through the thickness of the entire biopsy, is clearly shown. This is an example demonstrating that conventional microscopy techniques being limited to two-dimensional (2D) local information cannot often deliver a fully reliable quantitative analysis of the investigated constructs or, otherwise, require laborious 3D reconstruction of serial sections.

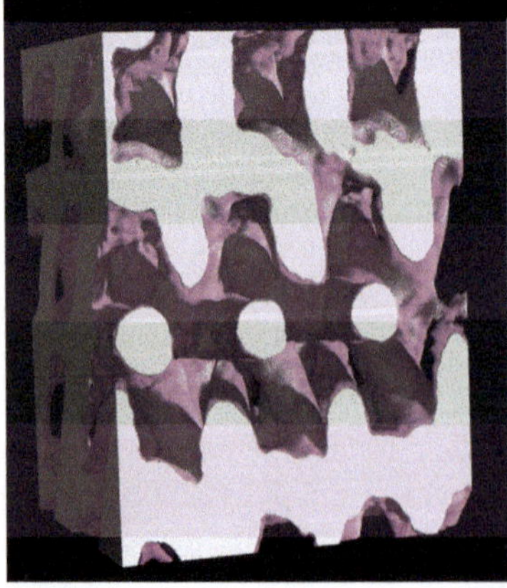

BV/TV (%)	MTh (μm)
34.9	61
23.2	34
12.5	19
7.2	13
4.8	12

Figure 12.1 Micro-CT 3D reconstruction (left) and newly formed bone quantitative analysis (right) of a biphasic calcium phosphate scaffold after 3 months of grafting in a maxillary sinus defect of a sheep animal model. White: residual scaffold; pink: newly formed bone; *BV/TV* = bone volume-to-total volume ratio; *MTh* = mean bone thickness.

Furthermore, conventional and digital X-ray radiology are imaging methods that present several important limitations linked, also in this case, to their 2D nature: anatomical structures may superimpose causing anatomical or background noises, possibly leading to misinterpretations of radiographs and preventing the revelation of soft-tissue to hard-tissue relationships [13].

In this scenario, the impact of the micro-CT technique has been revolutionary, enabling the observation of internal sample details with unprecedented precision, high resolution, and in a nondestructive way [14]. On the other hand, despite the high reliability of its ability to calculate the different morphometric parameters, the physical characteristics of the photon beam produced by laboratory X-ray sources often prevent reliable analysis of bone mineral densities and of the bone mineralization process itself. In fact, desktop micro-CT facilities do not allow the tuning of the selected photon energy, limiting the optimization of the contrast between bone volumes of different density.

Furthermore, even if there are several X-ray diffraction studies of the hierarchical structure of bone, the lowest hierarchical level, within the nanometer scale, is mostly still unexplored. It is indeed necessary to gain information also at this level in case of dental bone grafts because the distribution of organic collagen fibers and mineralized extracellular matrix has a major influence on the mechanical performances of the newly formed bone and of the whole graft.

In this direction, new possibilities can be offered by the third-generation synchrotron light sources. These large-scale facilities produce brilliant photon beams of spatial and temporal coherence properties at the sample stage, opening new solutions for advanced characterizations. Because of that, to efficiently study the dental bone grafts during mineralization process, the imaging quality and the quantitative analysis can be enhanced through the use of several synchrotron-based experimental methods, some of them described in the following paragraphs.

12.2 Synchrotron radiation and advanced physical techniques: a new approach

The researches carried out at synchrotron facilities have revolutionized, over the last 20 years, the modern science across a wide range of disciplines. But what is a synchrotron? First, it is an extremely powerful source of X-ray produced by highly energetic electrons moving in a large circular installation. The rationale behind the synchrotron science is linked to a single physical phenomenon: when a moving electron changes direction, it emits energy and this energy is in the X-ray range if electrons move at velocities close to the speed of light. Thus, a synchrotron facility serves to accelerate electrons to extremely high energy and then make them change direction periodically under the action of a magnetic field. The resulting X-rays are emitted and directed toward the different beamlines that surround the storage ring in the experimental hall. Each beamline is designed for use with a specific technique or for a specific type of research. The European Synchrotron Radiation Facility (ESRF) in Grenoble (F) is shown in Fig. 12.2.

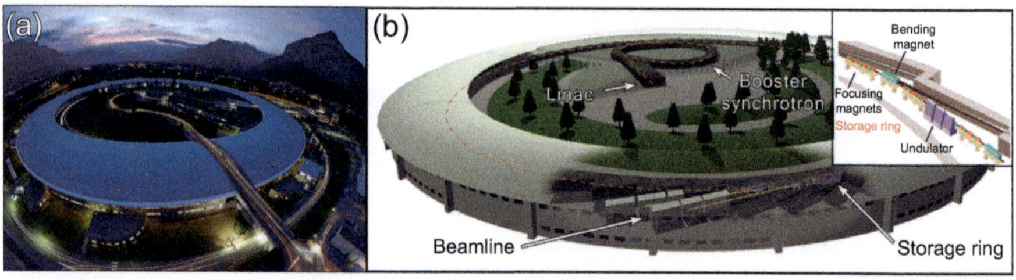

Figure 12.2 (a) ESRF synchrotron installation in Grenoble (France) *(Courtesy ESRF/Ginter)*; (b) schematic view of the ESRF synchrotron ring. In the Linac, the electrons for the storage ring are produced; in the booster, synchrotrons are accelerated to an energy of 6 billion electron volts (6 GeV) before being injected into the storage ring. The X-ray beams emitted by the electrons are directed toward "beamlines" that surround the storage ring in the experimental hall; (top-right inset) the storage ring includes 32 straight and 32 curved sections in an alternating order. In each curved section, two large bending magnets force the path of the electrons into a racetrack-shaped orbit; in each straight section, several focusing magnets ensure that the electrons remain close to their ideal orbital path. The straight sections also host the undulators, where the intense beams of X-rays are produced. *(Modified from ESRF Website—www.esrf.eu).*

Three successive generations of synchrotron radiation (SR) facilities have resulted in beam brilliances 12 orders of magnitude greater than the standard laboratory X-ray tubes; for this reason, the use of these beamlines by a continually growing community of users was the basis of the most advanced researches in a large number of scientific areas, including chemistry, physics, structural biology, medicine, earth sciences, materials sciences, and engineering, with a current interest in nanoscience.

SR produces X-rays of high energy, hard X-rays, with energies in the range 10−120 keV. Because of their higher energies, hard X-rays penetrate deeper into matter than soft X-rays, those with energy below 10 keV. Furthermore, in addition to being absorbed by a material, X-rays can also interact with the atoms, giving rise to diffraction or scattering of the X-rays. X-ray absorption can also be followed by re-emission of the energy absorbed, for example, as fluorescence. These interactions with matter are used to acquire data on sample composition, allowing to address fundamental research problems. Typical examples are (1) high pressure research, where equation of state, physical properties, and new materials are investigated also at extreme conditions; (2) highly correlated systems, which are studied with novel polarization-dependent scattering and spectroscopy techniques; and (3) time-resolved studies, addressing microscopic processes in the subnanosecond range. Furthermore, SR is strongly supporting the recent extraordinary revolution in biology, in particular, with protein structural studies [15].

The following sections are focused on some peculiarities and applications of SR sources. They illustrate some experiences and results of SR applications related to research problems dealing with bone tissue engineering with special reference to dental bone grafts studies. In particular, three techniques will be approached, namely microdiffraction, microtomography, and the innovative in-line holotomography (HT).

12.3 X-ray microdiffraction

X-ray diffraction is one of the most powerful techniques used to study the hierarchical structure of the bone. In particular, it plays a crucial role in studying the lowest hierarchical level, within the nanometer scale, where the distribution of organic fibers (collagen) and crystalline mineral nanoparticles (hydroxyapatite) has a major influence on the mechanical optimization of bone, especially in the case of newly formed bone in adhesion to different types of scaffolds.

The standard diffraction presents, however, some limitations due to the low spatial resolution imposed by the X-ray beam cross-section in the range between hundreds and several microns. Technological advances in X-ray optics, especially studied for SR, have recently and strongly improved the performances of this technique thanks to the new possibilities to focus the beam in the submicrometer range [16].

The X-ray microdiffraction combines the standard X-ray diffraction with X-ray focusing optics to highly improve the spatial resolution. This combination results in particularly interesting nonhomogeneous materials where the structural properties can change on a micrometer scale, as it is the case of dental bone grafts at the interface between scaffold and newly formed bone.

X-ray diffraction, being a scattering phenomenon, is characterized by a reciprocal law, with an inverse relationship between particle size and scattering angle [17]. In the bone and common polycrystalline scaffolds (especially ceramics), the lattice interplanar spacing parameter has a dimension comparable with the X-ray wavelength; consequently, the angular range of observable scattering results is correspondingly determined [wide angle X-ray scattering (WAXS)]. On the contrary, the colloidal dimensions (between tens and several thousands of Å) are enormously larger than the X-ray wavelength, which makes the angular range of observable scattering correspondingly small [small angle X-ray scattering (SAXS)].

WAXS of a polycrystalline material illuminated by a monochromatic X-ray beam appears with the typical ring pattern (Debye—Scherrer's rings—as shown in Fig. 12.3(c), which will be discussed in detail later on) due to all possible orientations of the microcrystals around the beam axis for each lattice plane family satisfying the Bragg law. After accurately measuring the detector-to-sample distance by calibration with a sample having a well-known structure, the corresponding lattice interplanar spacing parameter can be determined for each diffraction ring. Moreover, the azimuthal intensity distribution within a given ring supplies information on the grain orientation and on the axis along which a preferred orientation may occur in the case of texture in the material. Furthermore, the ring broadening gives information on both the crystal size and the eventual presence of strain, once an accurate data analysis is carried out by different procedures.

On the other hand, SAXS analysis [18] investigates the broadening of the primary beam to assess the crystallite dimensions, orientation, and arrangement whenever a discontinuity in electron density occurs in the sample, as in the case of hydroxyapatite crystals embedded in the organic bone tissue.

In this direction, it has been demonstrated [19—21] that the combination of WAXS and SAXS provides a complete quantitative description at the nanometric level of the

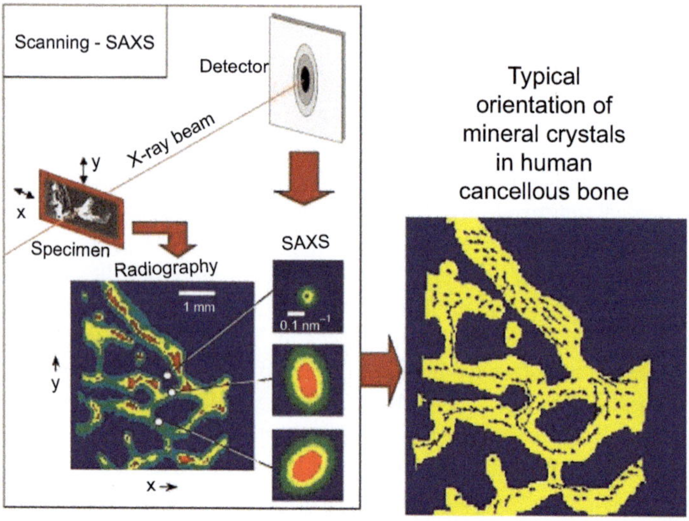

Figure 12.3 Scanning-SAXS investigation of the human vertebra. The specimen was a 200-μm-thick bone section embedded in the resin. It was well visualized by X-ray radiography (left) because, whereas transmission is high when the X-ray beam hits the organic resin, it is low when it hits the bone (being the bone a mixture of organic matrix and calcium phosphate). The orientation of the mineral particles is plotted by bars in the right side of the figure. Long bars mean high alignment, shorter bars mean pronounced alignment of the particles within the volume of each individual measurement.
From Cancedda R, et al. Bulk and interface investigations of scaffolds and tissue-engineered bones by X-ray microtomography and X-ray microdiffraction. Biomaterials 2007;28:2505–24.

bone, giving information (1) on the crystallographic orientation distribution; (2) on the morphological orientation distribution of the plate-shaped nanoparticles of bone; (3) on the texture of the crystallographic axes of the particles (WAXS); and (4) on the size, shape, and orientation of the mineral crystals (SAXS).

However, bone grafts and bone itself are nonhomogeneous composites where local characteristics change at the micrometer level; in such systems, the nanostructure has to be investigated by a position-sensitive method since it is necessary to relate the measurement to the exact position [14]. An important issue is the orientation relationship between the direction of the trabecula and the main direction of the long axis of mineral crystals [22–24]. For instance, the evaluation of the micro-SAXS patterns of human vertebra gives a high-resolution map of the thickness and the orientation of the mineral particles in the organic matrix, as shown in Fig. 12.3.

For these reasons an innovative X-ray focusing optics, delivering micrometer and even submicrometer-sized beams, was recently developed for combined scanning SAXS and WAXS setups. Indeed, acquisition of SAXS patterns usually requires dedicated experimental conditions, different from those used for WAXS experiments. However, the innovative setup [19], equipped with a beam having a submicrometer cross-section, produces a small beam size that, in turn, allows the use of a beam stopper small enough to work with a short sample–detector distance. In this configuration, the simultaneous WAXS and SAXS acquisition is achieved for each investigated point, ensuring that the complementary information is really referred to the same micrometer-sized sample area.

Fig. 12.4(a) [21] shows the optical microscopy image of a portion of a hydroxyapatite scaffold seeded with bone marrow stromal cells and ectopically implanted for 8 weeks in an immunodeficient mouse. The measured area is indicated by a rectangle. Three different regions are identified: (i) the soft tissue, (ii) the newly formed bone, and (iii) the hydroxyapatite scaffold. The microdiffraction patterns obtained in the three regions are shown in Fig. 12.4(b)–(d). As expected, the WAXS pattern from the fibrous tissue is essentially a diffuse ring, whereas the patterns corresponding to both newly formed bone and scaffold show diffraction signals due to the crystalline phase, i.e., the HA crystallites. However, these last two patterns are different because of the different dimensions of the crystallites: those of the scaffold are much larger, and comparable to the beam dimension, whereas those of the new bone are much smaller.

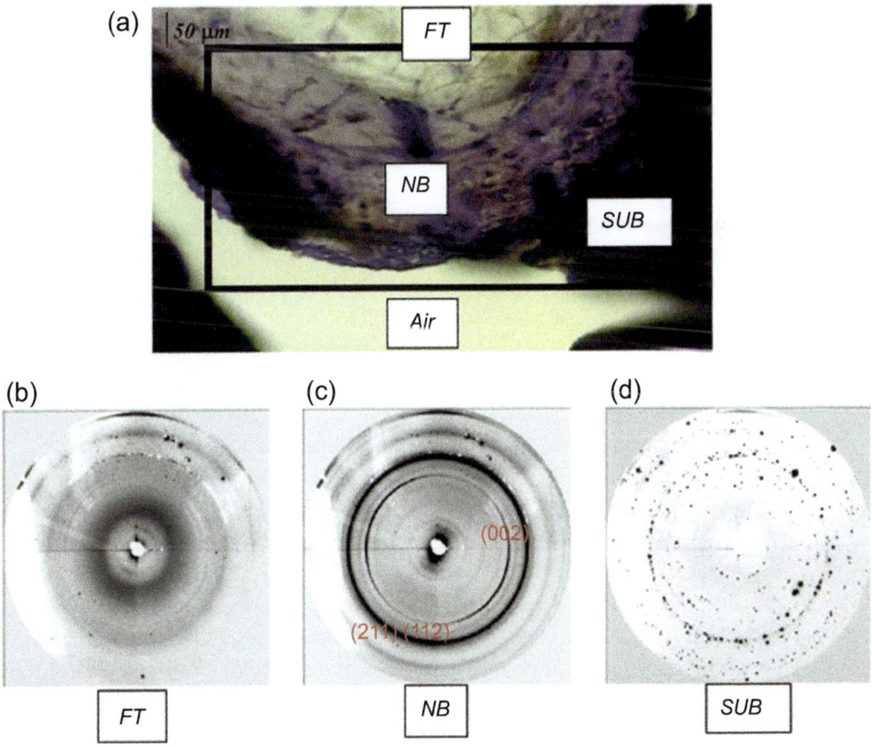

Figure 12.4 Scaffold seeded with bone marrow stromal cells and implanted for 8 weeks in an immunodeficient mouse. (a) Image of the stained section. Three different regions: NB corresponding to the newly deposited bone; SUB corresponding to the scaffold substrate; FT where a fibrous tissue is present. The *rectangle* indicates the analyzed sample area; (b–d) X-ray diffraction patterns recorded at the FT (b), NB (c), and SUB (d) regions.
From Cancedda R, et al. Bulk and interface investigations of scaffolds and tissue-engineered bones by X-ray microtomography and X-ray microdiffraction. Biomaterials 2007;28:2505–24.

The WAXS analysis, achieving to investigate the orientation of the crystallographic c-axis of the HA, also allowed to compare the growth model of the engineering bone to that of the natural bone. It was found that the c-axis orientation always remains parallel to the scaffold internal pore surface. Furthermore, derived from the SAXS signal, it was found that a pronounced anisotropic intensity distribution is evident.

The integral intensity of the black lobes, caused by X-ray scattered by the mineral bone crystals and adjacent to the white central shadow, is proportional to the density of the mineral bone (expressed in g/cm^3) in the investigated area. The pronounced anisotropy observed in the lobes indicates that the mineral bone crystals are elongated and have a predominant orientation, which follows the pore surface (data not shown). By combining the WAXS and SAXS information the authors concluded that the mean orientation of the crystallographic c-axis corresponds to the longest axis of the mineral crystals (as normally happens in the natural bone growth model [25]), that in turn, is parallel to the collagen fiber axis for all the patterns of the collection.

The microdiffraction technique, combining SAXS and WAXS signals, was also applied to resorbable porous ceramic scaffolds based on Si-tricalcium phosphate (Si-TCP), namely Skelite [26]. After seeding with bone marrow stromal cells (BMSCs), a progressive scaffold resorption was observed while new bone was deposited. The constructs were implanted subcutaneously in immunodeficient mice for 8 and 24 weeks. The WAXS analysis of the sample bone graft retrieved after 24 weeks in vivo showed the occurrence of two distinct and independent HA crystal sizes: micro-sized crystals for the scaffold and nanosized crystals for the newly formed bone. Quantification of the crystalline phases of interest (HA of the newly formed bone, HA and TCP from the scaffold) was obtained by applying the Rietveld method [27]. Furthermore, qualitative images were obtained by generating five diffraction patterns as signal models. Each pattern corresponded to one of the crystal structure occurring in the investigated area: HA, Si-TCP, and β TCP, for the microcrystalline scaffold phases, nanocrystalline HA for the newly formed bone, and an amorphous scattering curve for the soft tissue.

For the investigated sample, nanocrystalline HA and amorphous represented the highest signals, whereas the crystalline components of the original scaffold were vanishing almost everywhere. A quantitative characterization of the analyzed tissue was provided for each pixel, providing the spatial evolution of the materials belonging to the original scaffold and to the new bone tissue. This allowed the monitoring of the mineralization process with respect to the selective resorption of the original scaffold phases across any direction at the interface between the newly formed bone and the scaffold. The obtained data confirmed that at the interface between scaffold and newly formed bone the TCP component of the ceramic decreases much faster than the HA component.

12.4 X-ray microtomography

The introduction of the CT in medical imaging has revolutionized and strongly improved not only diagnosis but also research, with special reference to bone districts. CT avoids misinterpretations due to the superimposition inherent to radiographic imaging, and it nondestructively delivers volume reconstruction with contrast discrimination up to 1000 times better than that of a conventional radiograph [28].

Micro-CT is similar to conventional CT usually used in medical diagnosis but, unlike CT systems, which typically reach the spatial resolution of about 0.5 mm, micro-CT is capable of achieving a spatial resolution up to 0.2–0.3 μm, i.e., about three orders of magnitude lower [14].

In this context, SR offers the possibility to select X-rays with a small energy bandwidth from the wide and continuous energy spectrum and, at the same time, it guarantees a high enough photon flux for efficient imaging. Moreover, the use of SR allows tuning of the selected photon energy, with the aim to optimize the contrast between phases with different density in the investigated sample. This possibility is of great interest for micro-CT since it allows high spatial resolution images to be generated with high signal-to-noise ratio, permitting also to perform density measurements after several standard calibration measurements.

In this direction, allowing an accurate 3D examination of samples, SR-based micro-CT was first employed to reconstruct at high resolution the complex architecture of bone tissue [5] and now it is increasingly becoming a powerful tool for the engineered bone characterization, including the study of dental bone grafts.

In this context, interesting micro-CT studies have been performed on different biomaterials that have previously been indicated as bone-substitute optimal candidates in dental districts. In particular, successful bone regeneration using biphasic calcium phosphate materials has been reported in the recent literature in some clinical applications for maxillary sinus elevation [29,30]. Special morphologies of 3D scaffolds, in particulate or block formulations, potentially realize ideal systems to be used either in an acellular strategy (pure scaffold grafting and its colonization by endogenous cells) [29] or combining the biomaterial with cells in vitro [31]. Although these reported studies were based on a single time point (6 months), a quantitative kinetics evaluation of blocks versus granules in biphasic calcium phosphate scaffolds was carried out by SR X-ray micro-CT [32]. Twenty-four bilateral sinus augmentations were performed and grafted with HA/β-TCP 30/70, 12 with granules and 12 with blocks. The samples were retrieved at different time points and were evaluated for bone regeneration, graft resorption, neovascularization, and morphometric parameters by micro-CT. A large amount of newly formed bone was detected in the retrieved specimens, together with a good rate of biomaterial resorption and the formation of a homogeneous and a set of new vessels. The morphometric values were comparable at 5/6 months from grafting but, 9 months after grafting, this revealed that the block-based specimens mimicked the healthy native bone of the maxillary site slightly better than granule-based samples. This study is an example of the possibilities offered by SR-based micro-CT to accurately assess the kinetics on the long term of bone growth in dental bone grafts, thus achieving a detailed comparison between different morphologies of the scaffold.

In this context, there are several other studies in literature [14,33], demonstrating by micro-CT, the bioactive role of TCP or of TCP in combination with HA in bone regeneration.

Another example of ceramic material known for its ability to bond and to stimulate bone regeneration is the coralline-derived calcium phosphate [34,35]. SR X-ray micro-CT was recently used also to analyze the 3D porous architecture and microstructure of coralline-derived calcium phosphate scaffolds after long-term in vivo tests on humans [36]. Implant survival, bone regeneration, graft resorption, neovascularization, and morphometric parameters (including anisotropy and connectivity index of the structures) were evaluated after 6/7 months from grafting in human maxillary bone defects. A huge amount of bone was detected in the retrieved Biocoral-based samples, coupled with a good rate of biomaterial resorption and the formation of a homogeneous and rich net of new vessels. In Fig. 12.5, representative three-dimensional subvolumes are shown for the maxillary grafts obtained using porous Biocoral, bulky β-TCP, and HA(30%)/TCP(70%) scaffolds, respectively. In all the represented volumes, the vessel phase appears in green, the newly formed bone in pink, and the scaffold, independently from the specific biomaterial, in white. It was possible to detect newly formed vessels because the chosen experimental sample-to-detector distance, contained not only absorption but also phase-contrast signal, allowing also the visualization of these unmineralized tissues. The problem of the vascularization detection by micro-CT will be discussed later.

In any case, the sample referred to the Biocoral scaffold (Fig. 12.5(a)) presented a huge amount of newly formed bone with residual Biocoral, which was still not fully resorbed after 6 months from grafting. In the sample referred to the β-TCP block scaffold (Fig. 12.5(b)), the results were completely different: a small amount of regenerated bone, almost surrounding and in adhesion with the peripheral TCP grains, was detected. Finally, as shown in Fig. 12.5(c), the 70% β-TCP/30% HA sample, in analogy with the behavior of the Biocoral, presented a huge amount of newly regenerated bone. Morphometric 3D analysis confirmed these evidences showing that Biocoral microstructure is comparable to that obtained in the biphasic calcium phosphate-based control, with the exception of the connectivity index for which this control exhibited the most well-connected structure. On the contrary, the TCP block sample

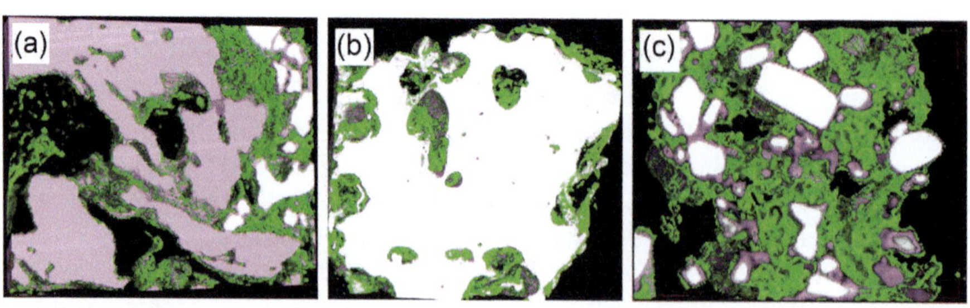

Figure 12.5 Regenerative properties of different scaffold grafts in human maxillary defects. Representative subvolumes (a) of the coralline-derived biomaterial (Biocoral) scaffold as retrieved from in vivo test after 6 months; (b) of the bulky sample made of β-TCP as retrieved from in vivo test after 6 months; (c) of the 70% b-TCP/30% HA sample as retrieved from in vivo test after 7 months. *Green phase*, regenerated vessels; *Pink phase*, newly formed bone; *White phase*, scaffold.

showed the worst morphometric characteristics in terms of newly formed bone due to its bulky shape with too low porosity. These morphometric data confirmed that despite the optimal performances of the β-TCP biomaterial for dental bone grafts, the particular TCP block morphometric characteristics do not favor bone regeneration.

As a general conclusion, micro-CT supported the finding that the implant success rate seems strictly dependent not only on biochemical properties but also on the morphology of the biomaterial [36].

In this context, the micro-CT capability of extracting morphometric parameters at the 3D level becomes of fundamental importance because, if on one hand, the histological results are greatly reproduced by micro-CT investigations. In this way, it is possible to overcome the histology limitation of not properly resolving the 3D structural information. Confirmation of the congruence between histological and micro-CT data is shown in Fig. 12.6, where a micro-CT and a histological image of the same collagenated cortico-cancellous bone graft in a human maxillary defect are reported. Micro-CT is able of discriminating (and quantify in 3D) all the mineralized phases shown in histological images: the residual scaffold, bone under remodeling, and also the fully mineralized bone.

However, it has to be stressed that third-generation synchrotron sources, such as ESRF or ELETTRA, produce brilliant photon beams with high spatial coherence properties, which are also suitable for application of phase-sensitive X-ray imaging methods. In particular, 3D imaging techniques based on phase-contrast detection offer an improved sensitivity compared to conventional attenuation-based techniques.

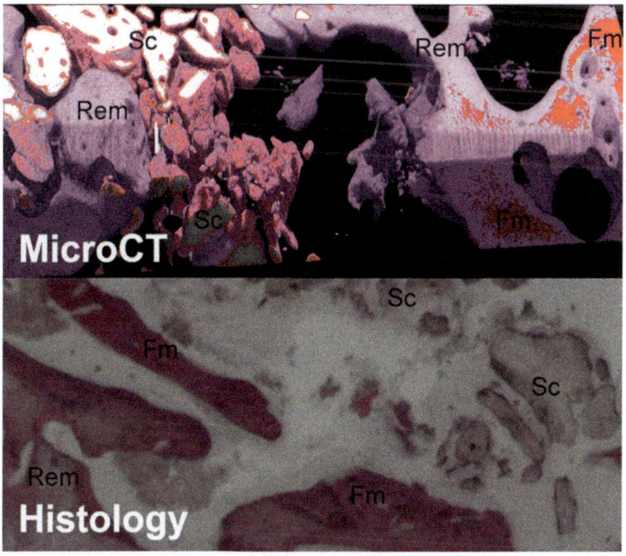

Figure 12.6 Micro-CT (top) and histology (bottom) images of collagenated cortico-cancellous bone grafts in human maxillary defects. Micro-CT ability to discriminate (in 3D) all the mineralized phases is shown, matching the histological information. *Fm*, fully mineralized bone; *Rem*, bone under remodeling; *Sc*, residual scaffold.

The phase-contrast approach differs from conventional X-ray imaging because the resulting images are not based solely on attenuation contrast. In fact, the effect of the X-ray beam going through the sample is usually described by the refractive index n:

$$n(r) = 1 - \delta(r) + i\beta(r), \tag{12.1}$$

where δ is the refractive index decrement and β is the attenuation index.

As δ is much larger than the imaginary part β, the phase approach provides greater sensitivity than the absorption approach. δ is actually proportional to the mean electron density, which in turn is nearly proportional to the mass density.

This gain in sensitivity can be several orders of magnitude for soft materials, which makes the phase-contrast micro-CT appealing for imaging of biological tissues, with special reference to dental bone grafts where we find osteocytes, bone under regeneration and remodeling, and the newly formed vascularization net.

Unfortunately, the simplest phase-contrast imaging arrangements do not automatically provide quantitative information, making the application of phase retrieval algorithms necessary. Satisfactory phase retrieval from a single-distance set of projections in free-space propagation in combination with the small exposure times due to large photon fluxes at synchrotron beamlines enable the quantitative analysis of these samples, thanks to the improvement in the segmentation of the different phases compared with conventional setups.

Typically, the phase retrieval implies the reconstruction of two different real-valued 3D distributions, $\delta(r)$ and $\beta(r)$; such reconstruction generally requires acquisition of at least two different 2D projections at each view angle. However, in some cases, it can be shown a priori that the distributions of the real and imaginary parts of the refractive index are proportional to each other:

$$\beta(r) = \varepsilon\delta(r), \tag{12.2}$$

where the proportionality constant ε does not depend on the spatial coordinates. This assumption is possible only for special classes of objects, such as *pure-phase* (i.e., very weakly absorbing) objects, or *homogeneous* objects, such as objects consisting predominantly of a single material (possibly, with a spatially varying density) [37]. This last case is represented by dental bone grafts, especially at the early stages of bone formation when there is a slow variation of the complex amplitude ("monomorphous" specimen). In this situation, a single projection per each view angle is sufficient for reconstruction of the 3D distribution of the complex refractive index [38].

This experimental protocol was used in a recent study of the early stages of in vitro bone formation in collagenated porcine scaffolds cultured with human periodontal ligament stem cells (hPDLSCs) [39]. The comparison between the osteogenic potential of this structure in basal and differentiating culture media was explored to predict the mechanism of its biological behavior as graft in human defect. In vitro cultures of human PDLSCs obtained by scraping of alveolar crestal and horizontal fibers of the periodontal ligament were seeded onto collagenated porcine blocks constituted by natural cancellous and cortical bone. 3D images were obtained by SR phase-contrast micro-CT and processed with a phase retrieval algorithm based on the transport of intensity equation [37,40]. From the second week of culture, a newly mineralized bone formation was observed in all scaffolds, both in basal and osteogenic media. It was shown that bone mineralization takes place preferentially in the trabecular portion of differentiating medium. In Fig. 12.7 a sample after 3 weeks of culture in osteogenic

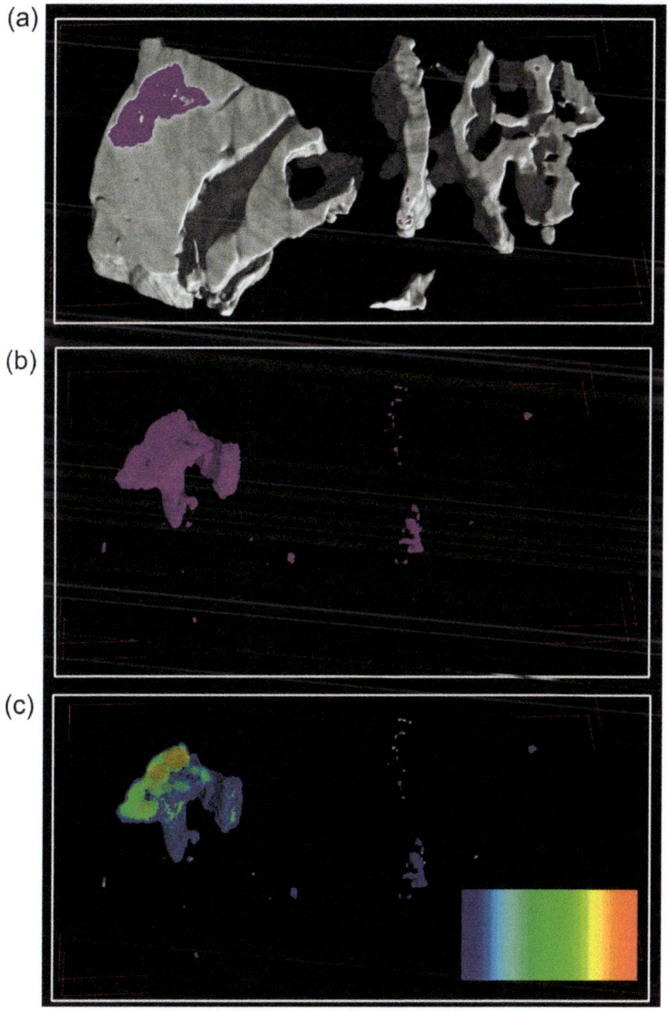

Figure 12.7 Collagenated porcine scaffolds and human periodontal ligament stem cells after 3 weeks of culture in osteogenic medium. The interaction between cells and scaffold produces 3D micro-CT images with two different phases, corresponding to different δ (refractive index decrement) values. The scaffolds are rendered in gray (a), whereas the contrast produced by cells—the newly formed bone—is colored in magenta (a and b). Color map of bone thickness distribution at week 3 is given in (c). Thickness scale on the right-bottom edge: from 10 μm (blue) to 390 μm (red).

medium, representing the mineralized portion, is shown in magenta (panels a and b) and shown using a color map for bone thickness distribution (panel c). Interestingly, micro-CT studies also revealed a mass density decrease in scaffolds seeded with hPDLSCs and in both media from the first to the second week of culture, whereas a slight increase was observed from the second to the third week. This seems to indicate that the scaffold bioresorption is more accentuated up to the second week of culture.

Looking at scaffold changes over time is still a challenging subject and needs a statistically consistent sample size with even more powerful detection systems (possibly increasing the spatial resolution and the signal-to-noise ratio) [41]. This will provide reliable quantitative data when micro-CT reconstruction histograms of biostructures undergoing remodeling (such as during cell adhesion, proliferation and differentiation on a bioresorbable scaffold) will receive a proper segmentation.

12.5 From micro-CT to HT: the new trends

The researches described in the previous paragraphs referred to SR-based microdiffraction and microtomography studies of bone grafts; they clearly indicate how both techniques complement each other in providing useful structural information on the newly formed bone at different hierarchical levels.

However, to do a reliable prevision on the life in service of a specific dental bone graft, it is not sufficient anymore to exclusively investigate the properties of mineralized tissues (such as the residual scaffold and the regenerated bone) but it is also fundamental to assess the presence, the distribution, and quantify unmineralized tissues (osteocytes, extracellular matrix, blood vessels, nerves, bone marrow, etc.) within the investigated specimens. In this direction, a growing interest is focused on the vascularization of the regenerated district [42,43].

In this context, a new SR-based physical technique was recently explored, namely the HT. HT physical principles are the same as those described for phase-contrast tomography in Eq. (12.1). Although phase-contrast tomography is based on a single distance between the detector and the sample, HT involves imaging at several distances, combining the phase shift information to generate 3D reconstructions. The HT setup at the ID19 beamline of the ESRF facility is shown in Fig. 12.8(a).

The imaging process, leading to the 2D phase radiographs, can be described as simple propagation, defocusing, or in-line holography and is done in two steps: in the first, the 2D distribution of the beam phase shift is retrieved; in the second, the 2D phase maps previously obtained are converted into a stack of 2D slices with the filtered back projection algorithm.

Thus, tomographic slices show the different physical densities of the analyzed samples. From these differences, we can evaluate the degree of mineralization. Furthermore, in the 3D reconstructions it is possible to observe also the presence of new vessels and extracellular matrix (ECM), which are transparent in conventional attenuation-based tomographic reconstructions because of their low attenuation coefficients.

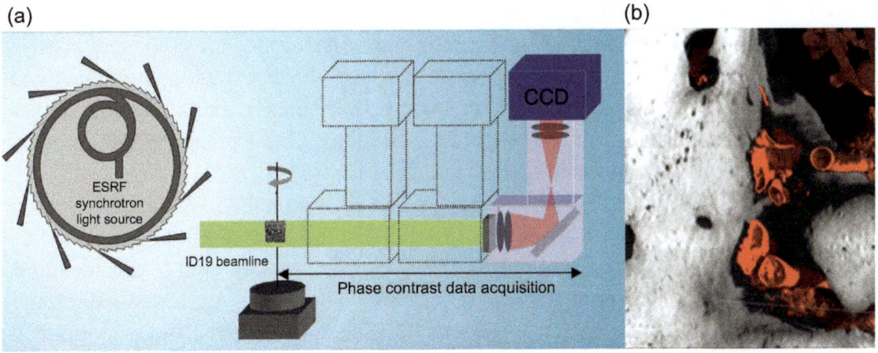

Figure 12.8 Synchrotron X-ray HT. (a) Setup at the ID19 beamline of the ESRF synchrotron facility *(Modified from ESRF Website—www.esrf.eu)*; (b) portion of a 3D reconstruction for a human mandible revealing the vascularization net. *(Modified from Giuliani A, Manescu A, Langer M, et al. Three years after transplants in human mandibles, histological and in-line HT revealed that stem cells regenerated a compact rather than a spongy bone: biological and clinical implications. Stem Cells Transl Med 2013;2:316–24).*

Hence, HT is helpful when the material of interest has very small variations in attenuation coefficients, which lead to unsatisfactory imaging results even with phase-contrast techniques based on a single distance between sample and detector. This is the case, as experienced and shown in Refs. [33,44], for fully and partially mineralized bones, such as those created by a regeneration process deriving from engrafted stem cells.

The first application of HT to study the angio- and microvasculogenesis process in a tissue engineered biological system (without any contrast agents to identify the microvasculature) was referred to Komlev [33]. In this work, 67% silicon-stabilized TCP/MSC composites were implanted subcutaneously on the back of immunodeficient mice. Mice were sacrificed 24 weeks after implantation and the extracted constructs were investigated by micro-CT and HT. Micro-CT 3D images were reconstructed from a series of 2D projections using a 3D filtered back projection algorithm, although "holographic" acquisitions were treated, at each sample-to-detector distance, with a phase retrieval procedure based on transport of intensity equation with a successive reconstruction of the 3D images by the filtered back projection algorithm. To combine both $\delta(x;y;z)$ and $\beta(x;y;z)$ maps, an optimized alignment procedure for one tomographic and three holotomographic (HT) volumes was used. Consequently, these volumes were aligned in one using the so-called, pseudo-HT process. Using this technique, soft tissue and vascular network were simultaneously imaged and quantified by using an adequately chosen algorithm and threshold value.

In a second work [44], the stability and quality of regenerated bone and vessel network were assessed, with conventional procedures and in-line HT, in mandible grafts (made of dental pulp stem cells seeded on collagen I scaffolds) 3 years after the grafting intervention. In this study, an innovative method for phase retrieval that was recently experimented and described by Langer [45] was explored. HT allowed not only to acquire qualitative and quantitative information on hard tissue, revealing that newly formed bone is of compact type (rather than a cancellous type that is physiological for the area), but also to assess the presence, the distribution, and quantification of unmineralized tissues (osteocytes, extracellular matrix, blood vessels, nerves, bone marrow, etc.) within the investigated specimens. One example of HT capacity to reveal the vascularization net is shown in Fig. 12.8(b).

Besides the specific results previously described, HT method is expected to be of much more general interest when considering dental bone graft engineering and stem cells therapeutic approach. In particular, the progress associated to this technique could be extrapolated to angiogenesis and microvasculogenesis studies in pathologies characterized by inflammation and tissue damage such as diabetes and osteoporosis.

This is of paramount importance and demonstrates that SR-based techniques, with special reference to HT, appear to be important ways to investigate the cellular events involved in bone regeneration and represent promising tools for future clinical investigations of the craniofacial tissues.

Acknowledgment

The majority of the research presented here is the result of collaborations created within the MPNS Action COST MP1005 “From nano to macrobiomaterials (design, processing, characterization, modeling) and applications to stem cells regenerative orthopedic and dental medicine (NAMABIO)” and/or was financed by the Program PRIN funds of the Italian Ministero dell’Istruzione, Università e Ricerca (Prot. 20102ZLNJ5).

References

[1] Karageorgiou V, Kaplan D. Porosity of 3D biomaterial scaffolds and osteogenesis. Biomaterials 2005;26:5474–91.

[2] Bostrom RD, Mikos AG. Tissue engineering of bone. In: Atala A, Mooney D, editors. Synthetic biodegradable polymer scaffolds. Basel: Birkhauser; 1997. p. 215–34.

[3] Middleton JC, Tipton AJ. Synthetic biodegradable polymers as orthopedic devices. Biomaterials 2000;21:2335–46.

[4] Wang M. Developing bioactive composite materials for tissue replacement. Biomaterials 2003;24:2133–51.

[5] Costa D, Lazzarini E, Canciani B, et al. Altered bone development and turnover in transgenic mice over-expressing lipocalin-2 in bone. J Cell Physiol 2013;228:2210–21.

[6] Hench LL. Bioactive materials: the potential for tissue regeneration. J Biomed Mater Res 1998;41:511–8.

[7] Klein C, et al. Osseous substance formation induced in porous calcium phosphate ceramics in soft tissues. Biomaterials 1994;15:31–4.

[8] Ripamonti U. Osteoinduction in porous hydroxyapatite implanted in heterotopic sites of different animal models. Biomaterials 1996;17:31–5.

[9] Barone A, Nicoli Aldini N, Fini M, et al. Xenograft versus extraction alone for ridge preservation after tooth removal: a clinical and histomorphometric study. J Periodontol 2008;79(8):1370–7.

[10] Orsini G, Scarano A, Piattelli M, et al. Histologic and ultrastructural analysis of regenerated bone in maxillary sinus augmentation using a porcine bone-derived biomaterial. J Periodontol 2006;77(12):1984–90.
[11] Piattelli M, Favero GA, Scarano A, et al. Bone reactions to anorganic bovine bone (Bio-Oss) used in sinus augmentation procedures: a histologic long-term report of 20 cases in humans. Int J Oral Maxillofac Implants 1999;14(6):835–40.
[12] Valentini P, Abensur D. Maxillary sinus grafting with anorganic bovine bone: a clinical report of long-term results. Int J Oral Maxillofac Implants 2003;18(4):556–60.
[13] Shah N, et al. Recent advances in imaging technologies in dentistry. World J Radiol 2014; 6(10):794–807.
[14] Cancedda R, et al. Bulk and interface investigations of scaffolds and tissue-engineered bones by X-ray microtomography and X-ray microdiffraction. Biomaterials 2007;28: 2505–24.
[15] Adams F, Van Vaeck L, Barrett R. Advanced analytical techniques: platform for nano materials science. Spectrochim Acta B 2005;60:13–26.
[16] Lagomarsino S, Cedola A. X-ray microscopy and nanodiffraction. In: Nalwa, editor. Encyclopedia of nanoscience and nanotechnology. Stevenson Ranch (CA): American Scientific Publishers; 2004.
[17] Ashcroft NW, Mermin ND. Solid state physics. Saunders College; 1976.
[18] Glatter O, Kratky O. Small angle X-ray scattering. New York: Academic Press; 1982.
[19] Cedola A, Lagomarsino S, Komlev V, et al. High spatial resolution X-ray microdiffraction applied to biomaterial studies and archeometry. Spectrochim Acta B 2004;59(10–11): 1557–64.
[20] Zizak I, Paris O, Roschger P, et al. Investigation of bone and cartilage by synchrotron scanning-SAXS and WAXS with micrometer spatial resolution. J Appl Cristal 2000;33: 820.
[21] Cedola A, Mastrogiacomo M, Burghammer M, et al. Structural study with advanced X-ray microdiffraction technique of bone regenerated by bone marrow stromal cells. Phys Med Biol 2006;51(6):N109.
[22] Camacho NP, Rinnerthaler S, Paschalis EP, et al. Complementary information on bone ultrastructure from scanning small angle scattering and Fourier-transform infrared microspectroscopy. Bone 1999;25:287–93.
[23] Fratzl P. Characterising natural fibre composites with hierarchical structure [Fibre Diffract Rev A, CCP13/NCD Publ, 10]. 2002. p. 31–9.
[24] Rinnerthaler S, Roschger P, Jakob HF, et al. Scanning small angle X-ray scattering analysis of human bone sections. Calcif Tissue Int 1999;64:422–9.
[25] Fratzl P, Fratzl-Zelman N, Klaushofer K, et al. Nucleation and growth of mineral crystals in bone studied by small angle X-ray scattering. Calcif Tissue Int 1991;48:407–13.
[26] Mastrogiacomo M, Papadimitropoulos A, Cedola A, et al. Engineering of bone using bone marrow stromal cells and a silicon-stabilized tricalcium phosphate bioceramic: evidence for a coupling between bone formation and scaffold resorption. Biomaterials 2007;28: 1376–84.
[27] Bish DL, Howard SA. Quantitative phase analysis using the Rietveld method. J Appl Cryst 1988;21:86–91.
[28] Claesson T. A medical imaging demonstrator of computed tomography and bone mineral densitometry. Stockholm: Universitetsservice US AB; 2001.
[29] Mangano C, Perrotti V, Shibli JA, et al. Maxillary sinus grafting with biphasic calcium phosphate ceramics: clinical and histologic evaluation in man. Int J Oral Maxillofac Implants 2013;28:51–6.

[30] Ohayon L. Maxillary sinus floor augmentation using biphasic calcium phosphate: a histologic and histomorphometric study. Int J Oral Maxillofac Implants 2014;29:1143–8.
[31] Barboni B, Mangano C, Valbonetti CL, et al. Synthetic Bone Substitute engineered with amniotic epithelial cells enhances bone regeneration after maxillarysinus augmentation. PLoS OneE 2013;8(5):e63256.
[32] Giuliani A, Manescu A, Mohammadi S, et al. Quantitative kinetics evaluation of blocks versus granules of biphasic calcium phosphate scaffolds (HA/β-TCP 30/70) by synchrotron radiation X-ray microtomography: a human study. Implant Dent 2016;25(1):6–15.
[33] Komlev VS, Mastrogiacomo M, Peyrin F, et al. X-ray synchrotron radiation pseudo-holotomography as a new imaging technique to investigate angio- and microvasculogenesis with no usage of contrast agents. Tissue Eng Part C Methods 2009;15(3):425–30.
[34] Soost F. Biocoral—an alternative bone substitute. Chirurg 1996;67(11):1193–6.
[35] Yukna RA, Yukna CN. A 5-year follow-up of 16 patients treated with coralline calcium carbonate (BIOCORAL) bone replacement grafts in infrabony defects. J Clin Periodontol 1998;25(12):1036–40.
[36] Giuliani A, Manescu A, Larsson E, et al. In vivo regenerative properties of coralline-derived (biocoral) scaffold grafts in human maxillary defects: demonstrative and comparative study with beta-tricalcium phosphate and biphasic calcium phosphate by synchrotron radiation X-ray microtomography. Clin Implant Dent Relat Res 2014;16(5):736–50.
[37] Gureyev TE, Pogany A, Paganin DM, Wilkins SW. Linear algorithms for phase retrieval in the Fresnel region. Opt Commun 2004;231(1–6):53–70.
[38] Gureyev TE, Paganin DM, Myers GR, et al. Phase-and-amplitude computer tomography. Appl Phys Lett 2006;89(3):034102.
[39] Manescu A, Giuliani A, Mazzoni S, et al. Osteogenic potential of dual-blocks cultured with periodontal ligament stem cells: in-vitro and synchrotron microtomography study. J Periodontal Res 2016;51(1):112–24.
[40] Gureyev TE, Mayo SC, Myers DE, et al. Refracting Röntgen's rays: propagation-based X-ray phase contrast for biomedical imaging. J Appl Phys 2009;105(10):102005.
[41] Giuliani A, Moroncini F, Mazzoni S, et al. Polyglycolic acid-polylactic acid scaffold response to different progenitor cell in vitro cultures: a demonstrative and comparative X-ray synchrotron radiation phase-contrast microtomography study. Tissue Eng Part C Methods 2014;20(4):308–16.
[42] Foster RD, Anthony JP, Sharma A, Pogrel MA. Vascularized bone flaps versus non-vascularized bone grafts for mandibular reconstruction: an outcome analysis of primary bony union and endosseous implant success. Head Neck 1999;21:66–71.
[43] Pogrel MA, Podlesh S, Anthony JP, Alexander J. A comparison of vascularized and nonvascularized bone grafts for reconstruction of mandibular continuity defects. J Oral Maxillofac Surg 1997;55(11):1200–6.
[44] Giuliani A, Manescu A, Langer M, et al. Three years after transplants in human mandibles, histological and in-line HT revealed that stem cells regenerated a compact rather than a spongy bone: biological and clinical implications. Stem Cells Transl Med 2013;2:316–24.
[45] Langer M, Cloetens P, Peyrin F. Regularization of phase retrieval with phase-attenuation duality prior for 3D holotomography. IEEE Trans Image Process 2010;19:2428–36.

Acoustic emission and ultrasound for monitoring the bone-implant interface

13

R.L. Reuben
Heriot-Watt University, Edinburgh, United Kingdom

13.1 Introduction: physical principles of mechanical monitoring of the bone-implant interface; vibration, ultrasound and acoustic emission

Ultrasound is widely used in medical applications, most notably in scanners for fetal monitoring, where contrast is achieved by differing scattering of components and reflection and transmission properties at boundaries between media with different impedances [1] thus generating an image. Such "active" ultrasonic probing also finds more quantitative medical application, for example, in soft tissue diagnostics, where it can be used to detect abnormalities (such as cancers), again using elastic transmission and reflection contrast, both of which are governed by differences in elastic modulus of the components of the tissue [2]. Variants on this technique include (sono-)elastography, which involves taking multiple elastographic images while deforming the target material [3] and using particular types of ultrasonic waves, such as surface acoustic waves [4] to enhance image contrast.

Acoustic emission (AE) is another technique that involves ultrasonic waves, although, in this case, the waves are self-generated, most commonly by microscale fractures. The term is something of a misnomer since the waves generally propagate at frequencies in the ultrasonic (rather than the conventionally "acoustic") range and are detected on the surfaces of the target material (and hence are not "emitted" in the conventional sense). AE has been very widely used in physical applications, including the detection of progressive fracture in composite materials [5] and even in machinery [6], and its applications in medicine, for reasons explained in Section 13.4, are only now evolving. Uniquely [7], researchers have applied the principles of traditional AE monitoring in an active mode to monitor the bone—dental implant interface using artificial AE sources in the mouth.

Palpation and vibration, unlike the two foregoing methods, do not use the transmission of mechanical waves, but involve either deformation of the target material (as in sonoelastograpy mentioned above) or the (forced or free) vibration of a surface of the target material at much lower frequencies than the ultrasonic or even the acoustic. Thus, for a given amount of energy (in the probe or the source), the surface movements are proportionately larger and hence can be detected using different types of

Bone Response to Dental Implant Materials. http://dx.doi.org/10.1016/B978-0-08-100287-2.00013-6

instrument. Because the governing physical equations are now the constitutive relationships of the material(s) involved, the quantities that need to be sensed are stress and strain, commonly measured as force and displacement. Palpation is used routinely by clinicians to assess various conditions, including looseness of teeth and dental implants, and, recently, a number of applications of "instrumented palpation" have been published [8] where the results can be correlated quantitatively with a clinical condition. The commonest application of vibration analysis in medical diagnostics is the assessment of stability of implants, reviewed in Section 13.2, although one group [9] have combined palpation with vibration in a technique they call "dynamic instrumented palpation."

A key difference between approaches based on deformation and wave propagation is the effect of aqueous components in the tissue. Although water (or a watery tissue component) allows the relatively free passage of elastic waves, deformation can be heavily influenced by the presence of watery components in soft tissue. For instance [8], researchers found that the periodontal regions around even cadaveric (porcine) teeth have a significant viscous component with time constants in the 1- to 10-s and 100-s orders. Since all implant materials, bonding agents, and dense bone behave, by comparison, in an elastic manner, differences in material and implant damping can, therefore, in principle, be used to monitor implant stability.

The mechanical stability of a dental implant depends critically on the integration of the metal with the bone into which it is inserted. Two broad regimes of stability are conventionally recognized; primary and secondary [10]. Primary stability is achieved on initial insertion by applying a suitable torque to a screw, which achieves contact by compression of (mostly cortical) bone. After about four weeks, cancellous bone grows around and into the implant, ultimately, it is hoped, leading to full osseointegration, where dense bone forms to an equilibrium depth within the surrounding cortical and cancellous bones, the degree to which this occurs being characteristic of the final stability [11].

Orthopedic implants, for example, the stem inserted into the femoral canal used in total hip arthroplasty, may involve osseointegration into textured implant surfaces, press-fitting or cemented fixation, which uses a (usually poly-methyl-methacrylate (PMMA)-based) cement placed into the canal prior to the installation of the implant [12]. Notwithstanding the different geometries and materials used, the basic principle of stability is the same for all implants, and so this chapter includes some reference to orthopedic implants, where relevant. Equally, a number of studies of both dental [13] (and orthopedic [12] implants) use physical models for all, or part, of the interface and surrounding hard and soft tissues.

Fig. 13.1 illustrates, schematically, the main modes of mechanical examination of the dental implant-bone interface. The first of these (Fig. 13.1(a)) is the most mature in terms of application and involves a vibrational (force) stimulus of the implant with the response (displacement) giving a direct measure of mechanical stability. The second (Fig. 13.1(b)) is derived from ultrasonic nondestructive testing and involves the injection of (usually) a pulse of ultrasound from a transponder. The pulse is reflected from the tooth-implant interface and the reflected pulse is read by the transponder, from which its quality can be deduced. The last two modes are perhaps the least

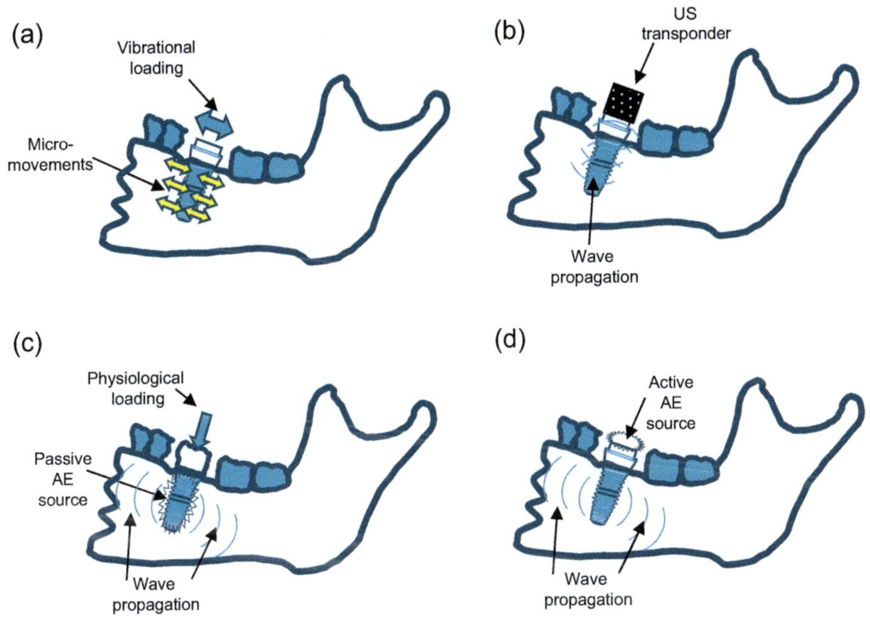

Figure 13.1 Schematic diagrams of the basic physical principles of mechanical implant stability monitoring. (a) Vibrational response, (b) ultrasonic probing, (c) conventional AE monitoring, (d) AE transmission.

clinically mature of the techniques, although conventional (passive) AE monitoring (Fig. 13.1(c)) has been used for many years to examine the degradation of the interface in the laboratory under simulated physiological loading. In this method, degradative events (such as microcracking) are detected on the surface of the specimen, subject or bone model by propagation of waves from the generation site to a transducer. The active technique (Figure 13.1(d)) is not unlike conventional ultrasonic testing, except that the source is usually a simulated one (avoiding the use of a transponder in the mouth) and it is the transmitted (as opposed to the reflected) ultrasound that is used as an indicator of interface quality.

These modalities are discussed in turn in Sections 13.2—13.4 and a summary of the state-of-the-art is provided in Section 13.5

13.2 Vibrational techniques

Following insertion, a dental implant fixity varies from the primary stability due to the mechanical engagement between the screw and the (mostly) cortical and cancellous bone (Fig. 13.2(a)) to a final equilibrium where (cancellous) bone remodeling and regrowth are complete (Fig. 13.2(c)). Both the primary stability and the secondary stability, as well as the intermediate stages (Fig. 13.2(b)), are patient specific, hence

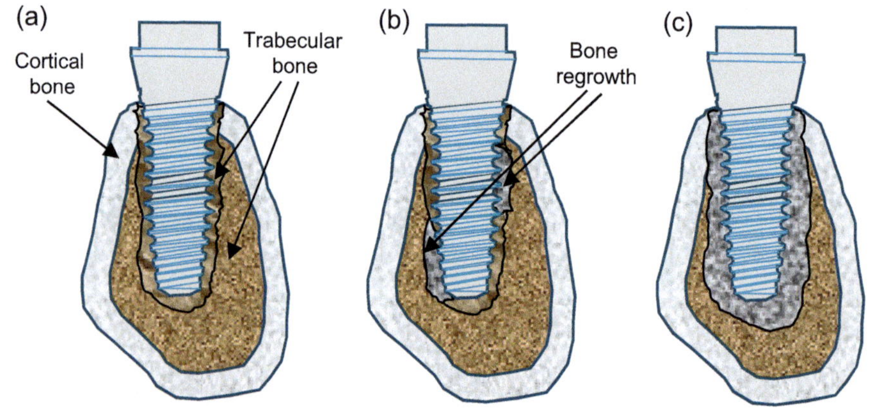

Figure 13.2 Phases of stability of implant fixity in a schematic cross-section of jaw bone. (a) Primary, (b) intermediate, and (c) secondary.

the need for monitoring to ensure acceptable function. A further complicating factor is that the implant design and surgical technique and follow-up can all affect bone remodeling because of its response to loading [11].

It is widely established that bone elastic modulus depends on bone density. Researchers [14] have carried out a systematic review of relationships between bone density and mechanical properties but found it difficult to draw a firm conclusion due to the wide variation in test conditions. After normalizing for strain rate and different density there was still a wide range in reported values of modulus, although it is clear from the data presented that compact bone (density of 1.8 g/cm^3) has a markedly higher modulus (10−18 GPa) than a typical trabecular bone (0.5 g/cm^3), showing a range of 0.2 to about 3 GPa. Given that the modulus of a typical implant material is in the order 200 GPa, the configurations represented in Fig. 13.2, even for full osseointegration, essentially constitute a column on an elastic support, so that the response to a force (irrespective of its direction) will be dominated by the stiffness of the support. It is, therefore, possible to calculate the response using elastic theory, although the calculations normally require numerical analysis, such as using finite elements (FE). For example, some researchers have used relationships for the modulus (E) of cancellous bone and cortical bone:

$$E_{\text{cancellous}} = 2.349\rho^{2.15}$$

$$E_{\text{cortical}} = -23.93 + 24\rho$$

with density (ρ), which is attributed to O′Mahoney et al. and Rho et al. [15,16], respectively, to model the response of an implant during osseointegration. Lin et al. calculated the implant neck displacement under a typical biting force to fall from around 0.05 mm to around 0.035 mm over the 48 months where the cancellous bone density increases (in a nonlinear fashion) from about 0.9 to 1.17 g/cm^3. The same model indicates a change in the first three natural frequencies of about 30%, mostly within the first 3 months, when the bone density increases from about 0.9 to 1.02 g/cm^3.

The above calculations and observations indicate the basis of implant stability monitoring, which essentially involves variants of methods that have been used widely in engineering and derive ultimately from what can be felt and heard by engineers and clinicians alike when testing the security of a foundation. All involve the application of an impulsive or modulated force to the abutment or the crown and the measurement of the resulting movement of the target. The movement is a time-varying function and can be interpreted in various ways, such as a frequency of resonance, which is then correlated with stability.

There are two main classes of clinical device for dental implant stability measurement, resonance frequency of the implant and impulse response [10]. There is much discussion about which is the more sensitive to stability, but this is probably a question of the engineering of the particular device rather than an inherent aspect of the method.

Stability measurements are often used to compare implant designs [17–19], interpatient variations [20], or surgical technique [21,22]. Researchers have specifically compared impact response (IR) and resonance frequency (RFA) measurements for a series of physical models made from polyurethane and polyurethane foam to simulate cortical and trabecular bone. They used a proprietary RFA instrument, which outputs an implant stability quotient (ISQ) related to the resonance frequency and used a proprietary impactor to excite the sample implants to which an inductively coupled transducer was attached to give the displacement response of the implant to the impactor as a function of time. This response was then analyzed to provide its frequency spectrum and the peak frequency chosen as the indicator of stability. They found that the two indicators were highly correlated and both changed in a similar way with changes in the model stability. They concluded that the peak frequency of the impactor response showed better consistency and differentiability over the range of stability studied, although this could be down to the detailed design of the two systems used rather than any inherent superiority of the technique. Certainly, the impulse-response technique holds more information since the response contains a range of frequency, although the use of the peak frequency narrows this potential advantage.

A growing proportion of the more recent published work involves joint clinical and engineering research and often includes mechanical (usually FE) modeling of the complex and evolving distribution of density (and hence modulus) around the implant, and/or development of techniques for improved resolution. In the former category is the work of Huang et al. [23] who investigated a FE model of an implant embedded in a square prism of bone in four configurations of systematically decreasing density; compact bone, dense trabecular bone surrounded by a thick layer of compact bone, dense trabecular bone surrounded by a thin layer of compact bone, and low-density trabecular bone surrounded by a thin layer of compact bone. The calculated resonance frequency ranged from around 32 kHz to around 10 kHz over the range of stability considered. In the latter category [24], researchers have introduced a method which uses a piezoelectric transducer to introduce multidirectional vibrations over a range of frequency, while measuring the mechanical resistance of the implant (what they term "electromechanical impedance"). In a later work, the same group [25] successfully simulated numerically the entire electromechanical system for a series of samples consisting of implants installed in bovine femur (cortical and trabecular bone) where the integration was simulated using root canal sealer.

Researchers [26] have considered the overall problem of implant stability modeling from a biomechanical perspective and have pointed out that both IR and RFA methods suffer from the potential disadvantages that the stimulus may be directional, thus interrogating only one aspect of the stability and, furthermore, that the surrounding bone, tissue, and even the implant design (e.g., length) can affect results (or at least calibration) and so detract from the monitoring of the interface between the implant and the bone. Vibration monitoring has also been advocated for detecting the loosening of hip prosthesis, where a stimulus, typically at a frequency of 100–2000 Hz, is introduced at the likely natural loading points, often a condyle of the femur, and the response measured at the other end of the femur (typically on the greater trochanter) [27,28]. Researchers have commented that the vibration response can be distorted by the surrounding soft tissue and have demonstrated, using a physical simulation, that an ultrasound probe to measure the response gave significantly clearer signals than the more conventional accelerometer.

13.3 Conventional ultrasonics

Researchers [26] have suggested that ultrasound, applied in pulse-echo mode at a convenient surface on the implant, will be sensitive to the interfacial region with relatively little sensitivity to the surrounding bone and tissue, thus offering better sensitivity than vibrational techniques. The essential physical basis is shown schematically in Fig. 13.3, where the outgoing pulse (of known speed, frequency and mode) from a transducer-sensor is transmitted through a couplant layer (which may be quite thin) to the implant, through which it travels relatively unattenuated until it encounters a boundary with another medium (material) where the wave speed is different. Some of the ultrasound is transmitted and some of it is reflected, a proportion undergoing what

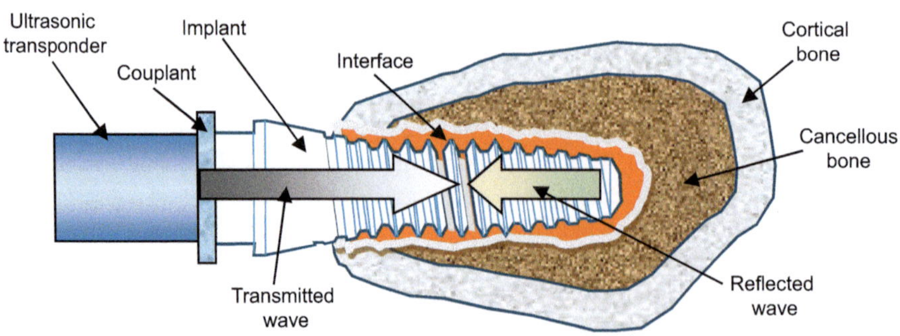

Figure 13.3 Schematic arrangement of pulse-echo ultrasonic testing of bone-implant interface.

is known as a mode conversion. Ultrasonic wave speeds depend on modulus and so the relative amounts of bone and fluid (i.e., bone density) at the interface will affect the amount of reflected ultrasound recorded. When the return wave reaches the couplant, some is transmitted back to the sensor and some is reflected back into the implant, so the same pulse may make many journeys to and from the interface.

The approach is very well established in engineering nondestructive testing to search, for example, for cavities in metallic castings. Some of the early works applied this principle to implants [29], where two slabs of bone cement were set up, one clamped and one bonded onto slabs of implant material to establish the characteristic return signals from the bonded and unbonded couples. They were then able to demonstrate that the same characteristic differences in return signals were seen with total hip femoral implants, which had been bonded into human cadaver femurs and the same implants, which had been removed and simply hammered back into their sockets.

Authors [30] went a step further, embedding a cylindrical implant model in ex vivo rabbit femurs using four different sized holes to represent a variation in primary stability. They then coupled an ultrasonic sensor/transducer to each implant surface and quantified the return echoes by adding the maximum amplitudes of the first 50 peaks. They found this indicator to be strongly indicative of the amount of simulated primary stability in their model. In later work, the same group [31] numerically simulated the pulse-echo wave propagation and successfully demonstrated that the return peaks could be classified as two types, which they termed "direct" and "transverse," the latter being a mode-converted reflection. By summing odd and even-numbered peaks, they were able to separate the diagnostic resolution of the two modes and found that the mode-converted indicator was more efficient. Further developments have included using the same approach to monitor rabbit femurs where a disc-shaped piece of implant material had been integrated in vivo to various degrees using a rabbit model [32] and where a cemented dental implant has been subjected to cyclic loading [33], both with some success.

These developments, along with others using different pulse inputs [12], have been quite successful, although there is a slight issue that the transducer/sensor can be quite sophisticated and its deployment in the mouth could lead to difficulties, including with coupling, and hence consistency of measurement.

13.4 Active and passive acoustic emission

Passive AE of implants requires the presence of a stimulus of the interface, usually brought about by artificial or natural loading (Fig. 13.4). The resulting reaction at the bone-implant interface can only be monitored if it leads to some kind of degradative event, such as microcracking of bone and/or cement. The technique has been used routinely to examine the behavior of new implant materials and designs. For example [34], researchers evaluated the adhesion strength of bioactive glass coating on titanium alloy oral implants and found AE to be useful in indicating the time and extent of cracking during force-displacement tests. Similarly [35], Santulli and Billi used AE

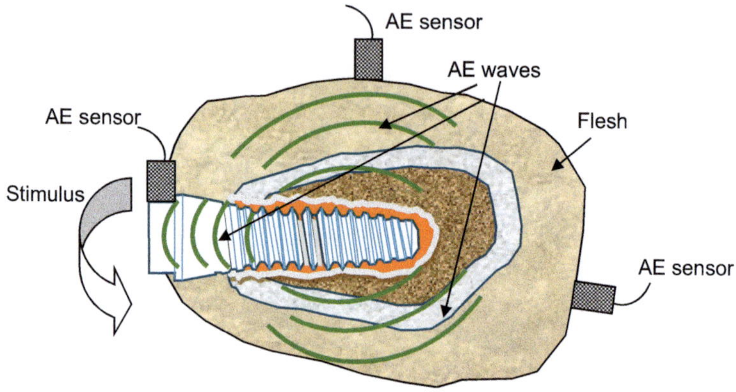

Figure 13.4 Schematic of passive AE monitoring of implants.

to monitor the failure of the implants under off-axis loading. The rather larger area and the use of cement in total hip prostheses have also led to AE being used to monitor the interface [36]. Researchers demonstrated that the accumulation of damage due to repeated loading in acrylic bone cement in hip stems could, in principle, be monitored using AE. They prepared cylindrical cement specimens and subjected them to various kinds of loading, assessing the cumulative AE counts (i.e., the summed number of significant events recorded at the sensors). Furthermore, they deployed two sensors on the specimens and used event correlation to locate the source of each event [37]. Researchers reviewed the role of AE in orthopedics and concluded that AE can locate and monitor bone cement damage in vitro and suggested, without being particularly specific, that "smart implants" could be developed to allow in vivo monitoring.

More recent developments by the same group include [38] various loading sequences of an idealized implant shape cemented into a bone analog material (Tufnol). Both embedded (in the implant) and surface (on the Tufnol) sensors were used and the events indicated by the AE sensors and parallel micro-CT scans. They concluded (with some qualification) that embedded sensors gave better correlations with the observed damage from the CT scans. Also, in the context of embedded versus surface sensors for monitoring the degradation of hip replacement stems [39], researchers have assessed AE attenuation in tissue by taking surface measurements on subjects with hip implants and asking them to perform a set of physiological tasks. However, they used sensors with a resonant frequency of 25 kHz, somewhat lower than that used by many other researchers. Nevertheless, on the assumption that the sources from the different trials and different subjects lie within a relatively narrow range of amplitude and frequency, they were able to establish the attenuation transfer functions for live human tissue. Although not associated with implants [40], researchers have assessed the use of AE to monitor disbonding of composite dental restorations during curing over a period of 10 min. The results were compared with micro-CT scans and with the shrinkage stresses, measured using a tensometer. They found a reasonable correlation between the cumulative AE on the one hand with shrinkage stress and cracking for the various types of restoration and specimen configuration on the other hand. Again relevant, although not directly related to implants [41], researchers have measured both ultrasonic transmission and fracture-related AE in bovine, ovine, and artificial bones. They report the relevant wave speeds (around 4000 m/s for surface transmission in ovine and bovine bone) as well as observe a relationship between cumulative AE events and bone microfracture [42]. They have also measured ultrasonic transmission speeds, this time in vivo and in human jaw bones for the purpose of using such measurements to quantify bone density before implantation. They found through-transmission speeds to be around 1700 m/s and concluded that some measurements might be usable for diagnostic purposes.

Recently, one group has combined some of the advantages of all of the aforementioned techniques, by introducing artificially induced AE into dental implants and measuring the proportion of the AE that is detected at a sensor placed on the bone or on the cheek of the patient (Fig. 13.5). The method relies on the use of a "standard" source, which is a reproducible ultrasound input generated from a physical phenomenon, such as a pencil-lead break (impulsive) or an air-jet (continuous). Artificial impulsive sources that do not involve fracture (or other phenomena undesirable in the mouth) are possible, although these are generally less easy to make reproducible. Using pencil-lead sources on implants installed in bovine rib bones [7], researchers have shown that the amount of AE transmitted to the surface of the bone is sensitive to the length and diameter of the implant as well as whether it is appropriately torqued (tight) or not (loose), thus making it a good indicator of primary stability. In a later work [43], they found that this relationship was affected by the hydration level of the bone but still gave a good indication of primary stability. To test the deployability of the technique in vivo, an air-jet source was developed and its sensitivity to primary stability cross-checked with the impulsive source. A small group of patients with fully osseointegrated implants was selected and air-jet transmission tests were carried out on these subjects; two indicators (transmitted energy and a measure of the frequency content of the transmitted AE) have been calculated for each patient. A score was devised for each patient based on qualitative observations, such as the amount of soft tissue between implant

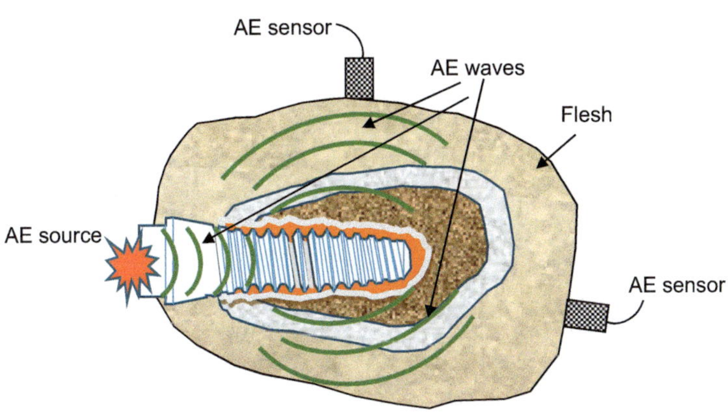

Figure 13.5 Schematic of active AE monitoring of implants.

and cheek, the movement of the patient, and more quantitative observations, such as implant size. Both transmission indicators were found to vary in a systematic way with score, suggesting that, with appropriate validation and calibration, the in vitro findings could be applied in vivo for a simple assessment of primary stability [44].

13.5 Summary of current state-of-the-art; dental and nondental implants

This section has illustrated the importance of mechanical stimulus response in the monitoring of dental implant primary and secondary stability. Broadly speaking, the higher the frequency of the mechanical stimulus, the less energy (and potential pain and/or damage) is involved. Also, when moving from low to high frequency, there is a move from whole-body vibration to wave propagation and in the essential physics of how the response is conditioned by the condition of the bone-implant interface.

A comparison has also been drawn with orthopedic implant monitoring as this has some common elements and has attracted considerable interest among the researchers. Because direct access to an orthopedic implant in situ is not normally possible, a number of devices have been developed with telemetry output, most of these for knee implants where force measurement is important in assessing the joint stability [45–47]. More significantly for this article [48], researchers have developed an oscillator that can be implanted in an endoprosthetic implant and actuated using an external magnetic field. They later demonstrated the system to detect loosening in vitro in a porcine foreleg using acoustic-mechanical frequencies over a wide range up to 350 kHz [49].

Clearly, the field of implant monitoring is continuing to develop and it can be expected that more and more information about stability in dental implants will be obtainable from relatively simple and noninvasive actuators and sensors.

References

[1] Wells PN, Liang H-D. Medical ultrasound: imaging of soft tissue strain and elasticity. J R Soc Interface 2011;8:1521–49.

[2] Zhang X, McKay CR, Sonka M. Tissue characterization in intravascular ultrasound images. IEEE Trans Med Imaging 1998;17(6):889–99.

[3] Pallwein L, et al. Sonoelastography of the prostate: comparison with systematic biopsy findings in 492 patients. Eur J Radiol 2008;65(2):304–10.

[4] Li C, et al. Laser induced surface acoustic wave combined with phase sensitive optical coherence tomography for superficial tissue characterization: a solution for practical application. Biomed Opt Express 2014;5(5):1403–17.

[5] Steel JA, Reuben RL, Hamlin M, Brown ER. Acoustic emission from the tension fatigue of glass fibre reinforced plastics. Proc Inst Mech Eng Part L J Mater Des Appl 2004;218(1): 9–17.

[6] Douglas RM, Steel JA, Reuben RL. A study of the tribological behaviour of piston ring/ cylinder liner interaction in diesel engines using acoustic emission. Tribol Int 2006;39(12): 1634–42.

[7] Ossi Z, Abdou W, Reuben RL, Ibbetson RJ. In vitro assessment of bone-implant interface using an acoustic emission transmission test. Proc IMechE 2011;226(1):63−9.
[8] Tohill R, Hien MR, McGuinness N, Chung L, Reuben RL. Short-term stress relaxation of porcine periodontal ligament—finding an appropriate visco-elastic model. IFMBE Proc 2009;25(11):335−8.
[9] Scanlan P, et al. Development of a novel actuator for the dynamic palpation of soft tissue for use in the assessment of prostate tissue quality. Sens Actuators, A Phys 2015;232:310−8.
[10] Atsumi M, Park S-H, Wang H-L. Methods used to assess implant stability; current status. Int J Oral Maxillofac Implants 2007;22(5):743−54.
[11] Lin D, Li Q, Li W, Duckmanton N, Swain M. Mandibular bone remodelling induced by dental implant. J Biomech 2010;43:287−93.
[12] Yang J, et al. Nondestructive evaluation of orthopaedic implant stability in THA using highly nonlinear solitary waves. Smart Mater Struct 2012;21:012002 (10pp).
[13] Vayron R, Haiat G. Assessment of the biomechanical properties of the interface surrounding a dental implant. IFMBE Proc 2014;49:5−8.
[14] Helgason B, Perilli E, Schileo E, Taddei F, Brynjólfsson S, Viceconti M. Mathematical relationships between bone density and mechanical properties: a literature review. Clin Biomech 2008;23:135−46.
[15] O'Mahoney A, Williams JL, Spencer P. Anisotropic elasticity of cortical and cancellous bone in the posterior mandible increases peri-implant stress and strain under oblique loading. Clin Oral Implants Res 2001;12:648−57.
[16] Rho JY, Hobatho MC, Ashman RB. Relations of mechanical properties to density and CT numbers in human bone. Med Eng Phys 1995;17(5):347−55.
[17] Friberg B, Sennerby L, Linden B, Grondahl K, Lekholm U. Stability measurements of one-stage Brånemark implants during healing in mandibles. A clinical resonance frequency analysis study. Int J Oral Maxillofac Surg 1999;28:266−72.
[18] O'Sullivan D, Sennerby L, Meredith N. Measurements comparing the initial stability of five designs of dental implants: a human cadaver study. Clin Implant Dent Relat Res 2000; 2:85−92.
[19] Elramady MM, Sayed AM, Awadallah MA, Naseef TM. Measuring primary stability for the inclined implants retaining mandibular overdenture using resonance frequency. In: 7th Cairo international biomedical engineering conference. IEEE; 2014. p. 83−6.
[20] Lopez AB, Peñarrocha-Diago M, Martínez-Cortissoz O, Mínguez-Martínez I. Resonance frequency analysis after the placement of 133 dental implants. Med Oral Patol Oral Cir Bucal 2006;11:E272−6.
[21] Lai H-C, Zhang ZY, Wang F, Zhuang LF, Liu X. Resonance frequency analysis of stability on ITI implants with osteotome sinus floor elevation techniques without grafting: a 5-month prospective study. Clin Oral Implants Res 2008;19:469−75.
[22] Kim D-S, Lee W-J, Choi S-C, Lee S-S, Heo M-S, Huh K-H, et al. Comparison of dental implant stabilities by impact response and resonance frequencies using artificial bone. Med Eng Phys 2014;36:715−20.
[23] Huang H-M, Lee S-Y, Yeh C-Y, Lin C-T. Resonance frequency assessment of dental implant stability with various bone qualities: a numerical approach. Clin Oral Implants Res 2002;13:65−74.
[24] Tabrizi A, Rizzo P, Ochs MW. Electromechanical impedance method to assess dental implant stability. Smart Mater Struct 2012;21:115022 (8pp).
[25] La Malfa Ribolla E, Rizzo P, Gulizzi V. On the use of the electromechanical impedance technique for the assessment of dental implant stability: modeling and experimentation. J Intell Mater Syst Struct 2015;26(16):2266−80.

[26] Mathieu V, et al. Biomechanical determinants of the stability of dental implants: influence of the bone-implant interface properties. J Biomech 2014;47:3–13.

[27] Rieger JS, Jaeger S, Schuld C, Kretzer JP, Bitsch RG. A vibrational technique for diagnosing loosened total hip endoprostheses: an experimental sawbone study. Med Eng Phys 2013;35(3):329–37.

[28] Rowlands A, Duck FA, Cunningham JL. Bone vibration measurement using ultrasound: application to detection of hip prosthesis loosening. Med Eng Phys 2008;30:278–84.

[29] Davies JP, Tse MK, Harris WH. In vitro evaluation of bonding of the cement-metal interface of a total hip femoral component using ultrasound. J Orthop Res 1995;13:335–8.

[30] Mathieu V, Anagnostou F, Soffer E, Haïat G. Ultrasonic evaluation of dental implant biomechanical stability: an in vitro study. Ultrasound Med Biol 2011;37(2):262–70.

[31] Mathieu V, Anagnostou F, Soffer E, Haiat G. Numerical simulation of ultrasonic wave propagation for the evaluation of dental implant biomechanical stability. J Acoust Soc Am 2011;129(6):4062–72.

[32] Mathieu V, Vayron R, Soffer E, Anagnostou F, Haïat G. Influence of healing time on the ultrasonic response of the bone-implant interface. Ultrasound Med Biol 2012;38(4):611–8.

[33] Vayron R, et al. Variation of the ultrasonic response of a dental implant embedded in tricalcium silicate-based cement under cyclic loading. J Biomech 2013;46:1162–8.

[34] Schrooten J, Helsen JA. Adhesion of bioactive glass coating to Ti6AlV oral implant. Biomaterials 2000;21(2000):1461–9.

[35] Santulli C, Billi F. Normal and off-axis compression tests of biocompatible titanium dental implants monitored by acoustic emission. J Mater Sci Lett 2002;21:727–30.

[36] Roques A, Browne M, Thompson J, Rowland C, Taylor A. Investigation of fatigue crack growth in acrylic bone cement using the acoustic emission technique. Biomaterials 2004; 25:769–78.

[37] Browne M, Roques A, Taylor A. The acoustic emission method in orthopaedics—a review. J Strain Anal Eng Des 2005;40:59–79.

[38] Mavrogordato M, Taylor M, Taylor A, Browne M. Real time monitoring of progressive damage during loading of a simplified total hip stem implant using embedded acoustic emission sensors. Med Eng Phys 2011;33:395–406.

[39] Khan-Edmundson A, Rodgers GW, Woodfield TBF, Hooper GJ, Chase JG. Tissue attenuation characteristics of acoustic emission signals for wear and degradation of total hip arthroplasty implants. In: Proceedings of the 8th IFAC symposium on biological and medical systems, BMS; 2012. p. 355–60.

[40] Li H, Li J, Yun X, Liu X, Fok AS. Non-destructive examination of interfacial debonding using acoustic emission. Dent Mater 2011;27:964–71.

[41] Stark F, et al. Investigation of failure processes in the human femur using signal-based acoustic emission techniques. In: Proceedings 30th European conference on acoustic emission testing and 7th international conference on acoustic emission, Granada, Spain; 2012. p. 175–84.

[42] Klein MO, Grötz KA, Manefeld B, Kann PH, Al-Nawas B. Ultrasound transmission velocity for noninvasive evaluation of jaw bone quality in vivo before dental implantation. Ultrasound Med Biol 2008;34(12):1966–71.

[43] Ossi Z, Abdou W, Reuben RL, Ibbetson RJ. Transmission of acoustic emission (AE) in bones, implants and dental materials. Proc IMechE 2013;227(11):1237–45.

[44] Ossi Z. Assessment of dental implant stability using acoustic emission analysis [Ph.D. thesis]. University of Edinburgh; 2012.

[45] Crescini D, Sardini E, Serpelloni M. Design and test of an autonomous sensor for force measurements in human knee implants. Sens Actuators A 2011;166:1–8.

[46] D'Lima DD, Townsend CP, Arms SW, Morris BA, Colwell CW. An implantable telemetry device to measure intra-articular tibial forces. J Biomech 2005;38:299–304.
[47] Arami A, et al. Instrumented prosthesis for knee implants monitoring. In: Proceedings 2011 IEEE international conference on automation science and engineering, Trieste, Italy; 2011. p. 828–35.
[48] Ruther C, et al. Investigation of a passive sensor array for diagnosis of loosening of endoprosthetic implants. Sensors 2013;13:1–20.
[49] Ruther C, et al. Investigation of an acoustic-mechanical method to detect implant loosening. Med Eng Phys 2013;35:1669–75.

A new approach for modeling bone response to dental implant materials

14

A. De Sanctis, S.A. Gattone
University "G. d'Annunzio" of Chieti-Pescara, Pescara, Italy

14.1 Introduction

Information geometry is a new research field that combines geometry and statistics [1]. It derives from Fisher information in inferential statistics. Rao proved it is a Riemannian metric in the family of probability densities. Information geometry can be used successfully in shape analysis [2] to describe mathematically patterns from complex systems and their changes in time. The aim of this brief note is to propose a novel framework to model medical imaging, such as that related to the bone response to biomaterials and implants.

14.2 The method

We deal with geometric objects such as a human head in the space. In the following, to simplify the analysis, we will consider only planar objects, such as a section of the skull. The shape of the object consists of all information invariant under similarity transformations, that is, translations, rotations, and scaling. Data from a shape are often realized as a set of points. Many methods allow us to extract a finite number of points, which are representative of the shape and are called landmarks. The choice of landmarks is crucial and different choices may lead to different results. To select them in a proper way, experts can suggest where to allocate the landmarks according to the specific application.

In Refs. [3–5], we proposed to model each landmark with a bivariate Gaussian model using means and variances as coordinates, the former ones reflecting the uncertainty in the landmark's placement and the latter ones reflecting the variability across a family of patterns.

Precisely the shape of a generic configuration may be represented by a $2K$-component Gaussian model, where the kth landmark, $k = 1,\ldots,K$, of the shape is given by the following:

$$f\left(x, \mu_k, \sum\nolimits_k\right) = \frac{1}{2\pi}\left|\sum\nolimits_k\right|^{-\frac{1}{2}} \exp\left\{-\frac{1}{2}(x-\mu_k)^T \sum\nolimits_k^{-1} (x-\mu_k)\right\}$$

Bone Response to Dental Implant Materials. http://dx.doi.org/10.1016/B978-0-08-100287-2.00014-8

under the condition

$$\sum_k = \sigma_k^2 I_2 = \mathrm{diag}\left(\sigma_{k1}^2, \sigma_{k2}^2\right).$$

In the model, the means $\mu_k = (\mu_{k1}, \mu_{k2})$ are the registered coordinates of the kth landmark of the shape, for $k = 1,\ldots,K$. The estimated covariance matrix $\sum_k$ is reduced to a diagonal one, through a suitable rotation of the landmark coordinates, with $\left(\sigma_{k1}^2, \sigma_{k2}^2\right)$ the vector of the variances of the kth landmark of the shape, for $k = 1,\ldots,K$. The main contribution is the relaxation of an isotropic covariance matrix as in Ref. [6], allowing the variances to vary among the landmarks and in time.

The shape representation with a Gaussian model allows the use of the Fisher–Rao metric. Within this framework, we can compute geodesic paths by minimizing the information in the Fisher sense. The length of the geodesic path connecting two shapes can be used for quantifying shape differences. It defines a distance called geodesic distance.

In particular, the geodesic distance, with respect to the Fisher–Rao metric, between a landmark of a shape S_1 and a landmark of a shape S_2, identified by two bivariate normal densities $\left(\mu_1, \sum_1\right)$ and $\left(\mu_2, \sum_2\right)$ with $\sum_1 = \mathrm{diag}\left(\sigma_{11}^2, \sigma_{12}^2\right)$ and $\sum_2 = \mathrm{diag}\left(\sigma_{21}^2, \sigma_{22}^2\right)$, can be computed as

$$d\left[\left(\mu_1, \sum\nolimits_1\right), \left(\mu_2, \sum\nolimits_2\right)\right] = \sqrt{d_1^2 + d_2^2}$$

where, for $i = 1, 2$,

$$d_i = \sqrt{2}\cosh^{-1}\left[\frac{(\mu_{1i} - \mu_{2i}) + 2\sigma_{1i}^2 + 2\sigma_{2i}^2}{4\sigma_{1i}\sigma_{2i}}\right].$$

The methodology is used to perform various type of analysis. In particular, geodesics can be used in the following:

- For cluster analysis of shapes, for example, distinguishing biological shapes in normal and pathological ones
- In the evolution, to reconstruct the shape in the intermediate times if it is known at two different times
- To predict, for a short time, the evolution of the shape from its past

The procedure of clustering was tested on the second thoracic vertebra T2 of mice, while the evolution was tested on a section of the rat skull. In both cases, we obtained very good performance to describe the real situation [3–5].

The approach allows also the analysis of the profile of the bone of a regenerated site, as shown in Figs. 14.1 and 14.2.

In particular, cluster analysis can be used to evaluate the effects of different biomaterials and implants on the shape of the bone, by selecting a group of people to whom different biomaterials are used to regenerate the bone. The evolution of the profile of

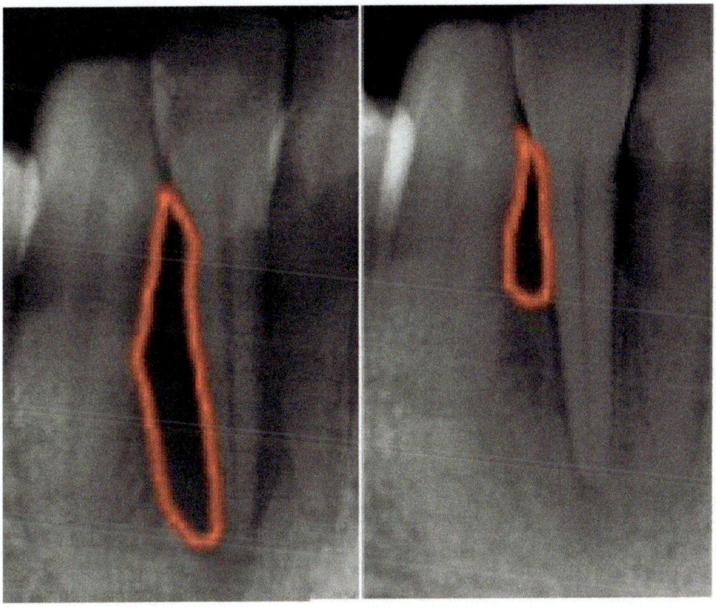

Figure 14.1 A regenerated site. On the left, the real initial profile, and, on the right, the real final profile.
Courtesy Dr. Antonio Barone, University of Pisa, Italy; Tuscan Stomatologic Institute, Lido di Camaiore (LU), Italy.

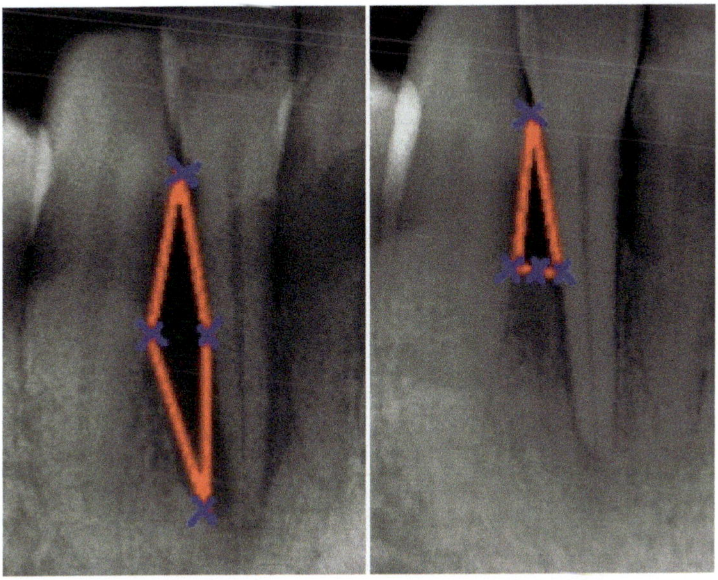

Figure 14.2 On the left: the initial shape as rhombus with four landmarks. On the right: the final shape as triangle with three landmarks on the base due to the floor elevation.
Courtesy Dr. Antonio Barone, University of Pisa, Italy; Tuscan Stomatologic Institute, Lido di Camaiore (LU), Italy.

the bone, during the regeneration period, can be reconstructed by the model, as well as a forecast in the short period.

This procedure could be used also with non geometric coordinates analogously to what we did with the cornea curvature in keratokonus [5]. It is possible to consider, for example, bone density to have a better description of bone response to dental biomaterials or implants.

References

[1] Amari S, Nagaoka H. Methods of information geometry, volume 191 of translations of mathematical monographs. 2000.
[2] Dryden IL, Mardia KV. Statistical shape analysis. London: John Wiley & Sons; 1998.
[3] De Sanctis A. Shape analysis for complex systems using information geometry tools. Nonlinear Phenom Complex Syst 2012;15:70–3.
[4] De Sanctis A, Gattone SA. A study of complex shapes using information geometry. Nonlinear Phenom Complex Syst 2015;18:70–80.
[5] De Sanctis A, Gattone SA. Methods of information geometry to model complex shapes. Eur Phys J 2016 (in press).
[6] Peter A, Rangarajan A. Information geometry for landmark shape analysis: unifying shape representation and deformation. IEEE Trans Pattern Anal Mach Intell 2009;31:337–50.

Index

Note: Page numbers followed by "f" indicate figures, "t" indicate tables.

CPI Antony Rowe
Chippenham, UK
2017-02-01 18:52